ORGANIC BRAIN SYNDROMES:
An Introduction To Neurobehavioral Disorders

ORGANIC BRAIN SYNDROMES:

An Introduction To Neurobehavioral Disorders

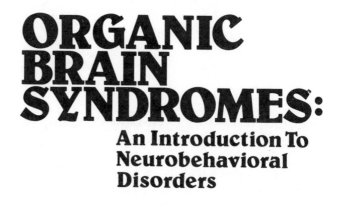

Richard L. Strub, M.D.
ASSOCIATE PROFESSOR OF NEUROLOGY
LOUISIANA STATE UNIVERSITY
NEW ORLEANS, LOUISIANA

F. William Black, Ph.D.
ASSOCIATE PROFESSOR OF NEUROLOGY
LOUISIANA STATE UNIVERSITY
NEW ORLEANS, LOUISIANA

Foreword by D. Frank Benson

Illustrations by Ann C. Strub

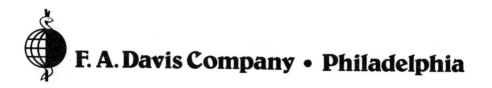

F. A. Davis Company • Philadelphia

Library of Congress Cataloging in Publication Data

Strub, Richard L
  Organic brain syndromes.

  Includes bibliographical references and index.
  1. Brain—Diseases.   2. Neuropsychiatry.
I. Black, F. William, joint author.   II. Title.
[DNLM: 1. Brain diseases.   2. Behavior.   WL 348 S927o]
RC386.S77   616.8   80–29400
ISBN 0–8036–8209–3

FOREWORD

The middle portion of the 20th century witnessed an almost complete separation of the previously related fields of psychiatry and neurology. Psychiatrists focused their interest, almost exclusively, on the effect that psychic background and current environmental pressure had on their patient's mental life. Abnormal brain function was rarely considered and an almost total eclipse of interest in organic mental problems resulted. At the same time, neurologists directed their interest towards the neurosciences with particular emphasis on the problems of the peripheral nervous system and basic-science related disorders, effectively ignoring behavioral abnormalities, even those with an obvious neurological basis. The resulting schism isolated (and ignored) an entire group of patients—those with behavioral problems based on organic changes within the nervous system. The number of patients with these problems has been and remains significant; it has been estimated that at least 10 percent of all patients in a general psychiatric practice will have organically based mental problems and that well over 50 percent of patients requiring hospitalization for psychiatric problems suffer from organically related problems. Thus, an enormous number of patients exist whose major disorder falls within this recently established no-man's-land between psychiatry and neurology. The number is sufficiently great that patients with these problems regularly come to the attention of all practitioners of medicine. In many instances, the patients need and deserve the attention of a specialist, but quite frankly, most patients with these disorders have been, and still are, mishandled.

In the last decade, there has been a moderate resurgence of interest in the neurologically based behavioral problem. Only in the past few years, however, has this reawakening reached significant dimensions. Research is now being conducted on behavioral problems, some individual practitioners claim a primary interest in these problems, and teaching programs are being organized to train specialists in the organic behavioral field. There is at least some return to the previous specialty of neuropsychiatry, although more often called neurobehavior now.

The upsurge in interest has been heralded by a considerable increase in the number of publications on the subject. Most major neurological, psychiatric, and psychological journals regularly include articles on organic behavioral problems, and a number of books discussing organic behavioral problems have appeared in the last few years. These publications are most noteworthy for their diversity. The articles are appropriately specialist oriented and most of the books have more than one author, featuring chapters on individual neurobehavioral problems written from idiosyncratic viewpoints. A single behavioral disorder may be described from a psychiatric, neurologic, psychologic, linguistic, philosophic, or physiologic viewpoint—the fact that the same disorder is being discussed may be obscured. While often of value, the diverse approaches have suggested an immensely complex group of problems and effectively discouraged involvement by most physicians.

The authors of the present volume set out to correct this difficulty by providing a textbook approach to organic behavioral problems that would fall within the scope of all physicians. Drs. Strub and Black have been eminantly successful in their task. They have presented a large number of common neurobehavioral problems in an authoritative, up-to-date fashion with superb reference selections for additional study. Most importantly, the entire production is comprehensible by clinicians without specialty training in neurology, psychiatry or psychology. While originally conceived for use by medical students and beginning neurobehavioral specialists, this volume actually provides an excellent introduction to behavioral neurology for all specialists in behavior (neurologists, neurosurgeons, psychiatrists, and psychologists) and a valuable source of information for all clinicians dealing with adult patients.

The authors have provided case histories of selected behavioral problems providing concrete, identifiable information. But the volume is much more than a compendium of case reports: rather, the case histories lead to the discussions and aid recognition of the disturbances under discussion.

From the low ebb of a decade ago, the interest in behavioral disorders has advanced considerably. The field has expanded rapidly and, simultaneously, investigations of the disorders are becoming more detailed. The authors have done an outstanding job of including recent references and have even included a large number of the currently novel hypotheses. While the up-to-date nature of the information offered in this volume enhances its quality, its greatest value lies in the introduction it provides to the problems of organic behavioral disturbances. From this point alone, this book will stand as a valuable contribution to the study of the neurology of behavior.

D. Frank Benson, M.D.
Professor of Neurology
UCLA School of Medicine

PREFACE

This volume presents a clinical discussion of the neurobehavioral changes seen as a sequel of brain damage or dysfunction. These behavioral syndromes are variously called the *organic brain syndromes, organic mental syndromes,* or more recently, *neurobehavioral syndromes.* These conditions taxonomically occupy the borderland between neurology and psychiatry. They have basically neurologic etiologies yet psychiatric manifestations. Long neglected, there has been a resurgence of interest in this area of clinical and research study on the part of neurologists, psychiatrists, and psychologists.

Our intention in writing this basic text is to acquaint physicians, nurses, physical and occupational therapists, psychologists, speech pathologists, and other persons working with the brain injured patient with the clinical features, diagnostic approach, and management plans for patients presenting with conditions within this vast spectrum of disorders. Where possible, we will also discuss the newer concepts of pathogenesis and hopefully provide the reader with a solid overview of the fascinating field of neurobehavior. The terminology, classification system, and the method of organization used in this text is discussed in Chapter 1, Introduction.

We would like to thank several individuals who have both encouraged and aided us in this endeavor: D. Frank Benson, M.D., Professor of Neurology UCLA School of Medicine, has been very kind in reviewing the entire manuscript and making substantive critical comments and has also written the foreward. Ann C. Strub generously applied her artistic talents to making the illustrations for the book. Carlos Garcia, M.D., neuropathologist at the Louisiana State University Medical Center, provided us with many of the photomicrographs and photographs of pathologic specimens and was also very helpful in discussing the sections concerning pathology in many of the chapters.

Richard L. Strub
F. William Black

CONTENTS

SECTION I

ANATOMY AND CLINICAL EVALUATION

1

INTRODUCTION

The organic brain syndromes are a commonly encountered group of diseases in clinical medicine in which either damage or dysfunction of the brain is manifested for the most part by an alteration in behavior. The behavioral change may be confined primarily to social or emotional behavior as in the remarkable personality change displayed by the patient with a frontal lobe tumor, or the change can be predominantly manifested in intellectual behavior as in the complex cognitive deterioration seen in the patient with dementia. Within the category of intellectual change, we include the selective defects of cognition such as aphasia, amnesia, alexia, and so forth, in which a focal lesion of the brain impairs a specific cognitive function; in the cases mentioned: language, memory, and reading.

The organic brain syndromes are acquired disorders that can occur at any age but are most commonly seen in adults. In this volume we will not discuss the behavioral syndromes that are developmental or congenital, such as mental retardation, learning disabilities, minimal brain dysfunction, and the like. In our opinion, current research indicates that most of these conditions have a basic organic etiology that is manifested as an alteration in the developmental process as the child matures as opposed to being the result of an acquired brain lesion. These developmental disorders are very important because of their frequency and social impact and will be discussed at length in a subsequent volume.[4]

We will also, by intention, exclude from our primary discussion the major psychiatric diseases of schizophrenia and manic depressive illness. Although recent advances in genetics, pharmacology, and neurochemistry have begun to provide strong evidence that these classic functional psychiatric disorders have, at least in part, an organic basis, we do not yet consider them to fall within the category of the organic brain syndromes.

TERMINOLOGY

We have chosen to utilize the term *organic brain syndromes* as it is a traditionally used and familiar term, both in the psychiatric nomenclature and common medical parlance. The American Psychiatric Association has consistently used this term and has continued its use in the third revision of the Diagnostic and Statistical Manual of Mental Disorders III (DSM III)[3]. This revision slightly amends the term to organic mental disorders and uses a double category, *organic mental disorders/ organic brain syndromes.* In recent years, neurologists have introduced the term *neurobehavioral disorders* to encompass this group of conditions, a term that stresses both the neurologic etiology of the diseases and their behavioral manifestations. However, while appealing in many ways, the newer terms of neurobehavioral disorders or organic mental disorders have the fault of introducing additional terms to a field in which inexact definitions and disparity in conceptual thinking already abound. We prefer to refine and expand the basic term *organic brain syndromes* so that those already acquainted with the term will more fully understand it and those who are new to this field will obtain a meaningful introduction.

CLASSIFICATION

After defining the general field of the organic brain syndromes and finding a suitable and acceptable term with which to label it, the next problem has traditionally been and still is, the classification of the different syndromes that constitute these organic behavioral disorders. In the past, the American Psychiatric Association has tried to divide these conditions into two major categories; in 1952[1] they utilized the terms, *acute* and *chronic,* and in 1968,[2] used *psychotic* and *non-psychotic organic brain syndromes.* Each individual disease (e.g., cerebral infection) became a subheading within the classification schema (i.e., organic brain syndrome with psychosis associated with cerebral infection). We have found these earlier classifications to be unworkable and to bear little relationship to the clinical syndromes themselves. We are very pleased that the revision of the organic classification within the DSM III,[3] largely through the influence and writings of Lipowski,[5,6] has adopted a much more phenomenologic approach and has divided the syndromes by their clinical psychologic features rather than by one isolated and offtimes vague feature such as chronicity or psychosis. Since this is the manner in which we have traditionally taught the symptoms, diagnosis, and management of these conditions to medical students and residents, we welcome this general trend and feel that the organization of this book will be in concert with the recent thinking of the psychiatric as well as neurologic community.[7]

The primary point which must be made in regard to the classification of these disorders is that there is not a single *organic brain syndrome;* this is a group of disorders, many of which have their own distinctive behavioral and pathologic features. There are, however, certain symptom clusters that correspond to rather specific disease entities and therefore the disorders within each group can be approached similarly from the standpoint of both diagnosis and management. The main categories of disorders in the classification system are: (1) *the acute confusional states* (delirium); these are in general, the acute, reversible, rather generalized behavioral disruptions that occur with temporary metabolic or toxic brain dysfunction. (2) *The dementias:* these are generally syndromes of slowly progressive deterioration in intellectual and adaptive social processes. Dementia is usually associated with atrophy or damage to brain that is irreversible; however, this is not invariably true as will be discussed in Chapters 5 and 6. Lipowski[6] has proposed combining delirium and dementia into a unifying category of "disorders of global cognitive impairment," but we feel that this move may be unnecessary lumping, since the two general conditions are so distinct in regards to pathophysiology, clinical picture, differential diagnosis, evaluation, management, and prognosis. (3) *Focal brain syndromes:* because of the complex, yet rather localized, anatomic substrate of intellectual, emotional, and social functions, lesions in disparate areas of the cortex and subcortex will produce distinct clinical behavioral syndromes. There are many such syndromes which are discussed in detail in Chapter 7.

A fourth category of organic syndromes, the "symptomatic functional syndromes," has been proposed.[3,6] These are organically based syndromes that clinically resemble functional psychiatric disease. For example, the schizophrenic behavior seen in some patients with chronic temporal lobe epilepsy, systemic lupus erythematosus, or chronic LSD use would be considered a schizophreniform syndrome within this classification. Other entities within this category are affectiform syndromes for organically based depression or mania and the organic personality syndrome for characterologic disorders of probable organic etiology. We personally have not embraced this last category and have chosen to discuss these functional changes within the specific disease categories under which they fall rather than as distinct clinical entities. The inclusion of these disorders as diagnostic categories is certainly defensible, but we have not utilized them in our classification system.

ORGANIZATION OF THIS TEXT

This book is intended to serve as a clinical guide to the diagnosis, evaluation and management of the organic brain syndromes, and we have organized it following the classification system discussed above. We have divided the material into four main sections. The first serves as an introduction to the relevant terminology and includes an overview of the neuroanatomic substrate involved in the production of human behavior. The third chapter in this section covers the clinical and neuropsychologic evaluation of these patients.

The second, and clinically most important section, discusses in detail the major clinical organic brain syndromes: confusional states, dementia, and focal syndromes. The typical clinical picture, the behavioral and medical evaluation, differential diagnosis, laboratory evaluation, management, and pathology of each syndrome are given. Wherever possible within each general syndrome, we have attempted to outline methods of making specific diagnoses on the basis of behavioral and other clinical grounds alone. This is generally impossible for most confusional patients but is more rewarding in the careful study of the clinical presentation of both the dementias and the patients with focal lesions.

The third section discusses the various neurobehavioral syndromes that are seen in patients with specific categories of disease such as head trauma, cerebrovascular disease, alcoholism, and so forth. This second method of classification is presented for several reasons. Firstly, a large number of neurobehavioral syndromes do not fall conveniently within the major clinical categories described in Section II and yet are of great practical importance in the day-to-day practice of medicine. An example is the patient who is having difficulty concentrating on his work after a relatively minor head injury. His alteration in behavior is subtle, possibly due to a focal brainstem dysfunction, but is so typically a transient sequela of head injury that we feel it is best discussed in a special chapter dealing with the problems resulting from trauma. Secondly, most textbooks and medical courses are organized around a disease or organ system approach, accordingly, the physician is accustomed to thinking in terms of the features and evaluation of specific types of disease (e.g., tumor, vascular disease). By discussing the behavioral disorders that occur with specific diseases we hope to alert the physician to possible behavioral sequelae that his patient with alcoholism, cerebrovascular disease, or epilepsy might develop during the course of his lifetime.

There is obviously considerable overlap in using two classification systems within a single book, but we have attempted to minimize redundancy. In those instances in which a specific disease (e.g., cerebrovascular accident) results in a specific neurobehavioral syndrome (e.g., Broca's aphasia), the behavioral syndrome will be discussed in the relevant chapter of Section II, while the specific disease will be mentioned in the relevant chapter of Section III. At this point in the evolution of our thinking about these diseases, we feel that this is the most satisfactory method of presenting these conditions to the clinician. In reality, patients present in two principal ways: either with a specific clinical syndrome such as dementia or with a specific disease process such as head trauma or toxic poisoning. The physician must be equipped to deal with the behavioral component associated with each mode of presentation; therefore, we feel justified in discussing the syndromes utilizing this double classification. The fourth and final section of this volume is a short discussion of some of the less distinctly organic syndromes (e.g., Gilles de la Tourette's syndrome, narcolepsy) and an overview of the clinical interactions of the fields of neurology and psychiatry.

ORGANIC BRAIN SYNDROMES IN MEDICAL PRACTICE

As a final point, we must stress the very real importance of these organic syndromes. They are extremely common in medical practice and constitute, in many instances, not only difficult medical diagnostic and management problems but also very complicated social problems. Over one-third of all beds in chronic psychiatric hospitals are occupied by patients with organic brain diseases. As the population of elderly individuals increases, this statistic will also climb. Stroke with its attendant behavioral sequelae such as aphasia is the third most frequent cause of death in this country and certainly one of the greatest causes of chronic disability. Brain damage secondary to head trauma, alcohol abuse, toxic exposure, and epilepsy produces large populations of patients with organically based behavioral disorders requiring appropriate medical care.

But despite the high incidence of such problems, organic brain syndromes receive little or no attention in many medical school and residency curricula. As a consequence, practicing physicians frequently fail to recognize the presence of atypical organic brain disease and even more frequently misdiagnose the symptoms as being purely functional. For example, we have seen many patients with infarcts, hemorrhages, and tumors of the dominant temporoparietal area who were initially misdiagnosed as functionally psychotic because of the clinician's failure to recognize the patient's abnormal speech as being aphasic rather than psychotic.

Beyond the clinical importance of recognizing such conditions, these diseases have a significant social impact which must concern all clinicians. Organic brain diseases frequently follow a long and complicated course. For instance, the patient with dementia may experience many years of declining intellectual capacity during which the family and eventually society become increasingly involved in providing medical and institutional care. The financial as well as emotional strain on such families is considerable, and in many cases, society must eventually assume total responsibility for the patient's care.

Caring for the patient with an organic brain syndrome is a multidisciplinary team effort. The physician must learn to enlist the assistance of family, nurses, physical and occupational therapists, speech pathologists, social service workers, psychologists, and other specialists within the medical profession. Only with the assistance of all of these varied specialists can the patient with an organic brain syndrome receive the best possible evaluation and management. This volume should serve as a significant aid to the clinician in dealing with the patient with an organic brain syndrome.

REFERENCES

1. American Psychiatric Association: Diagnostic and Statistical Manual of Mental Disorders I. Washington, D.C., 1952.
2. American Psychiatric Association: Diagnostic and Statistical Manual of Mental Disorders II. Washington, D.C., 1968.
3. American Psychiatric Association: Diagnostic and Statistical Manual of Mental Disorders III. Washington, D.C., 1980.
4. Black, F.W., and Strub, R.L.: The Developmental Disorders of Childhood. Philadelphia, F.A. Davis Co. In preparation.
5. Lipowski, Z.J.: Organic brain syndromes: Overview and classification, in Benson, D.F., and Blumer, D. (eds.): Psychiatric Aspects of Neurologic Disease. Grune and Stratton, New York, 1975, pp. 11–35.
6. Lipowski, Z.J.: Organic brain syndromes: A reformulation. Compr. Psychiatry 19:309, 1978.
7. Strub, R.L.: Toward a new classification of the organic brain syndromes (editorial). J. Clin. Psychiatry 40:2, 1979.

2

THE ANATOMY OF BEHAVIOR

To understand the changes in behavior that occur in patients with brain disease, it is important to have a working knowledge of the anatomy and physiology of those parts of the brain involved in the production and maintenance of normal behavior. Human behavior and its neurologic substrate are extremely complex and far from completely understood. Over the past hundred years, however, sufficient clinical and experimental material has been amassed to support a working hypothesis concerning the correlation between brain function and behavior. The schema presented here is simplified for clarity, but it does provide a model which will aid the student in understanding the neuroanatomic substrates of normal behavior and the alterations in behavior seen subsequent to brain damage and disease.

Behavior itself is multifaceted and can be broken down into two distinct, yet interrelated, categories. The first consists of emotional behavior: feelings, reactions to others in our environment, drives for survival, and desires to procreate. The emotional aspects of behavior serve as the background for the more elaborate social behaviors involved in developing an individual lifestyle, planning a career, or establishing a family and are under the control of the complicated, largely subcortical, limbic system. This system in its interaction with the cortex, especially the frontal lobes, is responsible for the development of personality and the establishment of elaborate social behavior.

The second major category is intellectual behavior; a complex very human quality which includes both the high level processes of verbal reasoning, calculating, and abstract thought and their building blocks: language, perception, and memory. The cerebral cortex is the principal structure responsible for these sophisticated functions, and a knowledge of cortical structure and functional organization is an important step in understanding normal behavior and in comprehending the behavioral syndromes seen with focal brain lesions such as stroke, tumor, or abscess.

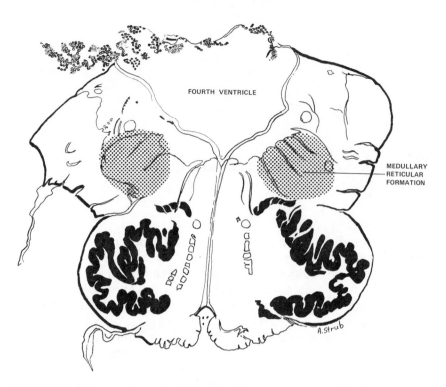

FOURTH VENTRICLE

MEDULLARY
RETICULAR
FORMATION

A.Strub

FIGURE 2–1. Cross section of medulla. Stippled area represents the reticular formation.

Underlying all behavior, whether it is emotional, intellectual, or a combination of the two, is the element of consciousness. Simply defined, consciousness is the state of awareness of both the environment and one's own thought processes. Man must be able to maintain a waking and alert condition in order to receive environmental stimulation and to initiate any meaningful mental or physical activity. Without such capacity, only sleep can occur. This rudimentary function is governed by the ascending activating system which consists of the brain stem reticular formation and its widespread projections to the thalamus, limbic system, and cortex.

ASCENDING RETICULAR SYSTEMS

Ascending Activating System

The ascending activating system is an arousal system whose activity maintains wakefulness and alertness and thereby allows the individual to interact with the environment. The ascending activating system

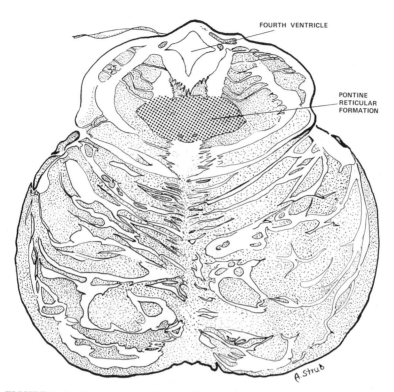

FOURTH VENTRICLE

PONTINE
RETICULAR
FORMATION

A. Strub

FIGURE 2–2. Cross section of pons. Stippled area is the pontine reticular area.

originates in the reticular cells of the brain stem. These cells lie in nuclear groupings in the perimedian areas of the medulla, pons, and midbrain (mesencephalon) (Fig. 2-1 to 2-4).

The medial group is gigantocellular and is the actual origin of the ascending and descending tracts. This effector zone receives its input from the lateral, small celled zone (parvicellular) which in turn receives its input from the ascending sensory pathways (with the exception of the medial lemniscus). Taken together, these cell groups are designated the *brain stem reticular formation.*

The most important fibers concerned with arousal are the ascending axons that originate in the gigantocellular zone of the pontine and mesencephalic reticular formation.[28] Fibers arising from the pontine neurons project to nonspecific nuclei of the thalamus (interlaminar nucleus, reticular nucleus, and midline nuclei such as the centrum medianum); these nonspecific nuclei then have diffuse projections to wide areas of brain. From these thalamic nuclei, there is also extensive interconnection with other thalamic nuclei, projection back to the pontine reticular cells, and a major outflow to the ventral anterior tha-

11

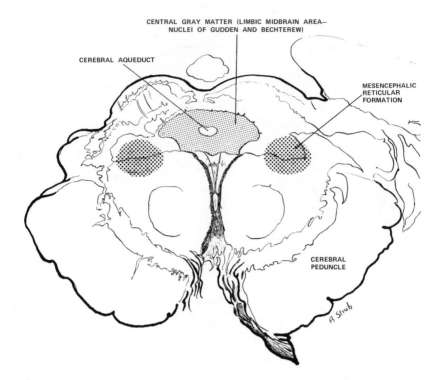

CENTRAL GRAY MATTER (LIMBIC MIDBRAIN AREA—
NUCLEI OF GUDDEN AND BECHTEREW)

CEREBRAL AQUEDUCT

MESENCEPHALIC
RETICULAR
FORMATION

CEREBRAL
PEDUNCLE

A. Strub

FIGURE 2–3. Cross section of mesencephalon (midbrain). The lightly stippled area surrounding the cerebral aqueduct (periaqueductal grey) is the caudal extension of the limbic system and has very extensive interconnection with the ascending activating system. The darkly stippled areas lateral to the periaqueductal grey represents the mesencephalic reticular formation.

lamic nucleus. This anterior nucleus sends diffuse projections to the cortex. These efferents from the thalamus are known as the *diffuse thalamic projection system.*

The mesencephalic reticular formation sends a significant number of ascending fibers to structures within the limbic system, principally the hypothalamus and the septal nuclei. Other reticular-limbic interaction occurs throughout the entire upper brain stem. In this area, reticular cells send a rich network of short collateral fibers to the central grey area of the pons and mesencephalon. This central grey substance represents the caudal extension of the limbic system into the brain stem[6] and, in essence, serves as a secondary arousal system.

The input to the reticular formation comes primarily from the ascending sensory tracts. Incoming noxious stimuli traveling through the brain stem in the spinothalamic tract are transferred to the lateral (small cell) zone of the reticular formation. Stimuli carried by the

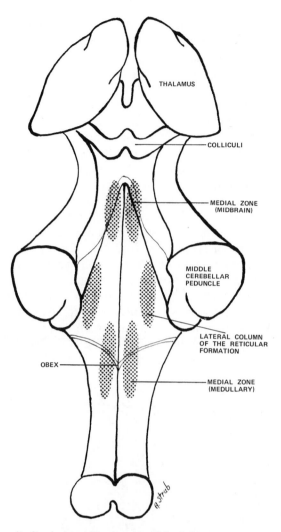

FIGURE 2–4. Longitudinal view of brain stem. Stippled areas represent the reticular nuclei.

paleospinal portion of the spinothalamic tract are transferred to the reticular formation via short collateral branches throughout the brain stem. Stimuli traveling via the primitive archispinal (spinoreticular) portion of the system terminate in the pontine and, medullarly, parvicellular reticular formation. In this way, a stimulus to the skin (e.g., a bee sting) will immediately arouse the activating system at all levels. Through the ascending pathways described above, arousal and basic alerting takes place throughout the thalamus, limbic system, and cortex. This arousal occurs at the same time the stimulus arrives at the

13

sensory cortex via the ventral posterolateral thalamus, and the final level of arousal produced by the painful stimulus is the combined effect of these inputs. Of course, all sensory input is not as intense as a bee sting, but it is largely through the constant flow of incoming environmental stimuli that arousal and alertness are maintained. Arousal, however, is not totally reliant on external stimulation; it can also be a self generated phenomenon (e.g., the student "forcing" himself to stay awake while studying in a warm quiet room). In most instances, arousal and the level of alertness result from a combination of environmental stimulation, the individual's need or desire to remain alert, and the reticular systems own intrinsic activity.

The arousal system can be adversely effected by a variety of disease processes. In cases of metabolic imbalance as with liver failure or diabetic acidosis, the entire system becomes depressed and the patient becomes lethargic or stuporous. A specific destructive lesion (such as, an infarction, hemorrhage, or traumatic contusion) involving the pontine or mesencephalic portion of the system (Fig. 2-5) will render the patient comatose, a state in which the patient is totally unresponsive to even the most vigorous stimulation. If, on the other hand, damage occurs in the projection system in the thalamus and subthalamus, there is a marked reduction in ascending activation and the patient, although appearing alert, can respond only minimally to stimulation.

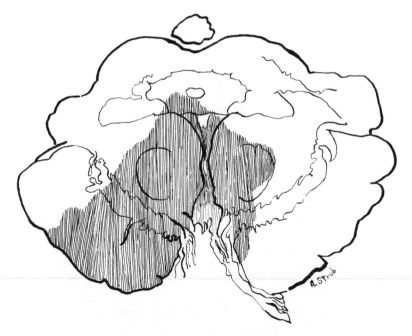

FIGURE 2-5. Shaded area indicates a typical coma producing lesion of mesencephalon.

Such patients can initiate eye opening, mumble a few words, and occasionally move but otherwise remain akinetic and mute.

The activation system can also respond with overactivity and a state of hyperalertness can be observed. This is seen in anxiety states or during fright; under such conditions the individual is acutely sensitive to any environmental stimulus. Such a hightened state of arousal may be beneficial (e.g., a soldier on patrol) or detrimental (e.g., a nervous speaker trying to deliver a speech in a noisy hall). Increased alertness can also be seen following use of such benign pharmacologic agents as coffee, tea, or cola. By use of such agents, man has learned to manipulate his level of arousal to suit his immediate needs.

Ascending Inhibiting System

The ascending activating system operates in concert with the ascending inhibitory system. It was previously thought that sleep, for example, occurred when there was a simple decrease in activation. Recent studies, however, have demonstrated that stimulation of the parallel inhibitory system can produce sleep rather than activation.[36] Accordingly, it appears that the clinical level of alertness is determined by a dynamic balance of activity in both ascending systems.

Damage can occur primarily to the ascending inhibitory system. As a result of the epidemic of influenzal encephalitis in 1918–1921, a number of patients developed a syndrome of hyperactivity that was called "organic driveness."[19] These patients had extensive lesions in the reticular formation, although the damage apparently affected primarily the inhibitory centers. This selective damage unbalanced the system and allowed an unbridled release of arousal activity.

In recent years, there has been considerable interest in young children who display hyperactive and/or distractible behavior. It is tempting to postulate that these hyperactive children may have some type of imbalance in the operation of these brain stem systems; but, with our current clinicopathologic knowledge, there is no evidence to support such a hypothesis.

The ascending brain stem systems are the anatomic substrate for the most basic levels of behavior: consciousness and alertness. Their primary function is to provide the level of arousal energy necessary to maintain normal functioning of higher centers in the limbic system and the cortex.

LIMBIC SYSTEM

The limbic system is composed of a ring of phylogenetically old cortex and a group of subcortical structures that serve as the anatomic substrate for survival instincts, emotions, and memory. Stimulation or destruction of specific nuclei or areas within the system can markedly alter such basic behaviors as eating, sleeping, or emotional response. The system is newer phylogenetically than the basic arousal system but is older than the neocortex. It is well developed in the rat, cat, and monkey and these animals have been used in much of the experimental study of limbic functions. In man, limbic activity is constantly modified by higher centers in the neocortex and basic instinctual behaviors are rarely seen in a pure form.

The limbic system is so named because its structures form a limbus or ring around the inner aspect of the cerebral hemispheres. This limbus originally was considered to consist of the cingulate and hippocampal gyri as they encircle the upper brain stem and diencephalon (Fig. 2-6). As knowledge of the physiology and functional significance of the limbic system has increased, the concept of the system has been expanded to include a large number of structures and fiber systems that appear to be involved in the elaboration of instinctual and emotional behavior. At present, its limits have become vague and the concept of a single limbic system is being questioned. However, although not an absolutely defined area, the limbic system is conceptually sound and most investigators are in agreement as to its basic structures and pathways. In this chapter we will not embroil the reader in the quibbling over semantics of those involved in limbic research but will discuss the major structures and connections usually included in the sys-

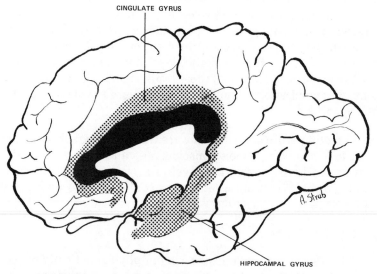

CINGULATE GYRUS

HIPPOCAMPAL GYRUS

FIGURE 2–6. Saggital cut of cerebrum showing limbic cortex.

tem and show how each structure contributes to the basic functioning of the entire system.

Anatomy

MAJOR STRUCTURES

The anatomy of the limbic system is complex and its principal structures have many interconnections. The central point of most limbic activity is the hypothalamus. The *hypothalamus* is that portion of the diencephalon lying anterior to the thalamus. It forms the floor and the ventrolateral walls of the anterior third ventricle and is directly superior to and intimately associated with the pituitary gland (Figs. 2-7 and 2-8). The hypothalamus has many nuclei, but the main areas of importance in regard to behavior are the ventromedial nuclear complex, the lateral hypothalamus, and the mamillary bodies.

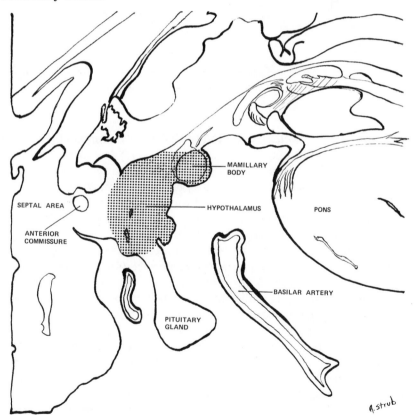

FIGURE 2–7. Saggital cut of brain, close up of upper brain stem, diencephalon and environs. Stippled area represents the hypothalamus.

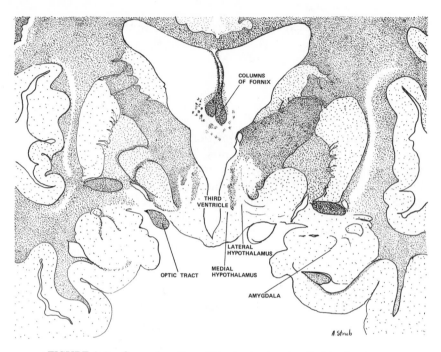

FIGURE 2–8. Coronal section of the brain showing limbic structures.

A limbic structure closely related to the hypothalamus is the *amygdala,* a large nuclear mass situated in the anterior and medial portions of the temporal lobe. Immediately posterior to the amygdala and in the medial temporal lobe itself is the *hippocampal formation;* this structure runs along the medial surface of the temporal horn of the lateral ventricle. The hippocampus is not seen on the medial surface of the hemisphere but is demonstrated after dissection into the temporal lobe (Fig. 2-9). Other nuclear structures intimately associated with limbic function are the *septal nuclei in the posteromedial frontal lobe* (Fig. 2-7), the *dorsomedial and anterior nuclei of the thalamus,* and the *limbic midbrain area.* The midbrain area is composed primarily of the *periaqueductal grey substance* and the *nuclei of Gudden and Bechterew* which lie in the midline ventral to it (Fig. 2-3).

The *hippocampal gyrus* and *cingulate gyrus* are the cortical aspects of the limbic system and form the limbus of cortex on the medial surface of the hemisphere (Fig. 2-6). Portions of the orbital and medial cortex of the frontal lobe are considered by some to be a part of the limbic system not only because of their rich anatomic connections with other limbic structures but also because of the emotional changes that occur if they are damaged or destroyed. There is also a significant amount of medial

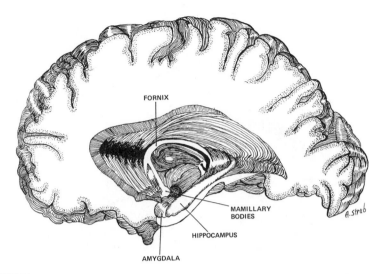

FORNIX

MAMILLARY
BODIES

HIPPOCAMPUS

AMYGDALA

A.strub

FIGURE 2–9. Dissection of cerebral hemisphere showing hippocampus and amygdala within temporal lobe.

temporal cortex (pyriform and entorhinal) that is also limbic. This cortex is associated with the olfactory system and is part of the old rhinencephalon. The rhinencephalon is of great importance in lower animals and remains an integral part of the limbic system in man.

FIBROUS PATHWAYS

There are many fibrous pathways associated with the limbic system, serving both as interconnections within the system and as connections between the limbic structures and other areas of the brain. As with most fiber systems in the brain, limbic pathways have fibers that go in both directions between any two structures. These reciprocating systems make constant feedback possible, and continuous adjustment of the system occurs.

The first limbic fiber bundle described and certainly the largest is the *fornix*. The fibers of the fornix originate in the cells of the hippocampus and are the major outflow from that structure. The fornix arches forward along the medial surface of the hippocampus, then curves to join the contralateral fornix beneath the corpus callosum. The columns of the fornix proceed ventrally in the septum pellucidum then divide to terminate both in the mamillary bodies of the hypothalamus and in the septal nuclei of the frontal lobe (Fig. 2-10).

A second major pathway originates in the mamillary bodies and terminates in the anterior nucleus of the thalamus; this is the *mamilo-thalamic tract of Vicq d'Azyr*. Fibers then project from the anterior thalamus to the cingulate gyrus (Fig. 2-10). This circuit from the hip-

19

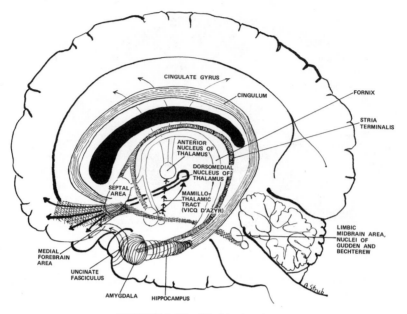

FIGURE 2–10.   Limbic structures.

pocampus to the mamillary bodies via the fornix then to the anterior thalami and cingulate gyri is known as the Papez circuit.[31] Historically, this was the first pathway hypothesized as a possible mechanism for the appreciation and expression of emotion in man.

A third important limbic pathway is the *stria terminalis* which runs almost parallel to the fornix in the lateral wall of the lateral ventricle. Its fibers originate in the amygdala and project to the ventromedial hypothalamus and the septal region (Fig. 2-10).

The fourth major fiber pathway is the *medial forebrain bundle*. The bundle originates in the inferior frontal cortex and septal nuclei. It passes through the lateral hypothalamus and continues on to the limbic midbrain area. Throughout its course it provides rich collaterals to the regions it traverses.

Other than these four major fiber systems, there are important connections from the hypothalamus and amygdala to the orbitofrontal cortex via the dorsomedial thalamus. The amygdala itself has three additional fiber connections: (1) the *ansa peduncularis,* that connects the amygdala directly with the hypothalamus, (2) the *uncinate fasciculus* that runs to the orbitofrontal cortex, and (3) the *stria medullaris,* a pathway connecting the amygdala, habenula, and septum. Again, it is important to mention that there are diffuse interconnections between the brain stem reticular formation and the limbic midbrain area. More extensive anatomic information is available and the interested student is referred to Isaacson[18] and to Crosby and coworkers.[8]

Function

Through stimulation and ablation studies in animals and the clinical study of humans with lesions in the limbic structures evidence has accumulated to support the hypothesis that the limbic system does serve as the substrate for innate drives, emotional behavior, and memory. The following pages provide a basic outline of the functional anatomy of the system and give specific examples of the relationships between the limbic system and these behaviors.

Basic to all behavior is a set of innate behavioral patterns that are instinctual. These instincts including eating, fighting, fear, and sexual desire are found in all animals and are vital to self-preservation and perpetuation of the species. The exact neuroanatomic substrate of such instincts is elusive, yet most can be identified as being predominantly localized within specific limbic structures. Limbic activity does not, however, operate in isolation and close interaction with the ascending arousal system, basal ganglia, and neocortex is critical. In man, the basic instincts are not expressed in pure form but are dramatically modified by the learned behavior patterns stored in the neocortex.

BASIC INSTINCTS

Feeding instincts seem to be primarily controlled by the hypothalamus. Excessive feeding, for instance, can be initiated in animals by stimulation of the lateral hypothalamus or destruction of the ventromedial hypothalamic nuclei.[18] This relationship of feeding behavior to hypothalamic function has also been verified in human cases with tumors destroying the ventromedial or lateral hypothalamus. Patients with lesions in the ventromedial zone show a marked hyperphagia as the primary symptom, whereas patients with lateral damage demonstrate anorexia and emaciation.[12,34,42] Both excessive eating and starvation have also been produced in animals by means of stereotactic lesions in the amygdala,[11] although no comparable human cases have yet been reported. It is possible that some of the lip smacking and chewing movements seen during temporal lobe seizures represent feeding behavior of purely amygdalar origin but this has not been supported by clinical evidence.

The *olfactory apparatus* is another part of the limbic system that is intimately associated with feeding activity. The olfactory system is sensory and its stimulation does not directly result in feeding behavior; however, olfactory inputs to the amygdala and hypothalamus will trigger an orienting response and a host of autonomic functions including salivation and changes in gastrointestinal motility. Occasionally, experimental amygdalar lesions in animals cause a very complex alteration in feeding behavior in which the animals actually display a violent attack behavior toward food.[32] This type of aggressive feeding behavior demonstrates the rather close association in the nervous system of such disparate functions as feeding and aggression. Among humans, eating is usually a calm and civilized activity, but in many carnivorous animals a close alliance between aggressive and feeding instincts is required to insure survival.

Aggressiveness (fighting) and knowing when to escape from danger (fleeing) are extremely important instincts in all animals. Man, through his elaborate civilizing process, has modified these instincts considerably, but they nevertheless remain present in cryptic form. In general, *fighting and fleeing behaviors* are controlled by the limbic structures in the temporal lobe, the amygdala and hippocampus. The relationship between aggressiveness and temporal-limbic structures was first recognized with the discovery that vicious monkeys were made calm and tractable by removal of both of their temporal lobes. This observation, by Drs. Klüver and Bucy,[20] was one of the milestones in elucidating the relationship of instincts and emotions to specific brain structures. Destruction of the temporal lobes can produce docility in some animals, whereas stimulation of the amygdala or hippocampus often causes violent attack behavior. The literature contains several clinical reports of violent or aggressive behavior in patients with epileptogenic lesions in the temporal lobes. (These cases will be discussed in detail in Chapter 11, Epilepsy.) Aggressive behavior has also been reported in patients with destructive lesions in the ventromedial hypothalamus[34]; this again points out the close interrelationship of the temporal and hypothalamic limbic structures in producing and modulating instinctual behaviors.

The neurophysiologic mechanisms by which an animal attacks and kills another animal for food are speculative; however, the following model hypothesizes a relationship between limbic structures and feeding behavior. Assuming that an animal first detects his prey by its scent, an olfactory stimulus would travel along the olfactory tracts to the amygdala and septal nuclei. These structures then cause an orienting response toward the stimulus and an arousal of aggressive gustatory feelings. The stimulus is then carried from the amygdala via the stria terminalis and ventrofugal fibers (ansa peduncularis) to the hypothalamus, caudate nucleus, and septum. From the hypothalamus and septum, stimulation passes via the medial forebrain bundle to the limbic midbrain area where interdigitation with the ascending arousal system occurs. At this point, arousal level is high, aggressiveness and feeding instincts are acute, and attack behavior is then integrated through basal ganglia, motor cortex, and other subcortical motor systems. This simplified model can also be applied to an animal's response to a food stimulus received through any sensory modality (e.g., the sight of food). Man's feeding and aggressive instincts are usually well controlled by learned cortical inhibitions, but these instincts do remain and may be seen in extreme situations, such as war and famine.

The final major instinct under limbic control is *mating*. Ostensibly present to insure that each species will procreate and thereby avoid extinction, sexual drives in man appear to have surpassed this basic need and have become an integral part of interpersonal relationships. Anatomically, the septal nuclei and the anterior cingulate gyri have the greatest role in sexual behavior. Stimulation of the septal area has been demonstrated to give a very pleasurable response in both animals and man, and subjects with experimentally implanted septal stimulators will repeatedly stimulate themselves without any other external source of reinforcement.[16,30,44] Because of this, the septal area is known as the pleasure center. Reports of clinical cases verify these experimental data. One female patient, who developed a tumor in the anterior cingulate gyrus, changed from modest sexual propriety to marked hypersexuality (erotomania).[10]

It is apparent from these studies and clinical cases that the limbic structures within the frontal lobes are very important for the maintenance of active sexual drives. Temporal lobe limbic structures on the other hand appear to have an inhibitory influence upon sexual behavior. Temporal lobe removal has been demonstrated to unleash very inappropriate and exaggerated sexual responses (e.g., the Klüver-Bucy syndrome), whereas patients with active temporal lobe epileptogenic foci often exhibit a remarkable global hyposexuality.[4] From available data, it appears that the mating drive originates in the deep frontal lobe structures of the anterior cingulate gyrus and the septal nuclei but is significantly modified by the inhibitory input from the temporal lobe limbic structures. In man, of course, the learned social behavioral patterns that develop in the cortex form yet another strong controlling influence upon sexual behavior.

EMOTIONAL BEHAVIOR

The innate limbic instincts discussed above form the basis of the survival drives that allow animals to satisfy their basic needs. In some animals, but particularly in man, the limbic system also serves as a substrate for emotional behavior. Emotional reactions, by definition, are not neutral experiences. They involve the appreciation and expression of positive feelings such as desire, joy, or love or the negative emotions of sadness, hate, or anger. Emotions have two distinct aspects, they are both felt internally and expressed externally. The conscious appreciation of an emotion is a cortical phenomenon that is probably subsumed by the cingulate and phylogenetically older limbic cortex of the temporal and frontal lobes. It seems justifiable to surmise that the temporal lobe cortex associated with the structures of the amygdala and hippocampus is concerned with the initial appreciation of negative emotions whereas the frontal cortex is associated with the septal nuclei and cingulate gyrus with positive emotions. Ultimately, however, the entire cortex will participate in the full emotional experience.

The outward expression of emotion is a rudimentary and basic process that seems to involve two levels of action. First, and concomitant with the appreciation of the emotion, the autonomic nervous system is stimulated, primarily by the hypothalamus, to change heart rate, respiration pattern, peripheral vascular tone, and a host of other endocrine and autonomic functions. Along with these changes in homeostasis, motor patterns are stimulated in the basal ganglia by the other limbic structures which initiate changes in such factors as facial expression (smile, frown, or fear) and body attitude (attack or flight postures).

A mechanism by which the appreciation and expression of emotions are integrated by the limbic system was first proposed by Papez,[31] and his hypothesis can still be used as a framework for understanding the function of the system. He suggested that the emotional information from the environment spreads to the hippocampus from the various cortical receiving areas. The fornix, being the major outflow of the hippocampus, carries the stimulus to the mamillary bodies. From the mamillary bodies (the posterior nuclear group of the hypothalamus), the stimulus spreads within the hypothalamus to initiate emotional expression. At the same time, the stimulus spreads to the anterior nucleus of the thalamus via the mamilothalamic tract (Vicq d'Azyr tract) and then through a diffuse projection in the internal capsule to the cingulate gyrus where the emotion is consciously appreciated. The stimulus then returns to the hippocampus via the cingulum, thus completing the circuit. This model became known as the Papez circuit and has served as a foundation for theorizing about the functional properties of the limbic system.

To synthesize all of the anatomic and clinical information thus far presented into a coherent functional concept, let us postulate what happens within the limbic system when a person encounters an emotionally charged situation, such as watching his parked car being smashed by a reckless driver. The visual and auditory perception of the crash enters the primary visual cortex in the occipital lobes and the auditory cortex in the temporal lobes. This input travels in two directions: first to the association areas within the neocortex where the event is perceived in an objective fashion ("A red car driven at a high rate of speed just demolished my car and is now leaving the scene"). In conjunction with this spread of the stimulus within the cortex, impulses are sent to the hippocampus and thence to the amygdala.[22] At this point, aggression is added to the input and sent along the Papez circuit via the fornix to the mamillary bodies, septum, anterior thalamus, and on to the cingulate cortex for the conscious appreciation of the associated affect (anger and aggression). There are other pathways from the hippocampus/amygdala that reach the hypothalamus via the stria terminalis and the direct amygdalohypothalamic pathway. The hypothalamus with the septal and frontal lobe inputs then initiates a discharge down the medial forebrain bundle into the limbic midbrain area where interaction occurs with the reticular system, thus adding a tremendous arousal and alerting to the entire brain. Rage is now truly beginning. Simultaneously, the hypothalamus initiates a massive autonomic response of hyperventilation, increased heart rate, and pupillary dilatation. Motor patterns of rage are expressed through various interactions within the cortical and subcortical motor systems and now the person looks angry as well as feels angry. How each person deals with this anger and aggression is a separate issue and results from a combination of the person's basic temperament and the way he has been taught to react to such situations (social learning). These learned behavioral patterns which constitute so much of our personality will be discussed later in this chapter.

TEMPERAMENT

Before leaving the topic of the limbic system, it seems justified to briefly postulate a possible substrate for individual differences in temperament. Temperament refers to that underlying basic and characteristic way in which an individual reacts in any situation; including the activity level expressed, the tempo of action, the degree of satisfaction or dissatisfaction that is felt in each situation, and the individual's general mood or emotional tone. Each person seems to be born with a basic temperamental pattern that remains relatively constant throughout his lifetime.[40,45] This temperament will determine to a great extent the fashion in which the individual will react to inner drives, environmental stimulation, and stress. An individual's temperament may be very different from that of the parents, and these differences in temperament within a family can cause considerable stress even before formation of basic personality patterns. For instance, an infant who is very difficult to satisfy, cries unless fed or held, and who has a high activity level may well be born to a calm, passive, somewhat sensitive and timid couple. The tension in that family will be much higher than if those parents had an easy, calm child who spent much of his time cooing, eating, and sleeping. This basic temperament is presumed to be constitutional and strongly influences the environment's responses and interactions with the developing personality. If we assume that each person is born with a specific temperament, we must postulate that temperament is the product of the person's individual brain structure and physiology. Accordingly, everyone must have a slightly different arousal system which gives each a different basic activity level, capacity for sustained attention, and sleep needs. At the extreme end of this spectrum are some children who are readily recognized as being markedly overactive, hyperreactive, and distractible. In many such cases there is no primary emotional problem, and the hyperactivity and distractability appear due to an organic imbalance between the arousal system and the inhibitory activities of the brain stem and cortex. This activity can often be controlled by some medications (amphetamines and methylphenidate [Ritalin]) and exacerbated by others (barbiturates). These responses are paradoxical to those expected in normal individuals which further suggests a physiological basis for these temperamental differences.

Temperament implies more than activity level alone. It also refers to drive level, need for attention, degree of satisfaction gained from rewards, and mood. These functions are in the province of the limbic system. Thus, it could be postulated that basic temperament is the product of each individual's limbic and arousal systems as they interact with the learning process and socialization.

MEMORY

The limbic system has one additional critical function that serves as a transition between innate and learned behavior. This function is memory: the basis of all learning. Experimental and clinical evidence has shown that many structures within the limbic system are essential for learning. The anatomy underlying the memory process will be reviewed here, while the clinical memory syndromes and case studies will be discussed in Chapter 7, Neurobehavioral Syndromes Associated with Focal Brain Lesions. It has been shown that removal of, or damage to, the hippocampi bilaterally significantly interrupts an individual's ability to learn.[38] It appears that sensory information (e.g., a person's name, a word, a face, or the street locations in a new city) must traverse the hippocampus for the data to be stored in recent memory. The mamillary bodies and dorsal medial thalami are also critical structures for the process of memory storage and retrieval. Combined damage to these structures will also block the memory process.[41] It is possible that areas in the limbic midbrain are also vital links in the complicated chain of limbic structures necessary to establish the permanent memory storage.[23]

Memory traces are probably complex patterns which are consolidated within the neocortex and not the limbic system. Exactly why the cortex is dependent upon these subcortical systems for memory storage and retrieval is uncertain. Since learning requires reinforcement or reward, the limbic system, through its role in the generation and satisfaction of both basic and socially learned needs, could logically serve as the essential link in learning (storage of memories). The limbic system very possibly assesses the reward values of each incoming stimulus. For example, there is a positive emotional reward for learning particular facts (e.g., the name of an attractive member of the opposite sex at a social affair). Conversely, negative emotional responses can also stimulate learning (e.g., the fear of not remembering an important lecture or neuroanatomic structure when a test is imminent). The limbic system serves to give all environmental inputs a relative value in terms of survival; factors with high survival value will be remembered, whereas factors with no personal relevance will not be learned efficiently.

This discussion of limbic functions is based solely upon an anatomic model. In recent years, neurochemical research has shown that many of the limbic circuits are composed of neurons which produce a single transmitter substance. Some neuronal systems are dopaminergic, others either serotonergic, cholinergic, or adrenergic. Someday it may be possible to further break down emotional, motivational, and learning functions to specific chemical subsystems rather than relying upon an anatomic model alone. Research into the relationship of cholinergic systems and learning and memory is currently in progress,[9] but data is too fragmentary at present to make the step from the anatomic bases of behavior to the chemical.

THE CORTEX

The neocortex is the most recently and highly developed portion of the central nervous system. In this area, all intellectual processes are carried out and refinements in personality and social behavior are developed. Our knowledge of higher cortical functions comes primarily from the study of the human brain, since man's use of language permits both clinical and experimental study. The cortex has been extensively studied anatomically and has been divided into many separate areas based on cytoarchitecture. Since the divisions described by Brodmann have been widely accepted we will employ that numbering system in our discussion[7] (Fig. 11).

Inherent in the cortex is the capacity for intellectual development. However, the actual functions of language, perception, abstract thought, and social interaction must be learned through the individual's day to day interaction with his environment. The raw material for this learning process comes to the cortex through the various sen-

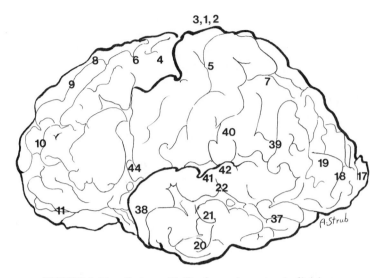

FIGURE 2–11. Cortex with Brodmann's anatomic divisions.

sory systems. The sensory input is constantly augmented by motor activity; this activity allows the individual to manipulate objects and move through the environment.

The basic sensory and motor systems have well established cortical representation. These are called the primary motor areas (areas 4,6, and 8) and the primary sensory receiving areas (area 17—visual area; areas 3,1, and 2—tactile; and areas 41 and 42—auditory). Our discussion of intellectual functions, although assuming the presence of intact basic sensory and motor areas, is primarily concerned with the association areas. Within these areas, the raw sensory and motor data are elaborated, compared with existing memory patterns, and then manipulated to meet environmental demands.

The visual system receives information through the primary visual cortex (area 17), these stimuli then spread to the primary and secondary association areas (areas 18 and 19). In these association areas, the basic visual sensations of light, dark, line, and position are transformed into forms or objects that can be compared with previous experience.[21] This sophisticated ability to discriminate between different shapes and to compare the present sensory pattern with past impressions is the basis of the visual perceptual process. The same type of process occurs in auditory perception. Sounds are first received in the primary auditory cortex (areas 41 and 42), then transferred to the primary auditory association area (area 22) and finally to the secondary association areas (areas 20, 21, 37, and 38). In the auditory association areas, sounds are appreciated as being specific types (e.g., boat whistles, cars starting,

28

human voices). As the stimulus spreads, human voice input can then be recognized as language.

Tactile perception and learning is analogous. Tactile stimuli spread from the primary receiving cortex (areas 3, 1, and 2) to the association areas (areas 5 and 7). The ability to discern objects placed in the hand (stereognosis) is localized in both the primary receiving areas and in the association areas. Accordingly, the primary tactile receiving cortex appears to be somewhat more highly developed than the primary visual and auditory cortex.[35]

In man there is a large, phylogenetically recent area of cortex called the inferior parietal lobule which serves as a tertiary association area (supramarginal gyrus—area 40 and angular gyrus—area 39). This third level association cortex receives the spreading sensory stimuli (of all visual, auditory, and tactile input) from the secondary association areas. By virtue of this confluence of all inputs, this area is capable of forming sensory associations (cross-modal association), allowing man to link visual, auditory, and tactile inputs in such a way that he is able to apply words to visual stimuli and describe what he sees or touches. This high level capacity to associate all inputs is the basis of most higher cognitive functions.

This section hypothesizes that intellectual functions develop through interactions among sensory inputs and their concurrent impact on motor learning. Each of these interactions occurs in a different area of the cortex and, accordingly, lesions in different parts of the brain will produce different clinical syndromes. A knowledge of the cortical localization of cognitive function is important because an examiner can then determine the location of a lesion such as a tumor or stroke by systematically testing a series of intellectual functions.

Localization of Function

Localization of function within the human cortex is made considerably easier by the fact that the two hemispheres subserve very different functions. The left hemisphere, in essentially all right-handed individuals (over 90% of the population), is dominant for the learning of skilled fine motor movements. This left hemispheric superiority for motor learning apparently is the neuroanatomic substrate for right handedness. Interestingly enough, the left hemisphere of the right handed individual is also dominant for the development of language. This remarkable lateralization of language is very probably a genetic trait that is based upon a structural asymmetry of the language cortex, although damage to the dominant hemisphere early in life can cause a transferal of dominance.[37] It has been demonstrated that the auditory cortex of the left hemisphere is larger and more developed in the right handed adult.[13] The asymmetry does not appear to be an effect of language exposure as it has also been observed in the brains of newborns.[43]

This strong left hemispheric dominance for language is not as pronounced in the left handed person; in fact only 60 percent of left handed individuals are strongly left brain dominant, while 40 percent have some right hemisphere dominance for language.[2] Lateralization for language in general is not as strongly established in the left handed person; 80 percent of the left handed population have some degree of language capacity in both hemispheres.[14] Because of this bilateral language representation, the localization of a lesion in the left handed patient should be made on grounds other than the presence of a language deficit alone.

LANGUAGE

Since the left hemisphere is dominant for language in the majority of the population, we will use left hemispheric function as the model for the discussion of the anatomy of language. Language and the ability to communicate our needs and thoughts are the bases for many of our intellectual processes. The complete use of language requires the following five basic processes: (1) comprehension of spoken language, (2) verbal reasoning, (3) production of speech, (4) deciphering written language, and (5) writing. Through the study of brain damaged patients with language disturbances (aphasia), many of these processes have been localized to general areas within the left hemisphere. The comprehension of spoken language occurs in the posterior area of the temporal lobe and adjoining parietal cortex (Fig. 2-12, area 1). The superior temporal gyrus (area 22) subsumes the most basic level of comprehension, whereas the association cortex (areas 20, 21, 37, 39, and 40) is more involved in higher level complex comprehension and verbal reasoning. The higher the level of the mental process (e.g., verbal abstract reasoning), the more widespread the cortical representation necessary for carrying out that process.

The actual production of speech is a motor act and, by virtue of this fact, is intimately associated with the area of the motor cortex responsible for the movement of the buccofacial apparatus. The actual cortical area necessary for producing speech is a sizeable region of the frontal lobe surrounding and including Broca's area (area 44) (Fig. 2-12, area 2).[27] The comprehension and production of spoken language, though not as discretely localized as some texts might suggest, does rely upon the posterior portions of the hemisphere surrounding the sylvian fissure for comprehension and the anterior portions for speech production.

For the individual to comprehend and discuss events occurring in the environment, a further step in language processing is required. This step is the integration of visual or tactile stimuli with the language system. Because there is an extensive overlap within the association cortex, verbal labels or names can be attached to visually presented objects or written symbols. In this way, language can be used to describe ongoing events within the environment. The same process pertains to the decoding of specific written symbols (reading). This overlap of vision and language occurs in the tertiary association areas of the left inferior parietal lobule (areas 39 and 40). This cortical localization of reading has been well established, as there have been many patients reported who have lost their ability to read and write with the destruction of areas 39 and 40.[3]

VISUAL PERCEPTION

Visual perception is a very important function that allows exploration of the environment and learning of relationships between various objects in space. In man, basic perceptual functions develop before the acquisition of verbal skills. The infant learns about his environment—the constancy of objects, certain laws of cause and effect, and a geographic plan of his life space—much before he utters his first intelligible word. As language develops, these visual perceptual processes become less apparent but are no less important. These processes are critically important to the child learning to write or to the architect who must be able to translate visual ideas to paper and then into structure. These basic perceptual skills are vital for our functioning but become so automatic that we are seldom aware of them. Visual perception and appreciation of spatial orientation in the environment is carried out almost exclusively in the parietal lobes. Here, visual input is manipulated within the visual association areas (areas 18 and 19) and compared with previous visual experiences. These visual skills are somewhat better developed in the right or nondominant parietal lobe. Accordingly, it is possible to say that the right posterior hemisphere is somewhat dominant for visual spatial tasks in the same manner that the left is more specifically specialized for verbal tasks. Language dominance, however, is much more strongly lateralized than is perceptual spatial dominance.

TACTILE PERCEPTION

Tactile perception develops in conjunction with the kinesthetic sensory system in much the same way as does visual perception. Basic tactile information concerning texture, weight, shape, and size of an object is processed in the sensory cortex (areas 3, 1, and 2) and adjacent association cortex (areas 5 and 7). This tactile information can then be compared with kinesthetic memories so that one can identify objects by touch alone. This comparison occurs in the parietal lobe; probably in areas 3, 1, 2, 5, and 7. Because of the rich overlap among tactile, visual, and language association areas, the individual is able both to use language to identify and name objects perceived tactilly and also to evoke visual memories from tactile stimulation (for example, recognition of eye glasses when touched in the dark or identification of a coin's denomination when felt in the pocket). Tactile-auditory associations are probably most highly developed in the blind since these individuals rely so heavily upon tactile input. Use of the Braille system demonstrates the high level to which this skill can be developed. Basic tactile skills are developed in both hemispheres and are primarily controlled by the cortex contralateral to the hand stimulated. When Braille is read with the left hand, the tactile images must be transferred from the right parietal lobe (tactile input) to the left inferior parietal lobe (association area) to be comprehended as language.

HIGHER INTELLECTUAL PROCESSES

The basic building blocks of man's intellect are language, perception (visual and tactile), and the motor skills that develop under the guidance of the basic sensory systems. Higher intellectual processes such as verbal reasoning, complex visual spatial problem solving (e.g., completing an architectural model), or higher skilled motor acts (e.g., replacement of a heart valve by a surgeon) all require the interaction and mental manipulation of stored language, visual memories, and tactile images. Man's ability to actively manipulate his store of information and to form different and novel combinations is the essence of thought and the creative process. This higher order mental activity is possible because of the rich association areas in the postrolandic cortex. Almost all nonemotional intellectual processes are carried out in this posterior region of the brain. Removal of both frontal lobes though causing distinct changes in personality, leaves basic thinking processes relatively intact.[15,24]

THE FRONTAL LOBES

While the parietal lobes and contiguous temporal and occipital lobes are the locus of intellectual processes and the limbic system is the substrate for instincts and emotions, the frontal lobes serve to mediate between the intellect and the emotions. These premotor frontal or prefrontal cortical structures (areas 9, 10, and 11) are both the most recent phylogenetic addition to the central nervous system and also the latest areas of the brain to mature in the child. Their architecture is distinctly granular, a feature that relates them more closely anatomically with the sensory than with the motor cortex. This association with the sensory cortex can be better understood after a discussion of the fiber pathways connecting the frontal lobe with the posterior sensory association areas.

The afferent and efferent connections of the frontal lobe are largely reciprocal. Afferents to the frontal lobes originate from two principal sources: the first is the sensory association cortex in the posterior hemisphere (inferior parietal lobule) via several pathways: (1) long chains of corticocortical neurons, (2) long association fibers (inferior and superior occipitofrontal fasciculi), and (3) the uncinate fasciculus from the temporal cortex. These pathways carry information concerning the external environment as well as data about thought processes being carried out within the parietal association cortex. These pathways project for the most part to the lateral convexity of the frontal cortex (areas 9, 10, and 11). The second major input comes from the limbic structures via several pathways: (1) the uncinate fasciculus from the amygdala, (2) the hypothalamus and amygdala via the internal capsule from the thalamic nuclei, (3) the limbic midbrain area and the hypothalamus via the medial forebrain bundle, (4) the cingulum, and (5) direct communications from the septal nuclei. This extensive limbic input is projected primarily to the orbitomedial or inferior surface of the frontal lobes. By virtue of this direct limbic connection, the prefrontal cortex receives continuous information concerning the individual's feelings and the state of internal needs.

Fears, threats, and desires for food, sleep, and sex are constantly communicated to the frontal granular cortex. All sensory and intellectual processing from the posterior cortex is also projected upon the frontal lobes.[29] This area of the cortex thus serves as the brain's final or quaternary association area. Within the frontal lobes, the interactions of inputs from the posterior centers and the limbic system allow basic emotional and intellectual behaviors to be synthesized and elaborated.

The prefrontal region does not have a major motor efferent pathway, rather the output of this region is reciprocal. The principal reciprocal paths to the limbic system are to the cingulate gyrus, hippocampus, septum, hypothalamus (via the medial forebrain bundle), and the amygdala (via the uncinate fasciculus and a pathway through the dorsal medial thalamus). The efferents to neocortical structures are to the temporal cortex (via uncinate fasciculus) and to the inferior parietal lobule (via fronto-occipital bundles). This reciprocal innervation of the frontal connections suggests that the frontal lobe acts to modulate the activities of the intellectual and emotional systems through the synthesis of both types of input. The function of reciprocal circuitry has been postulated to explain some of the subtle intellectual defects seen in patients with frontal lesions. For example, it has been demonstrated that the frontal cortex emits a preparatory discharge to the visual system prior to the movement of the eyes. This preparation stimulus insures that the individual will be prepared perceptually for the movement and not feel that the environment is moving when it is only the eyeball itself that is moving.[39] This preparatory process by the frontal lobes has been postulated to act as an active guidance system to control those environmental stimuli which will receive attention, those mental processes which shall be continued, and the time when change in any mental direction should be initiated.[33]

It has been amply demonstrated clinically that patients with frontal damage have great difficulty shifting mental processes from one concept to another. For instance, if a patient with damage to the frontal lobes is told to sort playing cards into piles and is rewarded when he places all hearts and diamonds in one pile and all clubs and spades in another, he will soon learn this task. If the examiner suddenly (without a change in instructions to the patient) begins to reward him only when he places odd numbered cards in one pile and even numbered cards in the other, he will be unable to make this shift efficiently.[26] This tendency to perseverate and inability to shift mental set efficiently is typical of the difficulty experienced by frontal lobe patients. The card sorting task relies heavily on the patient's desire to continue to be rewarded for his correct answers. The ability to learn from reward is a main function of the limbic system, and in the patient with frontal damage, the reward value from the limbic system has been disconnected from the sensory input from the parietal lobes and can no longer adequately interact with the now meaningless task of sorting cards. Accordingly the patient has no incentive or drive to alter his behavior on the task. Though subtle, this ability to actively shift mental sets and to adjust to changes in the environment is a very important aspect of higher cognitive processing.

Another cognitive activity directed by the frontal lobes is the ability to appreciate the temporal order of a series of events and the capacity to compare relative merit in importance of each event.[25] To compare specific alternatives and to keep all possibilities in mind, the individual must be able to actively shift attention from one alternative to another.

The basic functions of changing mental set, appreciating temporal order, controlling attention, and being able to compare various alternatives are all components of the more sophisticated and critical role that the frontal lobes play in making major decisions.[17] Major decisions are considered to be life or goal directed decisions such as the selection of a career, a spouse, or a school. Making of these decisions utilizes the ability of the frontal lobes to consider both the practical (parietal) and the emotional (limbic) aspects of the situation. In addition, the cortex draws upon its capacity to evaluate the probable outcomes of all possible alternatives to each decision. It then chooses the course of action that appears to best suit the individual's true needs. The frontal lobes allow the practical aspects of a situation to be projected against the emotional input from the limbic system permitting the positive and negative emotional and practical aspects of each alternative to be sampled. Internal emotional reactions are critical to reasoning applied to human situations. Without input from the frontal lobes, decisions are made without the advantage of emotional reflection (e.g., the patient who acts in a coldly intellectual fashion without any emotional concern for how his actions will affect others). Similarly the disconnection of limbic from cortical structures experienced in frontal lobe lesions may result in impulsive emotional behavior untempered by rational consideration.

The frontal lobes have another important role in behavior: that of utilizing the learned behavior of the intellect to modulate and control the forceful drives that emanate from the limbic system. In the absence of the frontal lobes, emotions and instincts may become dysinhibited. Patients with damage to the frontal lobes can demonstrate complete reversals in personality (e.g., ambitious, productive individuals can become apathetic and desultory while proper, reserved individuals can become euphoric, loud, and act completely inappropriately in social situations). While it is not possible to accurately localize specific emotional functions within the frontal lobes, some evidence indicates that damage to the lateral convexity results in an apathetic state whereas damage to the orbital/medial portion causes the more animated or manic type disturbance.[5]

Because frontal damage releases abnormal behavior, it has been assumed that in the intact individual the frontal lobes control and guide social behavior. Viewed developmentally, the child is born with many simple needs and instincts to insure survival. These needs are initially met by the environment. However, as the child grows he must learn that needs are neither always met immediately nor satisfied completely. This learning represents the process of socialization. This inculcation of social behavior is an example of the modification of basic instinctual behavior. It is within the frontal lobes that environmental experiences interact with the limbic drive system to produce the final and appropriate course of action in a given situation. Without this limbic/frontal interaction, an individual cannot properly learn from experience.[1] Clinical experience with patients with frontal damage supports the postulate that the frontal lobes are the place where temperament, drive, and experience interact.

SUMMARY

Human behavior is the product of many cortical and subcortical systems. Each individual's unique behavior and personality is the totality of his basic instincts, his constitutional temperament, and the sum of his learned experiences. Behavior relies upon an arousal system that allows the maintenance of alertness and upon the widespread inhibitory system in the cortex, limbic system, and brain stem that allows the individual to focus and sustain mental energy on an individual task or problem. The vast and complicated limbic system works in concert with the arousal system and the basal ganglia to provide an anatomic substrate for survival instincts, emotional expression and appreciation, and temperament. The limbic system adds reinforcement to learning and accordingly is vital to the acquisition and retrieval of memories. The cortex is the repository for the memories of all life experiences. The association cortex in the inferior parietal area has the capacity to actively manipulate in both familiar and novel ways the information stored therein. This active manipulation represents the basic physiologic process of thought and is the ground work of the intellect.

The intellect and instincts must be guided in order that activities will be productive, survival insured, and yet actions and behavior socially appropriate. It is these last elements that are the responsibility of the frontal lobes and are the final product of the brain's activity—human behavior.

REFERENCES

1. Ackerly, S.S., and Benton, A.L.: Report of case of bilateral frontal lobe defect in The Frontal Lobes. Ass. Res. Nerv. Ment. Dis. 27:479, 1947.
2. Benson, D.F., and Geschwind, N.: Cerebral dominance and its disturbances. Pediatr. Clin. North Am. 15:759, 1968.
3. Benson, D.F., and Geschwind, N.: The aphasias and related disturbances, in Baker, A.B. (ed.): Baker's Clinical Neurology, Vol. 1, Chap. 8. Harper & Row, New York, 1975.
4. Blumer, D.: Changes in sexual behavior related to temporal lobe disorder in man. J. Sex Res. 6:173, 1970.
5. Blumer, D., and Benson, D.F.: Personality changes with frontal and temporal lobe lesions, in Benson, D.F., and Blumer, D. (eds.): Psychiatric Aspects of Neurologic Disease. Grune & Stratton, New York, 1975, pp. 151–170.
6. Brodal, A.: Anatomical points of view on the alleged morphological basis of consciousness. Acta Neurochir. 12:166, 1965.
7. Brodmann, K.: Vergleichende Lokalisationslehre der Grosshirnrinde in thren Prinzipien dargestellt auf Grund des Zellenbaues. J.A. Barth, Leipzig, 1909.
8. Crosby, E.C., Humphrey, T., and Lauer, E.W.: Correlative Anatomy of the Nervous System. The MacMillan Co., New York, 1962.
9. Drachman, D.A.: Memory and the cholinergic system, in Fields, W.S. (ed.): Neurotransmitter Function—Basic and Clinical Aspects. Symposia Specialists, 1977.
10. Erickson, T.C.: Erotomania (nymphomania) as expression of cortical epileptiform discharge. Arch. Neurol. Psychiat. 53:226, 1945.

11. Fonberg, E.: The normalizing effect of lateral amygdalar lesions upon the dorsomedial amygdala syndrome in dogs. Acta Neurobiol. Exp. 33:449, 1973.

12. Fulton, J.F., and Bailey, P.: Tumors in the region of the third ventricle: their diagnosis and relation to pathological sleep. J. Nerv. Ment. Dis. 69:1, 1929.

13. Geschwind, N., and Levitsky, W.: Human brain: left-right asymmetries in temporal speech region. Science 161:186, 1968.

14. Gloning, I., Gloning, K., Haub, G., and Quatember, R.: Comparison of verbal behavior in right-handed and non-right-handed patients with anatomically verified lesions of one hemisphere. Cortex 5:43, 1969.

15. Hamlin, R.M.: Intellectual function 14 years after frontal lobe surgery. Cortex 6:299, 1970.

16. Heath, R.G.: Brain function and behavior I. Emotion and sensory phenomena in psychiatric patients and in experimental animals. J. Nerv. Ment. Dis. 160:159, 1975.

17. Hécaen, H., and Albert, M.L.: Disorders of mental functioning related to frontal lobe pathology, in Benson, D.F., and Blumer, D. (eds.): Psychiatric Aspects of Neurologic Disease. Grune & Stratton, New York, 1975, pp. 137–149.

18. Isaacson, R.L.: The Limbic System. Plenum Press, New York, 1974.

19. Kahn, E., and Cohen, L.H.: Organic driveness: a brainstem syndrome and an experience. New Engl. J. Med. 210:748, 1934.

20. Klüver, H., and Bucy, P.C.: Preliminary analysis of the temporal lobes in monkeys. Arch. Neurol. Psychiat. 42:979, 1939.

21. Luria, A.: Higher Cortical Functions in Man. Basic Books, New York, 1966.

22. MacLean, P.D., and Creswell, G.: Anatomical connections of visual system with limbic cortex of monkey. J. Comp. Neurol. 138:265, 1970.

23. McEntee, W.J., Biber, M.P., Perl, D.P., and Benson, D.F.: Diencephalic amnesia: a reappraisal. J. Neurol. Neurosurg. Psychiatry 39:436, 1976.

24. Mettler, F.A. (ed.): Selective Partial Ablation of the Frontal Cortex. Hoeber, New York, 1949.

25. Milner, B.: Interhemispheric differences and psychological processes. Br. Med. Bull. 27:272, 1971.

26. Milner, B., and Teuber, H.L.: Alteration of perception and memory in man, in Weiskrantz, L. (ed.): Analysis of Behavioral Change. Harper & Row, New York, 1968, pp. 268–375.

27. Mohr, J.P.: Broca's area and Broca's aphasia, in Whitaker, H., and Whitaker, H.A. (eds.): Studies in Neurolinguistics. Academic Press, New York, 1976, pp. 201–235.

28. Moruzzi, G., and Magoun, H.W.: Brainstem reticular formation and activation of the EEG. Electroencephalogr. Clin. Neurophysiol. 1:455, 1949.

29. Nauta, W.J.H.: The problem of the frontal lobe: a reinterpretation. J. Psychiatr. Res. 8:167, 1971.

30. Olds, J., and Milner, P.: Positive reinforcement produced by electrical stimulation of septal area and other regions of rat brain. J. Comp. Physiol. Psychol. 47:417, 1954.

31. Papez, J.W.: A proposed mechanism of emotion. Arch. Neurol. Psychiat. 38:725, 1937.

32. Pribram, K.H.: Languages of the Brain. Experimental Paradoxes of Principles in Neuropsychology. Prentice-Hall, Englewood Cliffs, New Jersey, 1971.

33. Pribram, K.H., and Melges, F.T.: Psychophysiological basis of emotions, in Vinken, P.J., and Bruyn, G.W. (eds.): Handbook of Clinical Neurology, Vol 3. Elsevier-North Holland Publishing Co., New York, 1969, pp. 316–342.
34. Reeves, A.G., and Plum, F.: Hyperphagia, rage and dementia accompanying a ventromedial hypothalamic neoplasm. Arch. Neurol. 20:616, 1969.
35. Roland, P.E.: Astereognosis. Arch. Neurol. 33:543, 1976.
36. Rossi, G.F.: Brainstem facilitating influences on EEG synchronization. Experimental findings and observations in man. Acta Neurochir. 13:257, 1965.
37. Satz, P.: Pathological left-handedness: an explanatory model. Cortex 8: 121, 1972.
38. Scoville, W.B., and Milner, B.: Loss of recent memory after bilateral hippocampal lesions. J. Neurol. Neurosurg. Psychiatry 20:11, 1957.
39. Teuber, H.L.: The riddle of frontal lobe function in man, in Warren, J.M., and Akert, K. (eds.): The Frontal Granular Cortex and Behavior. McGraw-Hill Book Co., New York, 1964, pp. 410–444.
40. Thomas, A., Chess, S., and Birch, H.G.: Temperament and Behavior Disorders in Children. New York University Press, New York, 1968.
41. Victor, M., Adams, R.D., and Collins, G.H.: The Wernicke-Korsakoff Syndrome. F.A. Davis Co., Philadelphia, 1971.
42. White, L.E., and Hain, R.F.: Anorexia in association with a destructive lesion of the hypothalamus. Arch. Path. 68:275, 1959.
43. Witelson, S.F., and Pallie, W.: Left hemisphere specialization for language in the newborn: neuroanatomical evidence of asymmetry. Brain 96:641, 1973.
44. Jacques, S.: Brain stimulation and reward: "pleasure centers" after twenty-five years. Neurosurgery 5:277, 1979.
45. Thomas A., and Chess, S.: Temperament and Development. Brunner/Mazel, New York, 1977.

3

NONMEDICAL EVALUATION

The organic brain syndromes are complex processes which often present a confusing picture to the inexperienced examiner. The symptoms are frequently overlooked or minimized (e.g., the vague anxiety and subjective complaints of memory difficulty in the patient with early dementia), misinterpreted as a functional psychiatric disorder (e.g., the agitated Wernicke's aphasic who is psychiatrically hospitalized because of his paranoid aggressive behavior and inappropriate speech), or unrecognized when associated with more striking physical findings (e.g., hemiparesis with associated aphasia). It is an unfortunate fact that even in patients with documented neurologic injury or disease, many subtle and some gross cognitive and emotional organic sequelae are unappreciated. The patient with mild aphasia, memory deficit, or constructional impairment after neurosurgical procedures; impaired attention and heightened irritability after head trauma; or mood fluctuations and emotional lability following central nervous system infection is frequently discharged from the hospital after recovery from the acute state of the injury or illness without recognition of the neurobehavioral changes. Such patients often have appreciable difficulty in readjusting socially and vocationally because of their deficits; they become frustrated, anxious, and depressed both because of their basic problems in adjustment and because of the inability of the physician to recognize and adequately explain their difficulties.

An early evaluation of neurobehavioral status in such patients will result in the documentation of any cognitive and emotional residual. Such documentation helps to delineate any subtle disability more fully and will serve as the basis for counseling both the patient and his family. This precludes the development of misunderstanding and promotes appropriate posthospitalization management. The data gained from a complete mental status examination is also a valuable aid to planning subsequent social and vocational rehabilitation if indicated.

All patients with known neurologic disease should receive a definitive mental status examination as outlined in the pages to follow. Those patients who demonstrate abnormal findings on the screening mental status exam should then be referred for more comprehensive evaluation by a consultant specializing in the area of the detected deficit (e.g., speech pathologist for the aphasic patient, psychiatrist for the individual with associated or reactive emotional disorder, neuropsychologist for the patient requiring more intensive comprehensive evaluation and rehabilitation planning, and so forth).

In our clinical practice, it has become increasingly apparent that there is a high incidence of demonstrable neurobehavioral disorders within the population of patients presenting with apparently functional complaints. Organic brain disease frequently presents initially in the guise of either subtle or not so subtle behavioral and emotional changes. This is particularly true of frontal and temporal lobe tumors, undetected temporal lobe seizures, hydrocephalus, and cortical atrophy. We have also repeatedly seen patients with acute focal left hemisphere strokes or subdural hematomas whose resulting receptive aphasias and associated agitation and paranoia were inappropriately diagnosed in the emergency room as "acute schizophrenic reaction." Patients with acute confusional states secondary to metabolic imbalance or drug toxicity are also prime candidates for misdiagnosis because of their frequent psychotic-like presentations. Only a thorough review of medical records and a carefully conducted mental status examination will reveal the organic nature of the disorder. Since neurologic disease so frequently masquerades as functional illness, we feel that all patients with a psychiatric diagnosis should be screened with a complete mental status examination. This is particularly true in those cases in which the psychiatric symptomatology is acute in onset or is superimposed upon a life history of relatively stable normal emotional functioning. It is far more efficacious in terms of time and money to spend 15 to 30 minutes additional time with the patient administering a complete mental status examination in search of possible organic etiology than to embark upon an expensive and lengthy regimen of psychiatric treatment. We have seen a number of patients who have undergone long periods of outpatient psychotherapy, psychotropic medication, electroshock, and psychiatric hospitalization, who, upon referral to the behavioral neurologist or neuropsychologist, showed clear evidence of primary central nervous system disease which was verified by neurodiagnostic procedures (CT scan, EEG, or pneumoencephalography).

Another group in which a complete mental status evaluation may prove invaluable is comprised of patients presenting with vague and subjective complaints such as anxiety, a lack of concentration, memory deficits, or a loss of interest in family or work. Any such complaint should alert the clinician to the possibility of organic disease, even in the absence of clear-cut physical findings. A number of neurobehavioral disorders, notably the early stages of dementia or the onset of a confusional state, initially present with primarily behavioral and cognitive symptoms. In such cases, the clinician must be prepared to make an oftentimes difficult differential diagnosis between functional and organic etiologies. The results of the mental status examination in such patients are often as valuable in making the correct diagnosis as are most other neurodiagnostic procedures including the CT scan, EEG, or pneumoencephalogram. Because the behavioral and cognitive findings often appear before overt physical symptoms, the mental status examination will often reveal diagnostic abnormalities prior to any indication of pathology on the standard neurologic examination.

In general, we feel that the following broad categories of patients should receive the benefit of at least a screening mental status examination:

1. Patients with documented central nervous system disease or injury of any type.
2. Patients with primary psychiatric diagnoses.
3. Patients with suspected neurologic disease, even (or especially) if the diagnosis cannot be made on the basis of a standard physical and neurologic examination.
4. Patients presenting with vague subjective behavioral, cognitive, or physical complaints which cannot be substantiated from physical and routine laboratory examination.

Although the examination as outlined in the following pages may appear to be lengthy and time consuming, with familiarity and experience it can be administered in 15 to 20 minutes. The value of the information it provides far exceeds the cost of the time expended in its administration.

The following pages provide a broad, yet relatively concise, outline of a medical history and mental status examination which has been specifically tailored for use with patients presenting with known or suspected organic brain syndromes. We feel that all neurologists, psychiatrists, and the well-trained primary care physician should be familiar with the administration and interpretation of these crucial techniques.

MEDICAL AND SOCIAL HISTORY

As in any area of medicine, the history is extremely important in the evaluation of patients with organic brain syndromes. This aspect of the

41

evaluation process should never be minimized in favor of the physical or laboratory examinations. It is often only from details in the history that organic disease may be accurately differentiated from functional disorders or from atypical lifelong patterns of behavior. As an example of the latter differential, we have not infrequently seen inexperienced residents make an initial misdiagnosis of dementia based upon abnormalities on the mental status examination, only to find after a careful social history that the patient had completed two years of formal education, had lived his entire life in a remote rural area, and had a number of relatives confined to institutions for the retarded.

If the patient is amenable to providing a history, even if memory problems and confabulation make the examiner suspicious of the obtained data's validity, an initial medical and social history should be obtained directly. This provides an opportunity to observe the patient's thinking and behavior under a situation of minimal stress and may offer historical information unavailable elsewhere (e.g., the family being unaware that the patient had contracted syphilis during an overseas military assignment and had been inadequately treated because of the pressures of combat necessities). In addition, the period of observation while the history is taken allows the careful observer to make a subjective assessment of the patient's interaction, attention, memory, language, and general behavior. Many patients are unable to provide a coherent and useful history; in these situations the history should also be taken from a reliable family member or friend. This is generally possible in the usual private practice or hospital. In many large public hospitals, however, there is often a surprising dearth of family or visitors for some patients. Unfortunately, these are often the patients with apparent chronic alcoholism, progressive dementia, or acute confusional states who find their way to public clinics and wards. It is virtually impossible to obtain valid histories from such individuals, but the history is often essential to making an efficacious differential diagnosis. In such cases, obtaining medical records from previous hospitalizations and telephoning the patient's family to determine the necessary medical and social information is required. Despite the apparent aversion of some young physicians to performing this type of "medical social work," the value of the obtained information to the patient's evaluation and management far outweighs the minor inconveniences involved. If available, medical social workers may be utilized to aid in the compilation of data from geographically scattered hospitals and family members.

Specific aspects of the medical and social history are especially important in the evaluation of patients with organic brain syndromes. Following the outline below ensures that the essential data are collected and recorded:

I. Medical history
   A. Family history
      1. Presence of neurologic or psychiatric disease in another family member. Obtain diagnosis and nature of the disease
      2. Familial neurologic disease (e.g., Huntington's chorea)
      3. Family predilection for a particular disease process that may involve the central nervous system (e.g., hypertension and cerebrovascular disease)
      4. Cause of and age at death of parents and siblings
   B. Birth and developmental history
      1. Prenatal, perinatal, or postnatal brain damage
      2. Delays in normal development
         a. Motor
         b. Language
         c. Intellectual
         d. Academic
   C. Past medical history
      1. Previous neurologic or psychiatric disease
      2. Significant head trauma
      3. Seizures
      4. Other medical diseases requiring hospitalization
   D. Description of present illness
      1. Nature of onset
      2. Duration of illness
      3. Characterization of the course of the illness
      4. Description of behavioral changes associated with illness
   E. Other relevant neurobehavioral data
      1. Memory difficulty
      2. Recent onset of reading, writing, or calculating difficulties
      3. Attention and concentration problems
      4. Recent onset of speech or language problems
      5. Unusual or bizarre behavior (e.g., nocturnal wanderings, paranoia, hallucinations)
      6. Difficulty with geographic orientation (i.e., getting lost or inability to find items)
II. Social history
   A. Social development
      1. Abnormalities in behavior
      2. Family and peer interaction
      3. Intellectual development
   B. Educational history
      1. Highest educational level attained
      2. Nature of any training following high school

43

3. Specific or general school problems (e.g., "slow learner," dyslexic)
4. Reason for terminating education
C. Vocational history
   1. Present occupation
      a. Length of current job
      b. Nature of job responsibilities
   2. Types of previous jobs. Note upward or downward mobility
   3. Frequency of job changes. Note reasons for leaving
   4. Any recent difficulties with work
      a. Type
      b. Severity
D. Other revelant data
   1. Adequacy of social adjustment
   2. Nature of specific social, behavioral, or emotional problems
   3. Use (duration, frequncy, and quantity) of:
      a. Alcohol
      b. Tobacco
      c. Licit and illicit drugs
   4. Family's description of the current problem

MENTAL STATUS EXAMINATION

Following completion of the medical/social history and the routine physical or neurologic examination, the physician should next administer the mental status examination. In some cases, a rapid screening evaluation will suffice, while with other patients a more comprehensive assessment of a wider range of functions is necessary. The brief exam stressing only the essential features can be easily administered in 10 minutes. In some complex cases, the physician may wish to spend a longer period with the patient in order to formulate a detailed description of cognitive and behavioral deficits and residual strengths. The evaluative material presented in the succeeding pages can be readily adapted to either the brief screening or a more comprehensive evaluation. Those items marked with an asterisk are considered critical and should be administered to all patients. The remaining items provide a means of more thoroughly evaluating a wider range of functioning.

The physician must recognize that the mental status examination is organized in a systematic and hierarchical fashion, in much the same way as any comprehensive medical examination. The higher cognitive functions (e.g., verbal abstraction or calculating ability) rely upon the integrity of more basic functions (e.g., attention or language). Thus, impairment demonstrated on early sections of the examination will make it difficult, if not impossible, to validly assess higher functions. For example, the patient with disturbed attention and vigilance secondary to an acute confusional state will be unable to perform validly on most parts of the mental status exam because of his inability to concentrate and assimilate details. Similarly, verbal memory or other functions relying upon language cannot be objectively evaluated in the patient with aphasia. Accordingly, the examiner must not haphazardly sample various aspects of neurobehavioral functioning as this will result both in confusing results and potentially erroneous conclusions. The mental status outline which follows has been placed in the hierarchical order which both neurobehavioral theory and clinical use suggests is most efficacious. Those readers desiring a more complete review of the administration, interpretation, and clinical implications of the mental status exam are referred to Strub and Black.[35]

Levels of Consciousness*

Before embarking upon any formal mental status testing, the physician must initially assess the patient's basic level of consciousness. This will determine the patient's capability of relating to the examiner and the general external environment. Anyone with an altered level of consciousness will inevitably demonstrate depressed functioning of some degree on various parts of the mental status examination.

TERMINOLOGY

Although many terms have been used to describe the basic states or levels of consciousness, we have found the following terms to be most appropriate descriptive labels.

Alertness. This state implies that the patient is awake and normally aware of both internal and external stimuli. He is able to respond to such stimuli except in cases of paralysis. In such situations, eye contact, eye movement, or similar signaling methods may be employed to establish the adequacy of interaction with the examiner.

Lethargy or Somnolence. In this state the patient fails to maintain normal alertness and will drift into sleep unless specifically stimulated. Both awareness of the external environment and purposeful spontaneous movements are considerably reduced. When aroused, the lethargic patient is generally unable to sustain a state of alertness, often fails to attend closely to the examiner, and will lose the train of thought in conversation. This impairment in the normal level of alertness will hinder, if not prevent completely, performance on the formal mental status tasks of memory, comprehension, calculations, and abstract rea-

---

*Administer to all patients.

45

soning. Accordingly, if the complete mental status exam is carried out with the lethargic patient, the results of specific findings must be interpreted with considerable caution and only in light of the patient's altered level of consciousness.

Stupor or Semicoma. This term is used to describe patients who are not self-alerting and respond only to rather persistent and vigorous external stimulation. The stuporous patient does not rouse spontaneously and when aroused by the examiner is incapable of normal alertness or interaction. Typically, they are able only to groan, move aimlessly in bed, and then lapse into their previous state upon cessation of stimulation.

Coma. The term coma has traditionally been reserved to describe the state of those patients who cannot be aroused. In this state, the patient is incapable of responding to any external stimulation and similarly does not respond spontaneously to an internal stimulus. Coma may be defined as a state in which there is a total absence of behavioral response to stimulation; in this sense it is an absolute end point on the continuum of consciousness or arousability. The reader interested in a more detailed discussion of the clinical, pathologic, and theoretical aspects of altered states of consciousness is referred to Fisher[7] and Plum and Posner.[22]

These four terms are general and qualitative in nature and encompass a wide range of possible points on the spectrum of consciousness. The use of such terms in isolation (e.g., "The patient was lethargic.") lacks the objectivity and reliability that can be achieved with a more complete assessment and rating scheme. We suggest that any qualitative term such as "stupor" be amended with a series of short, behaviorally related statements that more accurately document the patient's actual response.

EVALUATION

First, determine the intensity and nature of stimulation needed to arouse the patient by (1) calling the patient by name in a normal conversational tone, (2) calling in a loud voice, (3) lightly touching the arm, (4) vigorously shaking the patient's shoulder, and (5) use of painful stimulation. Second, describe the patient's behavioral response, including (1) degree and quality of movement, (2) content and coherence of speech, (3) comprehension, (4) presence of eye opening and eye contact with the examiner, and (5) quality of alertness and interaction. Finally, describe what the patient does upon cessation of stimulation. This qualitative and quantitative description provides much more usable data on the patient's level of consciousness, arousability, and capacity for interaction than the simple terms "lethargy" or "stupor." Charting

46

the level of consciousness in the progress notes allows both the medical and the nursing staff to assess and monitor rapid fluctuations in consciousness. These changes may often be of considerable clinical significance, as in the patient with a progressive subdural hematoma, with a stroke in evolution, or recovering from neurosurgery.

Attention

Having documented the patient's basic level of consciousness, the examiner must next make a careful assessment of the patient's ability to sustain attention over time. This must be determined before evaluating the more complex functions of memory, new learning, and problem solving as it is frustrating to both patient and examiner, as well as a waste of time, to attempt to assess higher cognitive functions in a patient who is continually distracted by cars in the street, the play of light and shadow on the office wall, or other irrelevant stimuli.

Attention refers to the ability to focus on a specific stimulus without being distracted by extraneous stimuli. Attention is quite different from alertness which is a more basic arousal state in which the patient is awake and responsive to *any* environmental stimulus. The patient who is alert but inattentive will tend to be attracted by any novel sound or movement in the room, but will be incapable of *sustaining* attention to the appropriate stimulus. Thus, attention presupposes alertness, while alertness does not necessarily imply attentiveness. Vigilance (or concentration) refers to the patient's ability to sustain attention over long periods of time. The ability to concentrate is quite important in carrying out intellectual tasks, in learning, and in academic situations especially. For the purpose of the mental status examination, testing vigilance for a period of 30 seconds is sufficient. Information regarding the environmental aspects of vigilance (e.g., ability to concentrate for extended periods on a demanding job) may be determined from the history and family information.

OBSERVATION*

Basic alertness has been evaluated during that part of the examination concerning levels of consciousness. A careful observation of the patient's general behavior, interaction with the examiner, and ability to maintain a logical conversation will provide valuable information regarding general attentiveness. Specifically note any evidence of distractability, difficulty in attending to the examiner, and inability to sustain attention over an extended period of time.

---

*Administer to all patients.

HISTORY*

Information regarding problems in concentrating on the job or upon routine tasks can generally be obtained from the patient or his family. In fact, this is often a presenting complaint as will be discussed in the clinical chapters. Simple questioning of the patient regarding difficulties in attending (attention) or concentrating (vigilance) often reveals evidence of problems even when the information is not spontaneously proffered.

DIGIT REPETITION*

A quantifiable measure of the patient's basic level of attention can be readily made by utilizing the digit repetition test. The use of this test, of course, presumes that the patient is alert, has sufficient comprehension to understand the task, and has language which is sufficiently intact to say the numbers. Adequate performance on this test indicates that the patient is able to attend to verbal stimuli and to sustain attention for the period of time necessary to comprehend and repeat the digits.

Directions. Tell the patient, "I am going to say some simple numbers. Listen carefully and when I am finished, say the same numbers after me." State the digits in a normal tone of voice at a rate of one digit per second. Take care not to group digits either in pairs (e.g., 2–4, 6–9) or in sequences which could serve as an aid to repetition (e.g., in the telephone number format, 376-8439). Numbers should be presented randomly without natural sequence (i.e., not 2–4–6–8). Begin with a two number sequence and continue until the patient fails.

Test Content

3 - 7
7 - 4 - 9
8 - 5 - 2 - 1
2 - 9 - 6 - 8 - 3
5 - 7 - 1 - 9 - 4 - 6
8 - 1 - 5 - 9 - 3 - 6 - 2
3 - 9 - 8 - 2 - 5 - 1 - 4 - 7
7 - 2 - 8 - 5 - 4 - 6 - 7 - 3 - 9

Interpretation. The typical patient of average intelligence can repeat five to seven digits without difficulty. Repetition of less than five digits by a nonretarded patient without obvious aphasia is strongly suggestive of defective attention.

---

*Administer to all patients.

"A" TEST FOR VIGILANCE

The random letter test is a simple test of vigilance which can be readily administered in the office or at the bedside. This test consists of a series of random letters among which a target letter appears with greater than random frequency. The patient is required to indicate whenever the target letter is spoken by the examiner.

Directions. Tell the patient, "I am going to read you a long series of letters, whenever you hear the letter A, indicate by tapping the desk with this pencil." Read the following list of letters in a normal tone of voice at a rate of one letter per second.

Test Content

L T P E A O A I C T D A L A A

A N I A B F S A M R Z E O A D

P A K L A U C J T O E A B A A

Z Y F M U S A H E V A A R A T

Interpretation. Although there are as yet no standardized levels of performance for this test, considerable clinical use suggests that the average person should complete the task without errors. Less than perfect performance raises the suspicion of impaired vigilance. Typical organic errors include: (1) failure to indicate when the target letter has been presented (error of omission), (2) indication made when a nontarget letter has been presented (error of commission), and (3) failure to discontinue tapping with the presentation of subsequent nontarget letters (perseveration).

Behavior*

During the examination, the physician should make a systematic observation of the patient's appearance, behavior, and mood. This is important because: (1) specific behavioral syndromes are associated with well-recognized neurologic disease processes (e.g., the denial and neglect syndrome associated with right hemispheric lesion), (2) behavioral observations are extremely helpful in making the differential diagnosis between functional and organic processes, (3) findings on the formal structured aspects of the mental status exam (e.g., memory or abstract reasoning) must be interpreted in light of the patient's behavior, including mood and cooperation, and (4) a significant behavioral disturbance will adversely affect formal testing (e.g., a floridly schizophrenic patient will perform poorly on structured memory

---

*Administer to all patients.

testing because of inattention, tangential thinking, and intrusions).

The purpose of this aspect of the evaluation is to provide an objective framework to aid the examiner in systematically observing behavior. Our primary concern here is with the identification and description of organically based behavioral changes; readers desiring a more extensive psychiatric orientation are referred to the many excellent texts in that field.

PHYSICAL APPEARANCE

Patients with either functional or organic disorders may demonstrate characteristic patterns of appearance. Classic examples range from that of the patient with unilateral neglect who neglects or denies one side of the body (failing to shave, wash, dress, or even recognize the presence of that side of the body) to the bizarre clothing styles affected by some chronic schizophrenics.

Assessment of the following aspects of physical appearance is crucial, and they should be systematically reviewed and recorded:

I. General appearance
   A. Appropriateness of appearance for age
   B. Posture
   C. Facial expression
   D. Eye contact
II. Personal cleanliness
   A. Skin
   B. Hair
   C. Nails
   D. Teeth
   E. Beard
   F. Indications of unilateral neglect
III. Habits of dress
   A. Type of clothing
   B. Cleanliness of clothing
   C. Care in dressing
   D. Evidence of unilateral neglect
IV. Motor activity
   A. General activity level
   B. Abnormal posturing (tics, grimaces, bizzare gestures, and other involuntary movements)

MOOD AND GENERAL EMOTIONAL STATUS

The term mood in this context refers to the prevailing emotional feeling expressed by the patient during the course of the mental status examination. Moods tend to be more persistent and are usually less intense than are the more specific emotional responses to particular situations. Emotional status is a term that encompasses the totality of the patient's emotional response and behavior. Both organic (e.g., frontal lobe disease) and functional (e.g., reactive depression) disorders may be manifested as a disturbance of mood and emotional status and can often be differentiated by their rather characteristic patterns. Significant disturbances of mood or general emotional status will adversely affect performance on the formal mental status exam. Such disturbances will similarly have an appreciable impact upon the patient's ability to function effectively in his day-to-day activities. Accordingly, a careful and systematic review of these behavior areas is important for the interpretation of mental status exam findings, for the identification of organically based behavioral change, and for assistance in the differential diagnosis of functional and organic disease.

The following outline provides a framework for a brief evaluation of emotional status.

I. Mood
    A. Mood normal to the situation
    B. Feeling of sadness or depression
    C. Feeling of elation
    D. Apathy or lack of appropriate concern
    E. Stability or fluctuations of mood
    F. Mood inappropriate to the situation, or mood expressed is not consistent with the patient's thought content

II. Emotional status
    A. Degree of cooperation with the examiner
    B. Anxiety
    C. Suspiciousness
    D. Depression
    E. Anger
    F. Insight
    G. Emotional responses inappropriate to specific situations
    H. Reality testing
        1. Delusions (false beliefs)
        2. Illusions (misperceptions of real stimuli)
        3. Hallucinations (modality and nature)
    I. Indications of specific neurotic symptomatology
        1. Phobias
        2. Chronic anxiety (object and degree)
        3. Obsessive-compulsive thinking or behavior
        4. Depression

J. Abnormalities in language or speech
 1. Neologisms (personal formation and use of a new word without meaning except to patient)
 2. Flight of ideas in thinking and speaking
 3. Loose (tangential) associations in thinking and speaking

Considerable interpretive material regarding the relationship of behavioral findings and clinical conditions is included in specific chapters of this book. Strub and Black[35] contains a greatly expanded review of this topic.

Language*

Language is the basic tool of human communication; as such it is crucial both to the patient's general functioning and in assessing most areas of cognitive functioning. Accordingly, the integrity of language functions must be evaluated early in the course of the mental status examination. Acquired language disturbances (aphasia) have been well-studied, as they are common sequelae of both focal and diffuse brain disease. The characteristic patterns of specific aphasic disturbances and their distinct neuroanatomic correlations are covered in Chapter 7, Neurobehavioral Syndromes Associated with Focal Brain Lesions.

This section deals with a systematic approach to the evaluation of language disorders. During this part of the examination, particular attention must be paid to spontaneous speech, language comprehension, ability to repeat, and facility in naming. Reading and writing are additional important areas of language functioning which may be assessed clinically after completion of the verbal language evaluation. The aphasic patient is always agraphic (loss of the ability to write) and is commonly alexic (loss of the ability to read); accordingly, in the aphasic, the reading and writing assessment may be abbreviated.

HANDEDNESS*

As handedness and cerebral dominance for language are closely related, the patient's handedness should be determined prior to language testing. Initially ask the patient whether he is right or left handed and whether he has been forced to change hands because of family or school pressure. Also, ask if he has any tendency to use the opposite hand for any skilled activity. Observe the patient using a paper and pencil, fork, stirring coffee, or carrying out other unilateral activities. A family history of left handedness or ambidexterity may be

---

*Administer to all patients.

important, as dominance is strongly affected by hereditary factors. There appears to be a spectrum of handedness ranging from strong right handedness to moderately strong left handedness, with weakly lateralized dominance, mixed dominance, and ambidexterity occupying central positions. See Chapter 7, Neurobehavioral Syndromes Associated with Focal Brain Lesions, for an extended discussion of this topic.

SPONTANEOUS SPEECH

The first step in formal language testing is to carefully listen to the patient's spontaneous speech. If he offers no spontaneous speech, ask relatively uncomplicated open ended questions which require more than a single word or phrase in response. Questions such as "Tell me why you are in the hospital," or "Tell me something about your work," should be used. Care must be taken to avoid questions which can be answered with a "yes," "no," or shake of the head.

In observing spontaneous speech, the examiner should note the following aspects:

1. Is speech output present?
2. Is the speech dysarthric?
3. Is there evidence of aphasia?

Aphasic language is characterized by some or all of the following errors: errors of grammatical structure, difficulty in finding and using the appropriate word (anomia), and word substitutions (paraphasia). The classic patterns of aphasia will be discussed in detail in Chapter 7.

COMPREHENSION*

The patient's ability to comprehend language must be assessed in a structured fashion without reliance upon his ability to produce speech. A frequent error made by inexperienced examiners is to evaluate language comprehension by asking complex or open ended questions. This type of evaluation taxes the entire language system and is not a measure of verbal comprehension in isolation. The two most efficacious ways of testing comprehension are to require the patient to follow pointing commands and to respond to questions that can be answered with yes or no.

Requesting the patient to point to single named objects in the room, body parts, or objects is an excellent way to quantify single word comprehension. If the patient is capable of performing on the single word

---

*Administer to all patients.

level, the task may be increased in complexity by gradually adding to the number of items in the sequence. After starting with single word items, increase the number of items until the patient consistently fails. The mildly aphasic patient may be capable of responding at the one or two word level with consistent accuracy but fail without exception at the three word level. This task makes it possible to evaluate single word comprehension, auditory retention, and memory for verbal sequences. As both the quality and nature of performance will vary among patients and oftentimes between examinations, for clarity the patient's responses should be reported as follows: "Patient consistently pointed to two items in series but failed all trials at three items."

Next, a series of questions requiring a simple yes or no response which gradually increase in difficulty should be asked. "Is it raining today?" or "Will a stone float on water?" are examples of the general type of question we suggest. Before beginning this task, ensure that the patient is capable of expressing both yes and no, either verbally, by gesture, or any other nonverbal means. The items should initially be quite simple to gain a baseline of comprehension; the task can then be made as complex as necessary to obtain a ceiling or consistent failure level or to determine that verbal comprehension is completely normal. A minimum of six questions should be used. The correct answers to the questions should alternate randomly from yes to no as perseveration is common in patients with brain dysfunction and it is not infrequent for a patient to respond "yes" to multiple questions without any conception of the correct answers. The examiner should make an effort to quantify the quality of the patient's performance if only to record that "The patient was able to respond to simple yes or no questions but consistently failed to give the correct response to more difficult items."

OBJECT NAMING*

The ability to name objects to visual confrontation is a very basic language function which is almost invariably impaired in most types of aphasia. Problems in word finding may be detected by listening to the patient's spontaneous speech, asking the patient to describe a picture, or by asking an open ended question. Anomia (loss of the ability to accurately name objects) is best tested by asking the patient to name specific items. If time allows, several categories of objects should be used as some aphasic patients show an interesting disparity between the ability to name items in various categories (e.g., colors, shapes). As the ability to name items is closely related to their frequency in language usage (e.g., *car* is far easier to name than *philodendron*), it is important to employ both common (high frequency) and uncommon

---

*Administer to all patients.

(low frequency) items in the confrontational naming test. Many aphasics will name common items with relative facility, only to have significant difficulty with less frequently used items, demonstrating hesitancy, paraphasic errors, and circumlocutions. The examiner should record both correct and incorrect responses as well as the nature of specific errors (e.g., refusal, paraphasic response, or circumlocution). A list of specific items for naming in order of frequency by object category are available in Strub and Black.[35]

Paraphasias are errors in word usage that are common in aphasia. They may be substitutions for the correct word (e.g., "I drove home my *pen*") or contain substituted syllables (e.g., "I drove home in my *lar*"). A third type of paraphasia is the neologistic (new word) paraphasia which is the substitution of a totally non-English word (e.g., "I drove home in my *burts*"). Paraphasic speech is easily recognized by the careful listener and can be evaluated during all aspects of the mental status examination. The examiner should note the frequency and type of paraphasic errors made by the patient.

REPETITION*

The ability to repeat spoken language is linguistically and to an extent anatomically distinct from other language functions. As this function may be impaired or spared in isolation, it is important to test it specifically. Dysfunction of any of the steps of auditory processing, verbal retention, disturbed speech production, or disconnection between the receptive and expressive language areas will disrupt the ability to repeat verbal material. Therefore, impaired repetition performance is clinically significant but not pathognomonic of a specific language disturbance.

Testing should be carried out with verbal material of increasing difficulty. Begin with single syllable words and proceed to complex sentences. We recommend the following items which provide an appropriate range of difficulty. Merely tell the patient to repeat the word or sentence after the examiner.

1. Ball
2. Help
3. Airplane
4. Hospital
5. Mississippi River
6. The little boy went home.
7. We all went over there together.
8. Let's go downtown for ice cream.

---

*Administer to all patients.

9. The short fat boy dropped the china vase.
10. Each fight readied the boxer for the championship bout.

Record the level of complexity at which the patient failed to repeat accurately. In addition, the examiner should listen and note any paraphasia, grammatical errors, omissions, and added material.

READING AND WRITING

After the evaluation of verbal language performance, a brief clinical assessment should be made of the patient's ability to read and write. Unless an objectively quantified measure of reading is necessary, the examiner can employ either words and sentences written on a sheet of paper or simple printed material. The initial reading evaluation should be made with single simple words, progressing to phrases and then sentences. Similarly, writing can be easily tested by having the patient write first words and then sentences on command. Assessment of these areas, of course, presumes that the patient has sufficiently intact language skills to understand the nature of the task and the verbal material.

Memory*

Because disturbances in memory are frequently the initial complaint of early organic brain disease and because they often have the most significantly disabling impact on the patient's ability to function effectively in society, careful attention should be paid to memory testing. Memory is not a unitary process and each of its various aspects must be assessed in some detail. From this evaluation, the examiner will be able to determine the type of memory disturbance (if any), the etiology of the disturbance (organic or functional), the degree of memory loss, and the probable impact of the deficit upon the patient's ability to function in a social or vocational role. Patients with language disorders cannot be validly tested with memory tests utilizing verbal material but must be tested using nonverbal material. The valid assessment of memory requires that any question asked by the examiner be verifiable from a source other than the patient. There is no use asking a patient what he ate for lunch, where he attended high school, or to name the mayor of his hometown if the examiner is unable to ascertain the accuracy of the patient's responses. Many patients with organic disease will deny their memory disorders and confabulate responses which appear perfectly appropriate to the naive examiner.

---

*Administer to all patients.

ORIENTATION*

The patient's ability to orient himself with respect to person (who he is), time (including day of week, date), and place (where he is) is important preliminary information. The examiner should note and record in a quantified way the integrity of the patient's orientation in each of these three major areas.

IMMEDIATE RECALL (SHORT-TERM MEMORY)

Immediate recall is traditionally tested by the digit repetition task which was covered in the section on Attention.

NEW LEARNING*

This section evaluates the patient's ability to actively learn new material, a process which requires establishing new memories. Normal performance requires the integrity of the total memory system: Recognition and registration of the initial verbal input and retention and storage of the information. An interruption of any one of these interrelated processes will impair new learning performance.

Four Unrelated Words*

Tell the patient, "I am going to tell you four words that I want you to remember. In a few minutes, I will ask you to recall the words." The four words we have used clinically because of their semantic, phonemic, and categorical diversity are:

1. Brown
2. Honesty
3. Tulip
4. Eyedropper

Ensure that the patient has understood and initially retained the four words by having him repeat them after presentation. Correct any initial errors he may make on this repetition. To eliminate the possibility of mental rehearsal (e.g., repeating the words to oneself mentally), provide verbal interference between presentation and requested recall. The examiner may wish to present the four words, conduct another verbal section of the examination, and then go back to this task and ask the patient to recall the four words. Five minutes should elapse between the initial presentation and the request for recall. If the patient is unable to recall any of the four words, it is often possible to obtain an indication of some memory storage by the use of either semantic

---

*Administer to all patients.

cues (e.g., "One word was a color"), phonemic cues utilizing syllabic components of the target word (e.g., "Hon. . . . , hones. . . . , honest. . . ."), or contextual cues (e.g., "A common flower in Holland is the_____?"). If even this degree of cueing does not result in recall, the examiner may resort to asking the patient if he recognizes the target word within a series (e.g., "Was the color red, green, *brown,* or yellow?").

Verbal Story for Immediate Recall

Tell the patient, "I am going to read you a short paragraph. Listen carefully, because when I finish reading, I want you to tell me everything that I told you." After reading the story, say, "Now tell me everything that you can remember of the story. Start at the beginning of the story and tell me all that happened." In the example below, the separate items in the story are indicated by slash (/) marks. As the patient retells the story, indicate the ideas recalled, errors, and confabulations.

A cowboy/from Arizona/went to San Francisco/with his dog/ which he left/with a friend/while he purchased/a new suit of clothes./Dressed finely,/he went back to the dog,/whistled to him,/ called him by name,/and patted him./But the dog would have nothing to do with him,/in his new hat/and coat,/but gave a mournful howl./Coaxing had no effect./So the cowboy went away/and donned his old clothes,/whereupon the dog immediately showed his wild joy/on seeing his master/as he thought he ought to be./

The story contains 23 relatively separate items of information. In our experience, the average patient should produce approximately ten of these items (or paraphrases of the items) on immediate recall.

Visual Memory (Hidden Objects)

Nonverbal memory testing is especially useful in evaluating the memory of aphasics. The examiner may utilize any four small, easily recognizable, objects which may be readily hidden in the patient's vicinity. The use of four objects provides a reasonable span for most patients; more items may be used for those who are relatively facile with four objects but in whom visual memory dysfunction is suspected. Hide the four items while the patient is watching, naming each object as it is hidden. This ensures that the patient is attentive to the task and is aware of what object was hidden in what area. After hiding the objects, the examiner should provide interfering stimulation by asking the patient routine questions or engaging him in general conversation. After a period of 10 minutes, ask the patient to find each of the hidden objects. If he is unable to recall the location of any object, ask him to name the hidden objects. If he is unable to perform this, ask him to find "the keys" or "the pencil." Cueing may be used if necessary ("It's somewhere on the table").

The averge patient should find each of the four hidden objects after a 10 minute delay without difficulty.

REMOTE MEMORY*

Tests in this section evaluate the patient's ability to recall events of both a personal and social nature from his store of remote memories. As has been previously emphasized, the answer to any question asked regarding personal events must be verified by a reliable source to ensure validity. This area of memory functioning is closely related to both premorbid intelligence and educational level. The following categories of questions are provided as representative samples, each clinician may assemble his own battery of questions appropriate to his sample.

I.   Personal information
II. Historical facts
     A. Name the last four presidents.
     B. What was the last war the U.S. fought?
     C. Who was:
         Lee Harvey Oswald?
         Patricia Hearst?
         Neil Armstrong?
         Henry Kissinger?

Constructional Ability*

Constructional tasks are frequently not included in the routine mental status examination despite their importance and proven clinical utility. Because problems in constructional performance are often present in the early stages of brain dysfunction and may appreciably aid in the differential diagnosis between organic and functional disorders, we strongly recommend their inclusion in the mental status examination of every patient with suspected organic brain disease.

Drawings to command and drawings reproduced from examples are the most easily administered and interpreted tests of constructional ability.

---

*Administer to all patients.

REPRODUCTION DRAWING*

We suggest that reproduction drawings be administered first when assessing constructional ability because of their apparent simplicity and familiarity. The drawings presented below are organized in order of increasing difficulty. Both two and three dimensional drawings are included because of the frequent discrepancies in the quality of performance on these two somewhat different tasks. Each design may be drawn carefully on a blank sheet of white paper. Under no circumstances should lined progress note paper, consultation forms, permission slips, and other readily available but visually confusing paper be used. The patient should be told to draw a design (or picture) that looks just like the one drawn by the examiner. The four designs that we have found to be most useful clinically are shown in Figure 3-1.

A formal scoring system for assessing the quality of the patient's constructional performance is available in Strub and Black.[35] The examiner should rate the quality of each design, preferably on a four point scale ranging from 0 (poor) to 3 (excellent).

Particular attention should be paid to any evidence of perseveration, rotations of more than 90 degrees, or "closing-in" (i.e., a tendency to either overlap a part of the stimulus design or to assimilate a part of the stimulus design into the reproduction).

DRAWINGS TO COMMAND*

Provide the patient with a *blank* sheet of paper and a pencil (or more ideally a felt tip pen) and ask him to draw a picture of a clock with the

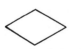
HORIZONTAL DIAMOND

TWO DIMENSIONAL CROSS

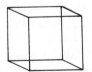
THREE DIMENSIONAL CUBE

THREE DIMENSIONAL PIPE

FIGURE 3-1. Test items for Reproduction Drawing Test.

---

*Administer to all patients.

numbers and hands on it, a daisy in a flower pot, and a house in perspective so that you can see two sides and the roof.

In general, any patient with evidence of perseveration, rotation, or rating scores of 0 on any of the reproduction drawings or drawings to command should be considered as demonstrating constructional impairment.

Higher Cognitive Processes

Basic attention, language, and memory are the primary processes upon which the higher intellectual abilities are developed. These basic functions are necessary but are not in and of themselves sufficient for the execution of more complex cognitive functions and the ability to function effectively within the environment. We include within the testable higher cognitive functions, the manipulation of well-learned material, abstract reasoning, problem solving, arithmetic calculations, and so forth. These complex functions represent the highest levels of intellectual functioning, their evaluation often demonstrates evidence of the early effects of cortical damage before the more basic processes are impaired. Important information regarding the patient's ability to function within his social and vocational environment is also gained from a careful examination of these higher processes.

The following tests are recommended to evaluate a spectrum of relevant higher cognitive processes:

1. Proverb interpretation. The patient is required to interpret well known proverbs (e.g., Rome wasn't built in a day.)
2. Similarities. The patient is required to explain the essential similarity between two overtly different objects (e.g., fly and tree).
3. Calculations. All basic arithmetic processes (i.e., addition, subtraction, multiplication, and division) should be tested in both the verbal and graphic modalities.

Following this mental status outline allows the clinician to systematically evaluate those behavioral and cognitive functions which accurately differentiate patients with organic brain disease from those with functional disorders. In the organic patient it is often possible to elucidate the type, locus, and degree of disease. The mental status examination provides an excellent, albeit brief, description of the individual's performance over a broad range of functions. Repeated examinations allow efficient comparisons for documenting improvement or deterioration. In some cases, the results of the mental status examination may be indicative or even pathognomonic of a specific neurobehavioral disorder (e.g., Wernicke's aphasia or Alzheimer's disease). In this way the mental status examination can be as efficacious as any other neurodiagnostic procedure.

We have emphasized throughout this section the need to record both how a function was evaluated (i.e., the question asked or the command given) and the patient's response to each item. A composite mental status recording form is included in Strub and Black[35] to aid in this data recording. The use of such forms allows more efficient documentation of changes in a patient's status over time and communication of findings to other professionals.

After completion of the mental status examination, the primary physician must determine if further specialized evaluation is necessary, and if so, which area should be emphasized.

CONSULTATIONS

When the primary care physician has diagnosed or suspects an organic brain syndrome from the complete basic medical evaluation and the initial mental status examination, consultation with additional specialized medical and ancillary professional personnel may be necessary.

Neurology

As the organic brain syndromes are, by and large, neurologic diseases; the neurologist is an extremely helpful consultant when the physician is evaluating the patient with altered mental function. The neurologist usually spends from 30 to 60 minutes taking an initial history and carrying out an extensive neurologic examination. With these standard data, he can make a specific neurologic diagnosis or plan a full neurodiagnostic evaluation.

Most neurologists are also willing and able to manage the short and long-term care of the patient with organic disease in conjunction with the patient's own physician. It is best to consult the neurologist early in the evaluation process before ordering a large and expensive battery of laboratory tests. We have seen all too many patients with a simple postoperative delirium who have been dragged screaming through a series of laboratories. After hundreds of dollars of testing, much of which is of questionable reliability because of movement artifact, the neurologist is finally asked to see the patient. In such cases the EEG, CT scan, skull x-rays, and so forth are unnecessary to make the clinical diagnosis. Confusional behavior (delirium) in the postoperative period is usually due to a medication or metabolic disturbance and not to structured brain disease. Valuable time and money may be unnecessarily spent if the physician attempts to "get all the tests done" before calling the consultant. The neurologic consultation is often the cheapest efficacious neurologic test and should yield the most pertinent information to the primary physician.

Neuropsychology

The neuropsychologist utilizes a wide variety of standard psychometric tests and specialized neuropsychologic evaluation procedures to provide an intensive and comprehensive evaluation of patients with organic brain disease. Although he is not medically trained, the neuropsychologist's academic background includes neuroanatomy, physiology, and basic clinical neurology in addition to the more traditional psychologic topics. The clinical neuropsychologist is primarily concerned with the identification, quantification, and description of changes in behavior which are associated with brain dysfunction. Because of their specialized training, the clinical neuropsychologist's primary areas of interest and expertise are the relationships between disturbance in human behavior and abnormal brain function. Accordingly, his activities can contribute to a variety of important clinical neurologic problems including differential diagnosis, lateralization and localization of lesions, and the establishment of baselines of behavior, emotional status, and intellectual functioning from which improvement or deterioration can be gauged. He can also contribute to the determination of mental and legal competency in the aged or demented, behavioral management recommendations, and development of specific remedial methods for the rehabilitation of the individual brain damaged patient.[21]

The neuropsychologic evaluation, briefly defined, is an objective comprehensive assessment of a wide range of cognitive, adaptive, and emotional behaviors which reflect the adequacy (or inadequacy) of cortical functioning. In essence, the neuropsychologic evaluation is a greatly expanded and objectified mental status examination. While the mental status examination is designed to briefly (within 15 to 30 minutes) screen a variety of critical areas, the neuropsychologic evaluation assesses a wider variety of performance, in more depth, and over a longer period of time (2 to 6 hours). It differs from the mental status examination in that it generally uses tests and evaluation procedures which have been standardized using samples from either normal individuals (e.g., Wechsler series of intelligence scales) or brain damaged patients (e.g., Memory for Designs Test or the Trail-Making Test). With use of these standardized measures, the individual patient's performance can be readily compared with that of normative groups. In addition, the adequacy of the same patient's performance in a variety of different cognitive functions and modalities can be assessed. The objective and highly quantified nature of most neuropsychologic tests aids in the detection of subtle changes in performance over time (e.g., the slow deterioration in dementia or improvements in specific cognitive functions after neurosurgery). Because of the wide range of performance assessed and the depth in which it is evaluated, the neuropsychologic evaluation may detect subtle deficits early in the course of a disease which are not apparent on the mental status examination.

The neuropsychologic evaluation has a number of advantages not shared by most standard neurodiagnostic techniques. It is a noninvasive procedure and has no risk of mortality or morbidity; these factors make the evaluation appropriate for patients for whom the risk of invasive procedures (pneumoencephalography or angiography) is too great or for whom the probability of positive findings is sufficiently small that any risk is too high (e.g., the child with questionable neurologic signs of minimal brain dysfunction on general clinical exam). The tests are inherently interesting to most patients and do not produce the possible adverse complications of anxiety and pain that result from some invasive procedures. The evaluation also provides important descriptive and prognostic information that other techniques cannot. This is especially true in the description of the effects of neurologic disease upon the patient as a person and its probable impact upon the patient's academic, social, and vocational adjustment.

The physician without ready access to a trained neuropsychologist may benefit from an evaluation performed by a clinical psychologist who has had some experience in evaluating patients with brain disease. This is especially true if the referring physician is familiar with the types of psychologic tests which are appropriate for use with such patients, understands the nature and limitations of the data which can be provided by the psychologist, and knows how to interpret both the objective and subjective aspects of the reports. A review of the information below should greatly aid in this familiarization and interpretation.

CRITERIA FOR REFERRAL

Patients for whom the physician requires further information concerning (1) diagnosis, (2) the effects of a well verified lesion upon behavior and social/vocational competence, and (3) prognosis and management should be referred for neuropsychologic evaluation.

Mild cognitive and behavioral disturbances frequently occur in the absence of any clear-cut physical signs of cerebral disease on the standard clinical neurologic exam; this is particularly true in cases of early dementia. Dementia typically presents with vague behavioral complaints such as mental dullness, concentration problems, increasing apathy and loss of interest in job or family, chronic fatigue without apparent organic etiology, depression, and subjective memory problems. Neuropsychologic evaluation of such patients can often contribute to an early diagnosis of dementia, help differentiate between dementia and depression, or determine the relative effects of organic and functional factors in a mixed disorder. The neuropsychologic evaluation may also provide strong supporting data for the presumptive diagnosis of brain disease and thus serve as a basis for ordering more extensive and specific neurodiagnostic procedures (e.g., a CT scan in the patient with only equivocal findings on physical examination but positive indications of cognitive deterioration during the neuropsychologic evaluation).

Any patient with a known brain lesion should receive a neuropsychologic evaluation as part of planning their rehabilitation program. The comprehensive nature of the evaluation provides valuable information regarding the effect of the lesion upon cognitive functioning, emotional status, behavior, and social adjustment. Both specific areas of impairment and residual abilities will be identified. This delineation of the patient's strengths and weaknesses is valuable in describing the effects of specific neurologic lesions upon the individual and provides information critical for vocational and social rehabilitation.

Serial testing can provide reliable objective information regarding the speed and degree of recovery after brain disease, injury, or neurosurgical procedures. Similarly, repeated evaluations can be used to quantify deterioration in cases of progressive disease or to rule out such progression in equivocal cases. Neuropsychologic evaluations conducted before and after neurosurgery will document effects of the surgery upon the patient's total functioning. The effects of any medical treatment (e.g., levodopa in parkinsonism or anticonvulsants in epilepsy) may also be readily demonstrated by neuropsychologic evaluations conducted before and after treatment is initiated. These changes over time are difficult to assess and impossible to quantify without an adequate initial baseline of data encompassing a wide range of cognitive functions and behavior.

It is apparent that in any case of trauma or suspected brain damage involving litigation or compensation, the objective data obtained from the neuropsychologic evaluation are of great value in documenting and describing the presence, absence, or degree of disability and vocational incapacity. There is considerable legal precedent for admission of the testimony of psychologists as expert witnesses in such cases.

THE NEUROPSYCHOLOGIC REPORT

The clinical information which the physician can expect to be provided by the neuropsychologist and which would appear in the psychologist's report is summarized below.

Categorization

The section of the report on categorization provides information as to the presence or absence of brain dysfunction as well as the presence or absence of significant emotional disturbance. The differential diagnosis between a primary organic or a primary functional disorder is made. If significant effects of both organic and functional components are present, the relative importance and impact of each will be discussed.

Localization

Typically, performance on the neuropsychologic test battery can be analyzed to determine if the brain dysfunction is diffuse or focal. Further analysis enables determination of the lateralization of the lesion to the right or left hemisphere and the localization of the lesion in the anterior or posterior regions of the hemisphere.

Description

The report will contain a comprehensive description of the patient's current level of functioning in a wide range of cognitive, adaptive, personality, and behavioral areas. From the academic and social history and an analysis of the variation of performance on various tests, it is generally possible to estimate the patient's premorbid level of functioning. By comparing the estimated premorbid level of function with current performance on standard tests, an accurate indication of deterioration in any of the areas assessed by the battery may be made. A comprehensive overview of the patient's deficits and residual abilities is made which describes current functioning, explains present behavior, determines the relative effects of organic and functional factors, and provides a baseline of data from which to judge future change. Documented statements should be made to help the primary physician determine the effect of the patient's current neurologic disease and its associated deficits upon his subsequent academic, vocational, and social adjustment. Answers to questions concerning mental competency and social independence can also be made in this section of the report.

Prognosis and Recommendations

Based upon the nature of the neurologic disease and the pattern and degree of deficits seen during neuropsychologic evaluation, a determination of the probability and degree of expected recovery or further deterioration can be made for most patients. As previously mentioned, serial evaluations some months apart aid greatly in the ability to make valid prognostic statements in cases of either deterioration or recovery. Finally, recommendations for further ancillary evaluations, including those of psychiatry, speech pathology, occupational therapy, and social service, are made when warranted. Recommendations regarding specific remedial methods or programs may also be made when requested or appropriate to the situation.

COMPONENTS OF THE NEUROPSYCHOLOGIC EVALUATION

Specific tests employed in a neuropsychologic battery will vary with the age of the patient, the nature of the medical problem, specific referral questions asked by the referring physician, and the particular training and experience of the psychologist. Virtually all such test batteries will, however, include objective tests of the following functions:

1. Behavior, attention, and mood
2. Intelligence, including general intelligence, verbal intelligence, and nonverbal intelligence
3. Language, including single word and sentence comprehension, auditory discrimination, and various aspects of expressive language
4. Memory, including verbal and nonverbal memory, short and long term memory, and new learning ability
5. Abstract ability, including verbal and nonverbal abstract reasoning
6. Constructional ability, including paper and pencil reproduction, construction, and reproduction from memory
7. Geographic orientation
8. Achievement, including reading, spelling, and calculations
9. Perceptual motor speed, including the ability to plan ahead and shift concepts rapidly
10. Motor strength and coordination
11. Personality

Some specific tests that are commonly used and reported upon in neuropsychologic evaluations are discussed below.

Halstead-Reitan Battery

This comprehensive neuropsychologic battery includes tests of general intelligence, concept formation, expressive and receptive language, auditory perception, time perception, verbal and nonverbal memory, perceptual-motor speed, tactile performance, spatial relations, finger gnosis, double simultaneous stimulation, and personality.

The basic elements of the battery are (1) Wechsler Adult Intelligence Scale (see p. 68), (2) Category Test (conceptual learning via trial and error, see p. 72), (3) Trail Making Test (see p. 72), (4) Aphasia Screening Examination (naming, spelling, expressive and receptive language, reading, arithmetic, drawing, and left-right orientation), (5) Rhythm Perception Test (perception of same or different tonal rhythms), (6) Speech Perception Test (discrimination of similar sounding words), (7) Finger Tapping Test (see p. 73), (8) Tactile Performance Test (formboard requiring performance by the dominant and nondominant hand, both hands, and drawing of the stimulus from memory), and (9) Perceptual Examination (including evaluation of double simultaneous stimulation, finger agnosia, discrimination of fingertip number writing and tactile form recognition). In many cases, the Minnesota Multiphasic Personality Inventory (see p. 74) is administered as well.

The battery is a complex and quite expensive set of tests and apparatus. Patient testing demands considerable effort from both the examiner and examinee and requires from five to ten hours of trained examiner time. Interpretation of the test results is typically carried out by a separate highly trained clinical neuropsychologist.

An Impairment Index is derived from the patient's overall performance; this score quite accurately differentiates most organic from nonorganic conditions. In the hands of a well trained examiner, the battery can also provide valuable information regarding the locus and nature of the lesion (e.g., intrinsic neoplasm vs. atrophy) and the effect of the neuropsychologic deficit upon the patient's subsequent functioning.

Initially devised by Halstead,[14] the battery has been subsequently revised and refined for many years by Reitan and coworkers[24–28] and has been statistically analyzed by Russell et al.[30] A recent publication by Swiercinsky[36] provides a relatively comprehensive manual for administration, scoring, and interpretation of most of the tests in the battery as well as other neuropsychologic tests. Golden[8,38] has written critical evaluations of the advantages and disadvantages of both the Halstead-Reitan Battery and other tests used to evaluate patients with suspected brain dysfunction while Anthony and associates,[39] Hevern,[40] and Lenzer[44] have dealt with its validity.

This battery is probably the best standardized and certainly the most widely reported neuropsychologic research battery in use in the United States at this time. The primary obstacles to its routine use are time and expense.

Wechsler Adult Intelligence Scale (WAIS)

The 1955 revision and restandardization of the original Wechsler Bellvue Scale, known as the Wechsler Adult Intelligence Scale, is one of the most commonly used psychometric tests and is probably the test of cognitive functioning that is most familiar to the practicing clinician. It is a well constructed and standardized test that is recognized as the standard measure of intelligence when time (1 to 1.5 hours) allows its use. Although standardized for use with the normal adult population, it has proven especially useful in the evaluation of patients with dementia and has also been employed successfully with a wide variety of neurologic conditions. The WAIS provides a Full Scale IQ (mean of 100 at any age) and both Verbal and Performance (nonverbal) Scale IQs. The results of six subtests make up the Verbal Scale: (1) Information (general stored knowledge; e.g., What is the capitol of Italy?), (2) Comprehension (social awareness and the ability to deal with hypothetical situations; e.g., Why should people pay taxes?), (3) Arithmetic (achievement in verbal arithmetic problems; e.g., A man with $18.00 spends $7.50, how much money does he have left?), (4) Similarities (verbal conceptualization; e.g., In what way are air and water alike?), (5) Vocabulary (verbal definition; e.g., What does *reluctant* mean?), and (6) Digit Span (repetition both forward and backward). The five primarily nonverbal subtests are (1) Digit Symbol (a perceptual motor speed writing task involving symbol coding), (2) Picture Completion (recognition of omitted details from pictured objects), (3) Block Design (reproduction of pictorially presented designs with multicolored blocks), (4) Picture Arrangement (visual sequencing of a series of pictures to complete a logical story), and (5) Object Assembly (construction of simple picture puzzles). Each subtest has a mean score of 10 at any age, this allows comparisons of the patient's discrepancy from the expected score for the normal population and assessment of the variations in performance among the various subtests. As a specific example, the WAIS performance of a patient with Alzheimer's dementia appears in Figure 3-2.

The Verbal and Performance Scale IQs and the scaled scores for the specific subtests do not vary appreciably in a normal individual. This is not as true for the patient with brain dysfunction. Discrepancies between the Verbal and Performance Scale IQs ranging from 10 to 30 or more points are not infrequent in such patients. Similarly, considerable variation in subtest performance may be seen in patients with organic disease (note the performance of the patient in Fig. 3-2) with the type of scatter being based upon the locus and nature of the brain lesion.

IQs within the range of 90 to 110 are classified as Average, between 80 and 89 as Low Average, between 70 and 79 as Borderline, and below 70 as Mentally Retarded. As there is a strong positive correlation between intelligence and educational level, historical information regarding achievement, as well as general social background and vocation must be considered when interpreting measured intelligence. An IQ within the Average Range may reflect the effects of a progressive dementing process in a patient with probable superior premorbid functioning. For example, we recently evaluated a 67-year-old physician whose performance on the WAIS resulted in a Full

Mrs. R. B.   Age: 55   Education: 17 years

TABLE OF SCALED SCORE EQUIVALENTS*

Scaled Score	Information	Comprehension	Arithmetic	Similarities	Digit Span	Vocabulary	Digit Symbol	Picture Completion	Block Design	Picture Arrangement	Object Assembly	Scaled Score
19	29	27-28		26	17	78-80	87-90					19
18	28	26		25		76-77	83-86	21		36	44	18
17	27	25	18	24		74-75	79-82		48	35	43	17
16	26	24	17	23	16	71-73	76-78	20	47	34	42	16
15	25	23	16	22	15	67-70	72-75		46	33	41	15
14	23-24	22	15	21		63-66	69-71	19	44-45	32	40	14
13	21-22	21	14	19-20		59-62	66-68	18	42-43	30-31	38-39	13
12	19-20	20	13	17-18		54-58	62-65	17	39-41	28-29	36-37	12
11	17-18	19	12	15-16	12	47-53	58-61	15-16	35-38	26-27	34-35	11
10	15-16	17-18	11	13-14	11	40-46	52-57	14	31-34	23-25	31-33	10
9	13-14	15-16	10	11-12	10	32-39	47-51	12-13	28-30	20-22	28-30	9
8	11-12	14	9	9-10		26-31	41-46	10-11	25-27	18-19	25-27	8
7	9-10	12-13	7-8	7-8	9	22-25	35-40	8-9	21-24	15-17	22-24	7
6	7-8	10-11	6	5-6	8	18-21	29-34	6-7	17-20	12-14	19-21	6
5	5-6	8-9	5	4		14-17	21-28		13-16	9-11	15-18	5
4	4	6-7	4		7	11-13	18-20	4	10-	8	11-14	4
3	3	5	3			10	15-17	3	6-9	7	8-10	3
2	2	4		1	6	9	13-14	2	3-5	6	5-7	2
1	1	3	1		4-5	8	12	1	2	5	3-4	1
0	0	0-2	0	0	0-3	0-7	0-11	0	0-1	0	0-2	0

SUMMARY

TEST	Raw Score	Scaled Score
Information	14	9
Comprehension	4	2
Arithmetic	7	7
Similarities	2	3
Digit Span	14	14
Vocabulary	53	11
Verbal Score		46
Digit Symbol	19	4
Picture Completion	5	5
Block Design	16	5
Picture Arrangement	2	0
Object Assembly	15	5
Performance Score		19
Total Score		65

VERBAL SCORE 46 IQ 90
PERFORMANCE SCORE 19 IQ 76
FULL SCALE SCORE 65 IQ 83

FIGURE 3–2. Performance on the Wechsler Adult Intelligence Scale of a female patient with Alzheimer's dementia.

Scale IQ of 103. Although this score was quite normal for his age, our patient's academic history, profession, and well-documented previous success as a surgeon strongly suggested a deterioration in intellectual functioning. His dementia was further indicated by impaired performance on more demanding neuropsychologic tests and was subsequently confirmed by CT scan and the progressive course of his deterioration.

In general, the existence of organic disease would be suspected in a patient when the WAIS results show:

1. A discrepancy between the current Full Scale IQ and that which would be predicted on the basis of premorbid historical information.
2. A Verbal-Performance discrepancy which is greater than expected (+15 points)
3. An appreciable degree of intersubtest scatter
4. Significantly impaired performance on areas of the test considered sensitive to the effects of organicity (i.e., Similarities, Digit Symbol, Block Design)

The discrepancy between Verbal and Performance Scale IQs and the variations among subtest scores may be used to determine the patient's specific areas of intellectual strength and weakness and, with some caution, to aid in cerebral localization.

Wechsler Memory Scale (WMS)

The Wechsler Memory Scale is a relatively brief (30 minutes) memory battery for clinical use. The WMS assesses a number of aspects of memory functioning including Personal and Current Information (e.g., In what year were you born? Who is the governor of your state?), Orientation to time and place (e.g., What is the month? What is the name of this place?), Mental Control (tested by counting backwards from 20 to 1, reciting the alphabet, and counting by serial 3s), Logical Memory (the immediate recall of paragraph length material read aloud by the examiner), Digit Repetition (both forward and backward), Visual Memory (paper and pencil reproduction from memory of simple line designs), and Paired Associate Learning (using three trial learning pairs, having both strong natural associations ["north" and "south"] and no logical association ["dig" and "guilty"]).

The test was standardized so that a Memory Quotient (MQ) is derived that is analagous to the WAIS IQ. Accordingly, a MQ of 100 is approximately equivalent to the same WAIS IQ. The WMS is the only objective memory test which provides a global assessment index, although there is some research evidence that the test should not be evaluated in this fashion.[29,38] Unfortunately, performance on the various components of the test cannot be easily compared by inspection (i.e., verbal vs. visual or new learning vs. long term memory) as is possible on the WAIS. However, a degree of familiarity with the test and clinical ingenuity does allow such comparisons to be made by interpolation or the use of clinically constructed charts.[41] Despite the continuing research controversy regarding the construction and basic factors implicit in this test,[4] the WMS remains the only widely available and widely used objective measure of memory functioning. Performance on the test can be compared with scores on standard intelligence tests (e.g., the discrepancy between a WAIS IQ of 94 and a WMS IQ of 69 may be very significant clinically). The WMS is often useful in providing a quantified measure of memory and in providing information to aid in differentiating between organic and functional memory disorders.

Bender Gestalt Test

The Bender Gestalt is a venerable test which is still commonly used to assess constructional ability. It consists of nine geometric line designs which the patient is asked to copy with paper and pencil. A memory component may be introduced after completion of the standard administration by requiring the patient to draw the designs again from memory. Errors in reproduction may be objectively scored,[18] with the primary pathologic features being (1) distortion or simplification of the gestalt, (2) failures in the integration of parts, (3) rotation of the reproduced design, and (4) perseveration. The stimulus designs are sufficiently simple that perfect reproduction is expected by age 12. Any errors by an adult which are unexplained by physical or sensory limitations, mental retardation, or lack of exposure to graphic tasks are assumed to reflect organic dysfunction.

Benton Visual Retention Test

In the Benton Visual Retention Test, a series of simple and complex line drawings are presented to the patient's view for periods of varying duration. The patient must then reproduce the design after different delay periods (direct copy, immediate reproduction from memory, and reproduction after a delay of 15 seconds). The patient's reproductions are scored for errors of omission, addition, distortion, rotation, perseveration, size, and misplacement. A relatively well-standardized normative system allows a quantified comparision of the patient's performance with that expected for age. This test was designed to assess visual perception, visuoconstructive ability, and visual memory. Its advantages are the objective scoring system and normative cutoff points for normal and brain damaged subjects, while its primary drawback in routine clinical use is the time required for administration, scoring, and interpretation (up to 30 minutes when all forms are used).

Trail Making Test

The Trail Making Test is a part of the Halstead-Reitan battery and involves two somewhat different tasks. In Form A, 25 small circles are randomly printed on a sheet of paper and numbered from 1 to 25. The patient is required to connect the numbered circles in sequence as rapidly as possible. In Form B, 25 randomly printed circles (the mirror image of Form A) are numbered from 1 to 13 and lettered from A to L. The patient draws a connecting line, alternating between numbers and letters (i.e., 1-A-2-B-3). Form A is assumed to be a right hemisphere task, primarily requiring perceptual-motor speed, while Form B is considered a left hemisphere task involving efficiency in conceptual shifting as well as perceptual-motor speed. The brief (5 minutes) test is reputedly sensitive to both diffuse and lateralized brain damage and is frequently useful in screening frontal lobe functions. Normative data is available.[25,33]

Category Test

This is a subtest of the Halstead-Reitan battery and is frequently used independently. It is generally considered to be a test of concept formation and abstract problem solving behavior. From a series of visually presented stimuli, the patient is required to abstract basic principles of similarity and difference and to learn sorting behavior based upon variables such as size, shape, number, brightness, color, and position. The Category Test is a very complex method of assessing abstract reasoning and learning under reinforcement conditions. Although brain damaged patients as a group do tend to demonstrate deficient performance,[27] factors such as intelligence, memory, and comprehension all impair performance and may be the crucial components in explaining discrepant scores.[36,38]

Proverbs Tests

There are probably as many forms of the proverbs test as there are examiners; each of us has a repertoire of familiar sayings that are brought out during the mental status exam. All are tests of verbal abstract ability and educational knowledge in which the patient either explains the meaning of proverbs or choses the best explanation from among a series of choices. Gorham[11] has devised a multiple choice proverb interpretation test with interpretations of each proverb ranging between the extremes of abstraction and concreteness. Proverbs of increasing levels of difficulty are also provided. Examples of responses of varying quality provided in the test manual facilitate an objective scoring of the degree of abstraction versus concreteness of the individual patient's performance. The use of this standardized test eliminates the need to rely on observation and the examiner's subjective impressions of the quality of the patient's responses. This allows a quantification of the individual patient's performance and a more systematic comparison with expected performance.

Finger Tapping Test

The Finger Tapping Test is commonly used in various forms in standard clinical neurologic exams and has been well standardized by Reitan[27] among others. The form of the test most commonly employed by neuropsychologists requires the patient to tap a mechanical counter with the index finger of each hand. Three trials of 10 seconds each are used, alternating between each hand. An averaged score is then obtained for each hand; these scores are then compared with norms for age and hand dominance. Significant discrepancies between expected norms and actual performance by either hand or discrepancies exceeding 10 percent between hands are considered diagnostic of organic brain disease.[26] The most commonly utilized expected mean scores for normal adults are 50 taps with the dominant hand and 45 taps with the nondominant hand. Somewhat slower performance is expected with older subjects, although standardized data regarding the quantification of the relationship between age and finger tapping speed is not yet available. Age related norms are available for children.[33]

Wide Range Achievement Test (WRAT)

The Wide Range Achievement Test is a briefly administered (15 to 20 minutes) test in reading (word recognition), spelling to dictation, and written arithmetic. The items in the WRAT are steeply graded in difficulty, allowing its use on all levels from kindergarten to college. It is a useful test when a standardized and more objective assessment of academic deficits is needed.[16]

Minnesota Multiphasic Personality Inventory (MMPI)

The most commonly used standardized test of personality, the Minnesota Multiphasic Personality Inventory consists of 566 statements (e.g., I seldom worry about my health) to which the patient responds true or false as they apply to him. The test is then objectively scored, with the resultant profile graphically showing performance in the clinical areas of hypochondriasis, depression, hysteria, psychopathic deviancy, masculinity-femininity of interests, paranoia, psychasthenia (obsessive-compulsive thinking), schizophrenia, hypomania, and social introversion. Validity scales L (lie), F (attempts to "fake bad"), and K (a suppressor variable reflecting attempts to "fake good") are also obtained. A number of guidebooks to aid the examiner in interpretation of the significance of individual MMPI configural profiles is available. There are some suggestions that the test may be useful in differentiating organic from functional states and as a lateralizing index for patients with organic brain disease[2,9,15] although others question this use.[42]

INTERPRETING AND OBTAINING THE NEUROPSYCHOLOGIC REPORT

A common feature of the psychologic reports of many clinical psychologists and even some neuropsychologists is the frequent reporting of so-called "organic signs." This may be difficult for the physician to interpret without some knowledge of the term. Such "organic signs" typically include the following:

Verbal-Performance Discrepancies. These discrepancies are appreciable differences between the Verbal and Performance Scale IQs on the Wechsler series of intelligence tests. Differences exceeding 25 points have consistently been shown to be statistically significant,[6] while differences of 15 points have been shown to be of clinical utility in identifying neurologic dysfunction.[1] Verbal-Performance discrepancies must be cautiously interpreted in the light of the overall psy-

74

chologic test profile, the patient's social and educational background, and the presence of any primary sensory or motor deficit (e.g., a visual impairment or cerebral palsy).

Scattering of Performance Levels.   A scattering of performance levels on the various subtests of the Wechsler tests or among any of the scores obtained on the full psychologic test battery (e.g., a subtest score of 12 on the WAIS Vocabulary subtest and 6 on the Similarities subtest or a WAIS IQ of 105 and a Wechsler Memory Scale Quotient of 67). Such difference in performance does indicate discrepant cognitive functioning which must be explained. The physician should recognize, however, that a number of factors (social, psychologic, and educational) as well as brain dysfunction may result in such subtest "scatter." Accordingly, this organic indicator should not be interpreted in isolation as an unequivocal sign of brain damage or dysfunction.

Sign of Visual Motor Dysfunction.   An indication of visual motor dysfunction as detected by any measure of constructional ability, including the nonverbal WAIS subtests, the Bender Gestalt, and Drawings to Command. The best predictors of brain dysfunction on constructional tests are the specific errors of rotation and perseveration. Errors related to the overall integration of separate parts or the distortion of the design gestalt often tend to be maturational rather than pathologic. Constructional ability and its impairment is covered in more depth in the section on the mental status examination in this chapter and in Chapter 7, Neurobehavioral Syndromes Associated with Focal Brain Lesions. Suffice it to say at this point, a wide variety of social, maturational, motor, and sensory factors as well as brain damage may affect constructional ability. Therefore, information regarding performance in this area must be evaluated within the context of the total neurologic and neuropsychologic evaluations and the patient's social and educational history.

Behavioral Findings.   Behavioral findings including hyperactivity, distractibility, mixed laterality, motor incoordination, clumsiness, and so forth are all regarded as signs of organic disease. It is well established that the incidence of such findings is higher in brain damaged individuals than in normals, especially among children. Because of the variability of maturation, the use of such behavioral indicators in isolation as diagnostic of brain damage is quite unwarranted.

In sum, the information provided by the clinical psychologist may be of significant value to the physician in describing the abilities and disabilities of the patient and in helping to make a diagnosis of brain dysfunction. The referring physician must, however, utilize the services of a well trained and experienced psychologist, understand something of the nature of the commonly employed psychologic tests, and be able to interpret both the utility and especially the limitations of the so-called brain damage indicators or "organic signs."

Those readers desiring more detailed information regarding specific tests and procedures included in the neuropsychologic evaluation are referred to the excellent reviews of Lezak,[19] Reitan and Davidson,[28] Small,[32] Golden,[8] and Swiercinsky.[36] Additionally, the publications of Hécaen and Albert,[13] Heilman and Valenstein,[43] and Walsh[37] provide very valuable overviews of the field of clinical neuropsychology and of specific topics within the field.

Clinical neuropsychology is a relatively new field with most of its practioners being located in universities or large medical centers. Accordingly, it may be necessary for the physician to utilize the services of a traditionally trained clinical psychologist. Many such psychologists have received some training in the administration of neuropsychologic tests and have an interest in the evaluation of patients with neurologic disorders. Before referring a patient to a clinical psychologist, the physician should ensure that the particular professional is in fact prepared to administer the type of evaluation necessary and to answer the specific neurobehavioral questions which have been raised. This can readily be accomplished through informal contact or a brief phone call.

Psychiatry

Many patients with organic brain disease have a commitant emotional disturbance which requires psychiatric consultation. Patients referred for psychiatric evaluation include (1) those with psychiatric disorders predating their neurologic problem, (2) those with emotional reactions to brain disease (e.g., reactive depression), (3) patients in whom an emotional reaction complicates dementia, or other organic conditions, and (4) those with functional disorders presenting as neurologic conditions (e.g., hysterical paralysis).

Emotional factors may be significant obstacles to the rehabilitation and social reintegration of any patient with organic disease. The psychiatrist should be consulted to aid in the management of the patient with an emotional disturbance sufficiently severe as to interfere with rehabilitative efforts or home adjustment.

REFERRAL

Because of the relatively high incidence of both mental illness and brain disease, many patients will have coexisting psychiatric and neurologic conditions (e.g., a brain tumor in a schizophrenic patient or a seizure patient with a manic depressive disorder). For example, we recently saw a 37-year-old woman with a 7 year history of schizophrenia. The patient was also an alcoholic and over the years had sustained several significant head injuries. After alcohol withdrawal, she had several grand mal seizures and was admitted to the neurology ward. As her postictal confusion cleared, she demonstrated gross delusional and aggressive behavior. After a complete history and medical evaluation, we determined that the patient had an acute neurologic condition which was superimposed upon a preexisting chronic schizophrenia. Because of the significant functional psychosis, psychiatry was consulted for treatment and long term management. In general, psychiatrists should be consulted on patients with preexisting psychiatric disease regardless of the nature of the coexisting medical disorder.

It is not uncommon for emotionally stable individuals to develop a significant emotional reaction to a recent neurologic or neurobehavioral disorder such as aphasia. Depressive reactions, anxiety, paranoia, and aggressiveness may all develop in response to brain damage. Such emotional reactions may significantly interfere with any rehabilitation efforts. For example, a 62-year-old woman developed right hemiplegia and anomic aphasia secondary to a left middle cerebral artery thrombosis. After the acute stage, she became increasingly depressed to a point of apathy, self depreciation, and constant crying. She would no longer actively participate in physical therapy and appeared to abandon any hope of improvement. When a serious emotional reaction such as this is superimposed on an organic deficit, the emotional component must be specifically treated in conjunction with the medical treatment. Psychiatric referral in the course of such cases will significantly aid the total rehabilitation program.

Demented patients present a particular challenge because they have both intellectual and emotional changes as a part of their disease. These changes produce a variety of difficult management problems which are often best handled with the aid of a psychiatrist. During the early stages of dementia, many patients retain considerable insight; this capacity to realize the seriousness of their condition often results in a profound reactive depression. Other patients with dementia become unaware of their deteriorating intellectual ability and often push themselves beyond their capability and develop frustration and severe anxiety. This situation was aptly illustrated by a recent case: A 58-year-old businessman was referred because of failing memory. Examination revealed a genuine memory deficit and other evidence of an early dementia. Severe anxiety was prominent and interferred with both specific test performance and his social and vocational life. This anxiety was greatly reduced by restructuring his lifestyle (e.g., his wife helped him with his business and he discontinued many civic duties) and the use of a mild tranquilizer to aid in sleeping. After several months, retesting showed improvement in many cognitive areas and he was better able to carry out his home and job responsibilities. Any degree of anxiety or depression can greatly exacerbate the mental and social disability experienced by the demented patient. The psychiatrist can provide great assistance through the use of psychotrophic drugs, family counseling, and general procedures of patient management.

The diagnostic problem of differentiating amongst dementia, depression, and dementia with depression is both common and often difficult in clinical practice. Because this differential diagnosis is critical in terms of patient management and treatment, the psychiatrist should be involved early in the evaluation process. Misdiagnosis of depression as dementia will deprive the patient of appropriate treatment and leave the family with the erroneous impression that the disease is progressive and irreversible. Conversely, the misdiagnosis of dementia as depression may lead to ineffective and costly psychotherapy, leaves the patient subject to social and vocational problems resulting from intellectual deterioration, and misleads the family as to the prognosis of the disease.

Psychiatric referral is also indicated for patients who develop depression in response to a chronic neurologic disease such as myasthenia gravis, epilepsy, multiple sclerosis, or parkinsonism. These patients can frequently live long and productive lives if they are able to accept and deal with their disability in a realistic fashion.

Many patients with chronic organic brain syndromes such as aphasia, dementia, traumatic encephalopathy, or Korsakoff's disease become management problems and eventually require long term care in a psychiatric hospital. Early referral to the psychiatrist or psychiatric social worker can help the family and the physician with the administrative and legal details involved in institutionalization.

A final group of patients who may initially be seen by the neurologist but require referral to the psychiatrist are those with hysterical conversion reactions. Many patients will present with symptoms which mimic neurologic disease (e.g., limb paralysis, loss of speech, or sensory loss), but which demonstrate no organic etiology. The treatment of choice for such functional disorders is psychotherapy.

EVALUATION

The psychiatrist utilizes psychiatric interview techniques, a psychiatrically oriented mental status examination, and personality tests in his evaluation. Information on specific interview and evaluation techniques is readily available in all major psychiatric texts.[3,12,17,20,34]

TREATMENT

Even though specific treatment is frequently unavailable for the primary brain disease, behavioral and pharmacologic treatment can often improve the lives of most of these patients. Medication is particularly useful in patients with preexisting psychiatric disease as the underlying psychiatric disorder will respond to a standard regimen of psychotrophic medication. Antianxiety or mood elevating drugs are effective in treating the anxiety or depression frequently seen as a reaction to organic brain disease. Major tranquilizers are often required to control the agitation and nocturnal wanderings of the deteriorated patient with organic brain disease.

Standard psychotherapeutic methods can be used in some patients with organic disease who retain comprehension, memory, and insight. On the other hand, insight therapy would be less than useful in many patients (e.g., severe amnesics, demented patients, those with significant frontal lobe behavioral changes, and Wernicke's aphasics). In this latter group of patients, behavior modification techniques to change specific behaviors are more appropriate.

Family counseling is often the most useful form of patient management. Through discussion, the psychiatrist is able to help the family understand the patient's problem and to offer suggestions on management. With the psychiatrist's help, the family can then restructure the patient's routine in an effort to minimize environmental stress.

The medicolegal aspects of organic brain disease are also very important and must be part of any long term management program. The patient's competence to make a will, to conduct personal financial affairs, and to enter into contracts such as marriage should be established in each case.

Finally, every treatment plan should include a consideration of possible eventual full time supervision if the patient becomes unmanageable in the home. The details of nursing home or institutional placement should be worked out with the help of the psychiatrist, social workers, and the patient's family. Such plans should be considered early in the course of the disease to allow time to assess family financial and personal resources; to determine the availability of home nursing services, nursing homes, and institutions; and to preclude the necessity of unsatisfactory and hasty decisions made at a time of crisis.

Speech Pathology

Patients with significant difficulty in communicating should be evaluated by a trained speech pathologist. All such patients will not be treatment candidates, but by means of a thorough language evaluation, the speech pathologist will be able to determine appropriate candidates for rehabilitation and provide other services to those patients and their families that are not selected for treatment. Patients with aphasia, apraxia of speech, or dysarthria are examples of patients with primary neurologic disease that should be referred. The speech pathologist is an important member of a comprehensive rehabilitation team; this is particularly true when the unit deals with a large number of stroke patients. Functional speech and language disorders such as elective mutism and hysterical aphonia are also ideal problems for speech evaluation and treatment. An evaluation by the speech pathologist provides a description of the patient's overall level of communication, the possible benefits of therapeutic intervention, and a plan for family counseling to facilitate alternate methods of communicating with the patient.

Virtually every physician has access to a speech pathologist, either in private practice or in hospital, university, or community clinics. The American Speech and Hearing Association and many states issue licenses or certificates of clinical competence to qualified clinicians. The referring physician should ensure the basic clinical competence of any speech pathologist he consults. Many speech pathologists will have specialized knowledge and experience in treating patients with delayed speech acquisition, articulation disorders, stuttering, or aphasia. The evaluation and treatment of aphasia and other acquired communication disorders is a very specialized field; the physician should determine the speech pathologist's competence in dealing with the specific disorder before referring his aphasic patients.

REFERRAL

The major reasons for referring patients to the speech pathologist are: (1) The mental status examination indicates the presence of a communication disorder that requires a more thorough evaluation, (2) Obvious communication disorders exist that require a detailed screening evaluation to determine the appropriateness of speech therapy, and (3) A significant communication disorder requires family counseling to inform the family members as to the patient's problem and to assist in maximizing communication within the home.

The physician will see the following general types of speech and language problems which will require more comprehensive evaluation than can be provided in his office:

1. Articulation disturbances such as the dysarthrias seen in pseudobulbar palsy, bulbar paralysis, neuromuscular disease such as myasthenia gravis, cerebellar disorders including cerebral palsy, and basal ganglia disease such as parkinsonism
2. Functional (hysterical) aphonias, especially in patients with a history of minor trauma or surgery to the throat or vocal cords
3. Elective mutism
4. Dysfluency (stuttering) is seen in both children and adults, and,

if untreated, may pose a significant obstacle to successful social and vocational adjustment.

5. Patients with acquired language disorders (aphasia, alexia, agraphia) deserve an initial speech and language evaluation, both to determine the potential for benefit from speech therapy and to aid the patient's family in understanding and dealing with the communication disorder. Because of the rapid changes in language which occur during the first two to four weeks following an acute cerebral lesion, speech evaluations will be most valid and prognostically useful if carried out after this initial period.

6. Patients with buccofacial apraxia in the presence or absence of aphasia may benefit from speech evaluation and therapy directed toward articulation and the intelligibility of speech, as well as other buccofacial activities such as drinking and swallowing.

SPEECH AND LANGUAGE EVALUATION

Features of the Evaluation

The comprehensive speech and language evaluation can be expected to provide information regarding:

Diagnosis. A definition of the primary language diagnosis (e.g., nonfluent aphasia, dysarthria, buccofacial apraxia) will be included.

Description. The evaluation will contain a comprehensive description of the type of language disorder, including all areas of deficit (e.g., word finding problems, alexia, or auditory comprehension problems) and residual language abilities. The description should contain some qualitative index of the degree of problem in each area assessed to allow comparison with subsequent evaluations. Some statement should be made as to the effect of the language deficit upon the patient's communicative ability in formal (test or interview) and informal (social) areas.

Recommendations. Recommendations will answer such specific questions as: Is speech therapy indicated and if so, what will be the emphasis of the therapy? What will be the frequency of therapy visits, what is the projected duration of therapy, and what are the specific plans for home therapy by family members and for family counseling?

Goals of Therapy and Prognosis. The establishment of goals will answer the questions of: What are the primary goals of speech and language therapy? What is the prognosis for language recovery? What will be the long term social impact of the language disorder?

Evaluation Components

There are numerous systems and methods of speech and language evaluation. The system and specific tests employed will be determined in part by the particular patient and partly by the individual speech pathologist's training and experience. As the enumeration of all of these methods is beyond the scope of this book, the interested reader is referred to the writings of Eisenson,[5] Goodglass and Kaplan,[10] Porch,[23] and Schuell.[31]

A comprehensive evaluation should include the following elements:

1. An examination of the oral physiology, including evaluation of the strength and alacrity of the muscles of articulation.
2. A description of the characteristics of speech articulation: dysarthria, dysfluency, and dysprosody.
3. A description of apraxias if present, both verbal (speech) and nonverbal (nonspeech facial movements).
4. An evaluation for aphasia, specifically including a description of spontaneous speech and an assessment of verbal comprehension, repetition, and word finding ability.
5. An assessment of reading and writing.
6. An evaluation of the adequacy of nonverbal communication, including an assessment of the ability to communicate utilizing gestures or other methods regardless of the language deficit.
7. A description of the patient's general behavior and specific behavioral responses to the stress of language items.

Treatment

Treatment is not universally efficacious in all speech and language disorders. The following is a general breakdown of the expected results with a number of patient types based upon our clinical experience.

Excellent results can often be produced in rehabilitating patients with: (1) functional voice disorders, exclusive of elective mutism (which is more resistant to traditional forms of speech therapy), (2) mild to moderate articulation problems, and (3) delayed speech in nonretarded children.

Good results can be expected in patients with: (1) anomic aphasia, (2) oral apraxia, (3) moderate articulation problems, and (d) developmental reading and learning disorders.

Fair results are generally obtained in patients with: (1) Broca's aphasia, (2) moderate to severe articulation problems, (3) aphasia with mild to moderate comprehension defects, (4) developmental aphasia, and (5) elective mutism (unless intensive behaviorally oriented therapy is employed, in which case the prognosis is improved).

Poor results typically result from therapeutic efforts with patients with: (1) global aphasia, (2) Wernicke's aphasia, (3) severe dysarthria and oral apraxia, and (4) language disturbances secondary to dementia.

We emphasize that these are only general rules of thumb; the individual patient with a particular language disorder will not always respond to therapy as projected. Accordingly, a complete speech and language evaluation of the patient with any developmental or acquired communication disorder is important to provide at least the consideration of therapy for those patients who may benefit from it.

SUMMARY

The management of patients with organic brain disease is a multidisciplinary effort. Physicians are strongly encouraged to acquaint themselves with the services offered by their colleagues in related specialized fields. By utilizing their resources, the physician will be better able to understand his patients and to provide them more comprehensive care.

REFERENCES

1. Black, F.W.: WISC verbal performance discrepancies or indications of neurological dysfunction in pediatric patients. J. Clin. Psychol. 30:165, 1974.
2. Black, F.W.: Unilateral lesions and MMPI performance: A preliminary study. Percept. Mot. Skills 40:87, 1975.
3. Detre, T., and Kupfer, D: Psychiatric history and mental status examination, in Freedman, A., Kaplan, H., and Sadock, B., (eds.): Comprehensive Psychiatry. Williams & Wilkins Co., Baltimore, 1975, pp. 724–736.
4. Dujoune, B.E., and Levy, B.I.: The psychometric structure of the Wechsler Memory Scale. J. Clin. Psychol. 27:251,1971.
5. Eisensen, J.: Examining for Aphasia. The Psychological Corporation, New York, 1954.
6. Field, J.: Two types of tables for use with Wechsler's Intelligence Scales. J. Clin. Psychol. 16:3, 1960.
7. Fisher, C.: The neurological examination of the comatose patient. Acta Neurol. Scand. (Suppl.) 36:1, 1969.
8. Golden, C.J.: Diagnosis and Rehabilitation in Clinical Neuropsychology. Charles C Thomas, Springfield, Ill., 1978.
9. Good, P., and Banter, J.: The Physician's Guide to the MMPI. University of Minnesota Press, Minneapolis, 1961.
10. Goodglass, H., and Kaplan, E.: The Assessment of Aphasia and Related Disorders. Lea & Febiger, Philadelphia, 1972.
11. Gorham, D.: The Proverbs Test. Psychological Test Specialists, Missoula, Montana, 1956.
12. Gregory, I.: Psychiatric interviewing and evaluation, in Fundamentals of Psychiatry. W.B. Saunders Co., Philadelphia, 1968, pp. 192–207.
13. Hécaen, H., and Albert, M.L.: Human Neuropsychology. John Wiley & Sons, Inc., New York, 1978.
14. Halstead, W.: Brain and Intelligence: A Quantitative Study of the Frontal Lobes. University of Chicago Press, Chicago, 1947.
15. Hathaway, S., and McKinley, J.: Minnesota Multiphasic Personality Inventory. The Psychological Corporation, New York, 1951.

16. Jastak, J., and Jastak, S.: The Wide Range Achievement Test. Guidance Associates, Wilmington, Delaware, 1965.
17. Kolb, L.: Noyes' Modern Clinical Psychiatry. W.B. Saunders Co., Philadelphia, 1968, pp. 147–158.
18. Koppitz, E.M.: The Bender Gestalt Test for Young Children. Grune & Stratton, New York, 1964.
19. Lezak, M.D.: Neuropsychological Assessment. Oxford University Press, New York, 1976.
20. Novello, J.: The psychiatric history and mental status examination, in Novello, J. (ed.): A Practical Handbook of Psychiatry. Charles C Thomas, Springfield, Ill. 1974, pp. 40–48.
21. Parsons, O.: Clinical Neuropsychology, in Speilberger, C. (ed.): Current Topics in Clinical and Community Psychology, Vol. 2. Academic Press, Inc., New York, 1970, pp. 1–60.
22. Plum, F., and Posner, J.: Diagnosis of Stupor and Coma, ed 3. F.A. Davis Co., Philadelphia, 1980.
23. Porch, B.: Porch Index of Communicative Ability. Consulting Psychologists Press, Palo Alto, Calif., 1971.
24. Reitan, R.: Investigation of the validity of Halstead's measures of biological intelligence. Arch. Neurol. Psychiatry 48:474, 1955.
25. Reitan, R.: Validity of the trail making test as an indicator of organic brain damage. Percept. Mot. Skills 8:271, 1958.
26. Reitan, R.: The effects of brain lesions on adaptive abilities in human beings (mimeo). Indiana University Medical Center, Indianapolis, Indiana, 1959.
27. Reitan, R.: A research program on the psychological effects of brain lesions in human beings, in Ellis, N. (ed.): International Review of Research in Mental Retardation, Vol. 1. Academic Press, Inc., New York, 1966, pp. 153–218.
28. Reitan, R., and Davidson, L. (eds.): Clinical Neuropsychology: Current Status and Applications. John Wiley & Sons, Inc., New York, 1974.
29. Russell, E.W.: A multiple scoring method for the assessment of complex memory functions. J. Consult. Clin. Psychol. 45:800, 1975.
30. Russell, E.W., Neuringer, C., and Goldstein, G.: Assessment of Brain Damage. Wiley-Interscience, New York, 1970.
31. Schuell, H.: Differential diagnosis of aphasia with the Minnesota Test. University of Minnesota Press, Minneapolis, 1965.
32. Small, L.: Neuropsychodiagnosis in Psychotherapy. Brunner/Mazel, Inc., New York, 1973.
33. Spreen, O., and Gaddes, W.H.: Developmental norms for 15 neuropsychological tests age 6 to 15. Cortex, 5: 170, 1969.
34. Stevenson, I., and Sheppe, W.: The psychiatric examination, in Asieti, S. (ed.): The American Handbook of Psychiatry, Vol. 1. Basic Books, Inc., New York, 1959, pp. 215–234.
35. Strub, R.L., and Black, F.W.: The Mental Status Examination in Neurology. F.A. Davis, Co., Philadelphia, 1977.
36. Swiercinsky, D.: Manual for the Adult Neuropsychological Evaluation. Charles C Thomas, Springfield, Ill., 1978.
37. Walsh, K.W.: Neuropsychology: A Clinical Approach. Churchill Livingston, London, 1978.
38. Golden, C.J.: Clinical Interpretation of Objective Psychological Tests. Grune & Stratton, New York, 1979.

39. Anthony, W.Z., Heaton, R.K., and Lehman, R.A.W.: An attempt to cross-validate two actuarial systems for neuropsychological test interpretation. J. Consult. Clin. Psychol. 48:317, 1980.
40. Hevern, V.W.: Recent validity studies of the Halstead-Reitan approach to clinical neuropsychological assessment: A critical review. Clin. Neuropsychol. 2:49, 1980.
41. Hullicka, I.M.: Age differences in Wechsler Memory Scale scores. J. Genet. Psychol. 107:135, 1966.
42. Dikmen, S. and Reitan, R.: MMPI correlates of adaptive ability deficits in patients with brain lesions. J. Nerv. Ment. Dis. 165:247, 1977.
43. Heilman, K.M., and Valenstein, E.: Clinical Neuropsychology. Oxford University Press, New York, 1979.
44. Lenzer, I.I.: Halstead-Reitan test battery: A problem of differential diagnosis. Percept. Mot. Skills 50:611, 1980.

SECTION II

MAJOR CLINICAL ORGANIC BRAIN SYNDROMES

4

THE ACUTE CONFUSIONAL STATE

T.H. is a 56-year-old right-handed businessman who had entered the hospital for cervical disc surgery. Because of his busy schedule and his anxiety relating to surgery, he had cancelled his admission on two previous occasions. The patient was a fairly heavy social drinker but not to the point of interfering in any way with his business performance. The surgery was uneventful and there were no immediate complications of the procedure. The patient was greatly relieved and seemed to be making a normal recovery until the third postoperative night. During that night he became quite restless and found it difficult to sleep. The next day he was visibly fatigued but otherwise normal. The following night, his restlessness became more pronounced, and he became fearful and anxious. As the night progressed, he thought that he saw people hiding in his room, and shortly before dawn he reported to the nurse that he saw some strange little animals running over his bed and up the drapes. At the time of morning rounds, the patient was very anxious and frightened. He was lethargic, distractible, and quite incoherent when he tried to discuss the events of the night before. He knew who he was and where he was but did not know the date or when he had had his surgery. During that day his mental status fluctuated, but by nightfall he had become grossly disoriented and agitated. At this point, psychiatric consultation was obtained.

The consultant's diagnosis was acute postoperative confusional state. The cause was probably due to a combination of factors: withdrawal from alcohol, fear of surgery, use of strong analgesics, stress of the operation, pain, and the sleepless nights in an unfamiliar room. The treatment consisted of a reduction in medications for pain, partial illumination of the room at night, and a family member in attendance at all times. These simple changes in conjunction with 50 mg. of chlorpromazine (Thorazine) three times daily and 500 mg. of chloral hydrate at bedtime reversed his confusional state within two days, and he was able to return home in a week with no residual evidence of abnormal behavior. To date there has been no recurrence of these problems.

The above case is a typical acute confusional state. This condition is encountered frequently in the routine practice of medicine and surgery and should be readily recognized by any physician.[26] The confusional state is usually of medical origin and due to a metabolic imbalance, adverse drug reaction, head trauma, or alcohol or drug withdrawal; or as in the case above, a combination of these factors. The abrupt change in behavior can be most upsetting to family and physician alike, but with prompt evaluation and therapy, the condition is usually completely reversible. If the physician fails to appreciate that this acute behavior change is caused by a primary medical problem and is not a functional psychiatric disorder, the patient's condition will worsen. Ultimately, the untreated patient can slip into coma and die. It is because of the frequency, seriousness, and reversibility of this problem that the confusional state is the most important of the neurobehavioral syndromes for the primary care physician to recognize.

All patients do not present with the same clinical picture and that is why the plural, confusional states, rather than confusional state is used. The behavior of some confusional patients is very bizarre, with agitation, shouting, and active hallucinations dominating the clinical picture. Other cases present primarily with lethargy and incoherent speech. Because of this diversity of clinical presentation, no single term has been universally adopted in the literature to indicate these conditions. The neurologic literature most commonly uses the terms acute confusional states, delirium, or toxic or metabolic encephalopathy; while psychiatrists at various times have employed the terms toxic psychosis, acute brain syndrome (Diagnostic and Statistical Manual of Mental Disorders I), psychosis associated with organic brain syndrome (Diagnostic and Statistical Manual of Mental Disorders II), and delirium (Diagnostic and Statistical Manual of Mental Disorders III). Each of the above terms emphasizes a specific aspect of the syndrome and all have been used interchangeably as a denotation of cases such as the one presented at the beginning of the chapter.

We prefer the term *acute confusional state* because it stresses both the acuteness of the process and the principal mental change seen. Simply defined, an acute confusional state is a rapidly developing, reversible change in behavior that is characterized by a clouding of consciousness, incoherence in the train of thought, and difficulty with attention and concentration. No definition can possibly include every aspect of each clinical case, but this one contains the essential features of the clinical syndromes.

DESCRIPTION OF THE CLINICAL SYNDROME

The major diagnostic feature of the confusional states is a clouding of consciousness. Level of alertness and arousability are affected as well as the content and coherence of thought processes. These alterations of consciousness may be subtle and present only during a portion of the day; such intermittent clouding is typical early in the course of the illness. If, however, this sign is not fully appreciated and the underlying condition progresses, the more dramatic behavioral changes of lethargy, disorientation, or agitation will develop. These alterations in consciousness and the tendency to fluctuate during the day are critical in identifying this as an organic condition and not primarily psychogenic. The schizophrenic may present with incoherent thought processes and the outward appearance of confusion, but his level of consciousness is normal and does not vary over time.

In the early stages, patients are frequently restless, particularly at night. Sleep is disturbed and mild behavioral changes such as anxiety or depressive feelings may appear. The patients experience difficulty concentrating and their conversation tends to drift from the subject. As the condition progresses, they become unable to think clearly and efficiently and their thoughts lack their accustomed coherence. Patients often lose track of the temporal sequence of recent events and will describe events as having happened that day that actually occurred in the recent past. All of these symptoms fluctuate but are usually accentuated at night.

In later stages, inattention and distractibility become prominent, speech is less coherent, and the patients appear confused and bewildered. They are unsure of the date and gradually show disorientation for place as well as time. Activity level changes. In some patients restlessness may be accentuated to the point of agitation and hyperactivity, whereas in the majority of patients the level of consciousness decreases and psychomotor retardation and lethargy are evident. The agitated patient may show swings from hyperactivity to lethargy during each 24 hour period. In this more severe stage, abnormalities in perception can occur and patients frequently misperceive unfamiliar people in their environment as being familiar. It is not uncommon for a patient in the incipient phase of delirium tremens to steadfastly hold to the belief that the doctor is his brother or other close relative. This is quite a different situation from that seen in the schizophrenic. To them, the familiar figure is often felt to be a stranger and in some way threatening.[12,32] Such delusions and illusions may be accompanied by frank visual or tactile hallucinations.

Eventually, confusional patients lose touch with reality; they are grossly disoriented, incoherent, and hallucinatory. Fluctuations in level of awareness are more dramatic, and the patients are totally unable to sustain attention. At this point the behavioral disorder can be classified as psychotic in degree. If the disease process is not reversed, the patients will rapidly become stuporous. Patients who have been grossly agitated may present with a muttering stupor (i.e., requiring vigorous stimulation to arouse, yet emitting constant muttering noises).

The total clinical picture of most patients in the acute confusional state falls into two main categories: lethargic or agitated. In some patients the picture is consistent throughout the course of the acute episode, whereas in others, it varies from lethargy to agitation during the same day. Often the lethargic patient can become very anxious and agitated when the lights are turned off in the room at night and he is left alone with reduced sensory stimulation. The following case exemplifies this point.

A 72-year-old woman suffered an episode of confusion during a transient global amnesic episode. The next morning the patient was clear mentally, but somewhat lethargic. Her daughter stayed with her throughout the day and reported that the patient had only several short periods when she was unsure of why she was in the hospital. Early in the evening the patient was sleeping; the daughter turned out the room light and went home to clean up and have supper. She returned three hours later to find the nurses greatly disturbed because the patient had pulled out her intravenous infusion, tried to climb over the side rails of the bed, and was shouting violently that everyone was trying to kill her.

When a patient becomes agitated and hyperactive as did this woman, it is proper to consider her confusional behavior as delirious. The agitated confusional state or classic delirium, in addition to having the behavioral changes seen with any confusional state, also has the added feature of autonomic overactivity with pupillary dilatation, flushed facies, tachycardia, and tachypnea. Delirium can be a phase of any confusional state or can be the predominant behavioral pattern, as in cases of delirium tremens from alcohol withdrawal. Regardless of the mode of presentation and activity level, the basic features of the acute confusional syndrome (e.g., clouding of consciousness, fluctuating course, incoherent and slow thinking, inattention, and disturbance of perception) are common to all such patients.

One additional feature of these states which is often useful in differentiating them from the dementias or the schizophrenias is their rapidity of onset. Confusional behavior develops over a period of hours to days rather than over months or years. In taking the history from the family of a demented or schizophrenic patient, many clues of dis-ordered behavior slowly developing over a long period of time are found. The family of the confusional patient is frequently very upset and distraught because of the sudden appearance of bizarre and un-characteristic behavior in a previously normal individual.

THE NEUROBEHAVIORAL EVALUATION

The acute confusional state can readily be diagnosed at the bedside and all physicians should train themselves to become sensitive to each of its clinical features.

Acuteness of Onset

The acuteness of onset can be readily evaluated by clinical observation of the patient if the confusional state developed in the hospital or by the history obtained from family members if the condition arose at home. The evolution of confusional behavior over a course of hours to days is strongly suggestive of an acute organic etiology, whereas a history of months to years of progressively confused behavior raises the question of an underlying functional disorder or a progressive de-mentia.

Clouding of Consciousness

Evaluation of the clouding of consciousness involves the assessment of both the level of alertness and the content of thought processes. The level of alertness is determined by the quality of the patient's response to environmental stimulation. When evaluating the patient, the exam-iner should utilize graded levels of stimulation to quantify the patient's responsiveness. The initial stimulation should consist of calling the patient's name in a conversational tone. If the patient fails to respond at this level, a louder and more persistent tone of voice should be used. Next, gentle shaking of the patient's arm should accompany the vocal stimulation. Finally, more vigorous stimulation (auditory and tactile) should be applied. Patients who respond only to vigorous stimulation or who fail to respond at all are classified as stuporous or comatose and do not fall within the category of the acute confusional state. The confusional patient is typically lethargic and responds to a loud spoken voice with minimal tactile stimulation. The agitated confusional (delir-ious) patient on the other hand is hyperresponsive to environmental stimuli and because of this, responds readily to any attempt at stimula-tion. Despite their alertness, these agitated patients are distractible and fail to sustain attention to the examiner.

The level of alertness of the acutely confusional patient fluctuates during the course of the day and night. Such patients are often lethargic and sleepy during the day while becoming agitated at night. In the early stages of the confusional state, the patient may appear normally alert and respond appropriately much of the time. However, there will be periods when the patient becomes lethargic or agitated. Because of these fluctuations, the physician must carefully evaluate the level of alertness on a number of occasions during the day and question nurses and visitors concerning variations in the patient's responsiveness.

Recognition of the clouding or impairment of thought processes requires careful observation of the patient's behavior and conversation. It is important for the physician to actually converse with the patient several times a day to determine if he is thinking clearly and coherently. It is surprising how many doctors enter the patient's room after a review of the chart and say, "How are you today? Things seem to be going well; the heart test was normal and you will be having some x-rays today." The patient is frequently given time only to say, "Hello, I'm fine," and then nod in agreement with the day's plan before the busy physician, with a stack of charts in hand, is off to the next room. From this cursory glance, things seem to be all right, but the patient has not been allowed to demonstrate if he can think and talk coherently. It is useful to ask the patient about what he has been doing in the hospital and particularly to have him review the tests that he has had and laboratories to which he has been taken. This information is known to the doctors, and it is easy to verify if the patient is fully aware of what is transpiring.

If the nurse or family has reported an episode of confusion, ask the patient about it. One of our patients questioned after being missing from the ward for two hours, reported that he "got up to see a friend in the lobby and could not see what all the fuss was about," failing to see the inappropriateness of wandering about the hospital lobby at 2:00 A.M. in an open hospital gown. Such inconsistencies in the patient's logic and the abnormal behavior are important bits of evidence in diagnosing an early confusional state. When listening to the patient, it is important to look for signs of slow and imprecise thinking. This is very easy to recognize if the physician has known the patient for some time but is more difficult for the consultant seeing the patient for the first time. It is, therefore, very important for the primary physician to listen carefully to the patient's conversation. Any sign of incoherent thinking should alert the examiner to the fact that mentation is becoming confused. It is useful to ask basic questions concerning orientation (e.g., date, time, place, and person). Many hospitalized patients have difficulty with exact dates, but the confusional patient demonstrates more flagrant disorientation.

Attention

The next step in the mental status evaluation is the assessment of attention. Throughout their course, confusional patients have difficulty with attention and concentration. This problem may not be obvious to the casual observer, although the patient himself may complain of difficulty in concentrating. During the examination the physician should look for signs of inattention or distractibility. If it is not obvious that the patient is inattentive, specific tests of attention and concentration should be administered. The best and most commonly used is the digit repetition test. The average nonaphasic person should be able to repeat 6 to 7 digits forward, and any difficulty with this task suggests inattention. A more complicated yet better test of vigilance or concentration is the "A" test (see Chap. 3) in which the patient must signal whenever he hears the letter "A" in a verbally presented random series of letters. The serial subtraction test (the patient is asked to subtract 7s serially beginning with 100 (i.e., 100 − 93 − 86 − 79) is a complex yet commonly used test of concentration. This test can be failed for numerous reasons other than inattention and concentration (e.g., aphasia or calculation problems), so we prefer to use the digit repetition and "A" tests as measures of attention.

Perception

Disorders of perception (illusions, delusions, and hallucinations) are evaluated by carefully observing the patient's behavior, questioning him about any strange or unusual feelings or sensory experiences, and asking the nursing staff and visitors if they have observed any indications of these misperceptions or hallucinations. The patient may not overtly display this behavior and often will not report such events spontaneously. We recently saw. an elderly patient with parkinsonism who was apparently doing well on levodopa. During one office visit, the patient's wife asked us if her husband had told us about the animals that he reported seeing. He had not told us about this experience, but when asked, he described "nice little rabbits and other furry animals climbing over the bed and TV set at night." When asked why he had not reported these before, he replied simply, "I kind of liked them and didn't think that it was important to tell you." Other confusional patients, particularly those in acute delirium tremens, actively hallucinate and frequently become paranoid, shouting at the object of their hallucination (e.g., blue spiders crawling on the skin or snakes infesting their bed).

Disorientation

Disorientation is another typical feature of the more florid confusional patient and may readily be assessed by asking the patient the date, where he is, who he is, and what he is doing here. Frequently such patients will insist that they are at home or in some other familiar place and that the medical staff are all personal acquaintances. Disorientation to person is relatively infrequent and is indicative of the most severe stage of confusion.

Fluctuations in Behavior

As previously mentioned, it is important for the physician to note any fluctuations in the patient's mental status during the course of the day and night. Since there is a great diurnal variation of behavior in the confusional state, it is not unusual for the night nurse to report that a patient is agitated, confused, and wandering; yet on morning rounds, the patient is alert, bright, and capable of carrying on a normal conversation. Nocturnal peregrinations and confusion are frequently the first sign of an impending confusional state and must be recognized as such by the physician. Although confusional behavior is more typical at night, fluctuations may also occur at any time during the day.

In summary, the evaluation of the acute confusional state relies heavily upon the examiner's ability to observe and elicit the various behavioral abnormalities that comprise the syndrome. No simple physical or neurologic signs can establish the diagnosis; the diagnosis must be made on behavioral grounds alone.

Differential Diagnosis

Although there is usually no difficulty in identifying confusional behavior as being of organic origin, it is necessary to consider those functional psychiatric disorders whose behavioral features may resemble the acute confusional states. In their most florid stages; acute schizophrenic episodes, acute mania[36] (manic-depressive illness, manic-type), severe psychotic depressive reactions with marked psychomotor retardation, and the severe adjustment reaction of adulthood (acute panic state) may demonstrate some of the behavioral features of acute confusional states. Both the organic confusional states and the above psychiatric conditions have an acute onset, an alternation of activity level which may be either to restlessness and hyperactivity or lethargy and hypoactivity, disordered thinking, and inattention and distractibility.

Despite these similarities, the organic and functional conditions can usually be readily differentiated by careful observation and examination. The findings which allow the examiner to make the differential diagnosis include:

CLOUDING OF CONSCIOUSNESS

The most important differential feature between organic and functional conditions is the presence or absence of alterations in the level of consciousness. Organic patients typically have a decreased but fluctuating level of awareness. The level of awareness can vary from patient to patient; ranging from relatively subtle decreases to stupor. In contrast, the patient with a functional illness maintains a constant and normal level of consciousness. The use of major sedating medication in the psychiatric patient will, of course, result in a decrease in the level of awareness, thereby making the differential diagnosis more difficult.

COGNITIVE IMPAIRMENT

The organic patient demonstrates a global impairment of cognitive functions. Psychiatric patients, conversely, show little evidence of true cognitive deficit, although their inattention and disordered thought processes cause them to make errors on mental status testing, particularly on measures of memory, calculation, and complex reasoning.

NATURE OF INCOHERENT THOUGHT PROCESSES

The thought processes of the organic patient tend to be fragmented, slow, and disordered. Their language is often circumlocutory, and sometimes aphasic. Paranoid ideation and delusions may be present in both the patients with organic and those with functional conditions; however, symbolic and systematized delusions are more typical of the functional psychotic disorders. Manic and acutely anxious (panic) patients have a press of thought, flight of ideas, and a very rapid production of speech; these features are not seen in the typical organic confusional state. In psychotic depression, the thought processes are slowed but only infrequently are they incoherent. The speech production in such patients tends to be laconic and measured, a feature not found in acute confusional patients.

QUALITY OF DISORDERED PERCEPTION

Although both organic and functional patients may have delusions and/or hallucinations, the nature of the perceptual disturbance is usually different. The organic patient experiences primarily visual and tactile hallucinations, whereas the functionally psychotic patient more commonly has auditory hallucinations. The delusions of the organic patient are characterized by the misperception of the unfamiliar as familiar, while the reverse is true in the functional patient (i.e., the familiar as unfamiliar).

MEDICAL EVALUATION

The diagnostic challenge presented by the confusional patient is similar to, and equally as critical as, that presented by the patient in coma. A systematic and deliberate evaluation is imperative. The first step, as in any diagnostic problem, is to obtain the available historical data from family, friends, or the nursing staff in cases where the patient has developed confusional behavior while in the hospital. Following the history, a careful physical and neurologic examination is necessary. Table 4-1 lists the most important factors to consider in taking the history, performing the examination, and choosing the appropriate laboratory tests.

Differential Diagnosis

There is a myriad of medical illnesses that can present with acute confusional behavior. It is impossible to discuss each in detail; however,

TABLE 4–1. Medical Evaluation of the Confusional Patient

History

1. Medications: Particularly psychotropic, antiparkinsonism, diuretic, anorexic, or sedative

2. Illicit drug use

3. Medical illness:
   Heart disease
   Diabetes
   Liver or kidney disease
   Hypertensive or arteriosclerotic vascular disease
   Thyroid disease or previous thyroid surgery
   Other endocrine disturbances

4. Alcohol use

5. Neurologic disease:
   Epilepsy,
   Evidence of early dementia (e.g., memory failure, difficulty doing job)
   Recent onset of neurologic symptoms (e.g., visual disturbance, gait difficulty)

6. Psychiatric illness (e.g., anxiety, depression, psychosis)

7. Recent trauma

8. Recent surgery

Physical Examination

Parameter	Finding	Clinical Implication
1. Pulse	Bradycardia	Hypothyroidism Stokes-Adams syndrome Increased intracranial pressure
	Tachycardia	Hyperthyroidism Infection Heart failure
2. Temperature	Fever	Sepsis Thyroid storm Vasculitis
3. Blood Pressure	Hypotension	Shock Hypothyroidism Addison's disease
	Hypertension	Encephalopathy Intracranial mass
4. Respiration	Tachypnea	Diabetes Pneumonia Cardiac failure Fever Acidosis (metabolic)
	Shallow	Drug or alcohol intoxication
5. Carotid vessels	Bruits or decreased pulse	Transient cerebral ischemia
6. Scalp and face	Evidence of trauma	
7. Neck	Evidence of nucal rigidity	Meningitis Subarachnoid hemorrhage
8. Eyes	Papilledema	Tumor Hypertensive encephalopathy
	Pupillary dilatation	Anxiety Autonomic overactivity (e.g., delirium tremens)
9. Mouth	Tongue or cheek lacerations	Evidence of grand mal seizures
10. Thyroid	Enlarged	Hyperthyroidism
11. Heart	Arrhythmia	Inadequate cardiac output, possibility of emboli
	Cardiomegaly	Heart failure Hypertensive disease

TABLE 4–1. *Continued*

Parameter	Finding	Clinical Implication
12. Lungs	Congestion	Primary pulmonary failure Pulmonary edema Pneumonia
13. Breath	Alcohol	
	Ketones	Diabetes
14. Liver	Enlargement	Cirrhosis Liver failure
15. Nervous system		
a. Reflexes-muscle stretch	Asymmetry with Babinski's signs	Mass lesion Stroke
	Snout	Preexisting dementia Frontal mass Bilateral posterior cerebral artery occlusion
b. Abducens nerve (6th cranial nerve)	Weakness in lateral gaze	Increased intracranial pressure
c. Limb strength	Asymmetrical	Mass lesion Stroke
d. Autonomic	Hyperactivity	Anxiety Delirium

we will try to cover those conditions which are most frequently encountered in clinical practice to enable the physician to develop a systematic approach to the investigation of an individual case.

Before considering specific etiologies, it is important to recognize that several significant factors predispose patients to develop confusional behavior. Advancing age or existing brain disease are by far the most prominent. The elderly and particularly those showing evidence of early senility (dementia) are unusually susceptible to any physiologic or environmental disruption. The mentally retarded also have a greater probability of developing a confusional state.[26] A history of alcohol or drug abuse or recent sleep or sensory deprivation can all be contributory. In fact, sleep or sensory deprivation alone can cause concentration difficulties, perceptual distortions, and decreased reasoning ability.[30,31]

Another factor about which there has been considerable disagreement is the role of premorbid personality.[22] It is generally agreed that anyone can develop a full blown confusional state if the brain's physiology is sufficiently disturbed.[25] It is also true that each person has his own threshold for the development of confusional behavior.[13] Major psychiatric disease, either in the patient or his family, however, does not appear to be the factor establishing that threshold.[8] Stress and the anxiety generated by a serious illness do seem to have a significant disrupting effect on some patients and may precipitate confusional behavior.

Awareness of all of these predisposing factors not only helps the physician understand the confusional behavior in a specific patient but also alerts him to watch the confusion-prone patient very carefully when he develops minor illness, has surgery, or uses a new medication.

When confronted with a patient in a confusional state, the physician must be able to logically determine its etiology. Occasionally the offending agent is obvious, for instance, the confusion that occurs following a grand mal seizure, but frequently the cause must be carefully sought. The following factors should be considered in the differential diagnosis.

MEDICATIONS

Barbiturates; tranquilizers such as diazepam (Valium) and chlordiazepoxide (Librium); antiparkinsonism drugs, particularly levodopa, trihexyphenidyl HCl (Artane), benztropine mesylate (Cogentin), and amantadine (Symmetrel); and digitalis are all medicines routinely used in medical practice that are known to precipitate confusional behavior in some patients. Atropine and scopolamine are other common offenders and need not be given in large doses to cause a toxic response as the following case history demonstrates.

A 42-year-old oil-field worker was given a premedication of 0.6 mg of atropine sulfate prior to a cardiac catheterization. The procedure went smoothly with no suggestion of arrhythmia or anoxia. As the premedication sedative wore off, however, the patient became extremely agitated. He pulled out his intravenous needle, started climbing over the side rails of the bed, and began talking in a loud voice about a recent sexual escapade. He was bewildered, disoriented, and inattentive. The patient was then sedated with chlorpromazine (Thorazine) for 12 hours and the delirium passed without recurrence.

Atropine opthalmic solution contains 0.75 mg of atropine sulfate per drop and sufficient absorption can occasionally occur to cause toxicity.[24]

Although toxic reactions can occur at therapeutic dosages of these medications, many patients who develop confusional behavior have either misused prescribed medication or have been placed on multiple medications whose combined effect is adverse. Some patients increase dosages in an effort to gain additional effect; this is most frequently seen with analgesics, psychotropic drugs, and anorexics (diet pills). This polypharmacy is often the cause of confusional behavior and can be corrected by tailoring and monitoring the patient's drug regimen. The elderly patient with memory difficulty is particularly at risk because of a tendency to forget prescribed dosages at times of administration.

The abrupt withdrawal of certain medications can also precipitate a confusional state. Barbiturates, alcohol, opiates, and psychotropic drugs are the most frequent offenders, but others have been known to demonstrate this effect.

NONMEDICINAL SUBSTANCES

Acute alcoholic intoxication as well as acute alcohol withdrawal in the heavy drinker can cause confusional behavior. Recently, cases of confusion have been reported with excessive coffee intake in otherwise normal young adults.[4,15]

One of the most frequent causes of acute confusional behavior in young patients is use of the illicit drugs that are now available almost everywhere. Opiates, cannabis, amphetamines, and hallucinogens have been implicated. Exposure to the hallucinogenic drugs in particular can cause an acute psychotic delirium that is not unlike an acute schizophrenic state. Usually the patients have bizarre hallucinations (e.g., hearing colors), vivid visual illusions, and distortions of perception rather than the auditory hallucinations typically seen in schizophrenia. The schizophrenic is usually more withdrawn and autistic in his behavior and thinking than the drug user.[1,33]

ELECTROLYTE IMBALANCE

Electrolyte imbalance can develop in any patient and particularly in those using diuretics. Any medical condition in which gastrointestinal function is abnormal (e.g., vomiting, diarrhea, fistulae, or obstruction) can lead to marked shifts in electrolytes and subsequent dysfunction of the brain. Patients taking intravenous fluids are an obvious group at risk for developing electrolyte problems. Water intoxication, though rare, can occur and will cause an acute confusional episode until corrected.

METABOLIC DISEASE

Several metabolic diseases cause sufficient disruption in cerebral metabolism to produce confusional behavior. Diabetes is by far the most common. Hyperglycemia with or without acidosis (nonketotic hyperosmolar state) or hypoglycemia, primarily in the treated diabetic, can all cause a clouding of consciousness and confusion.

Thyroid disease with either hyperthyroidism or myxedema is another common cause of confusional behavior. In thyrotoxicosis, the patient becomes very agitated and hyperactive, but beneath this agitation may be elements of mood depression. We saw a 58-year-old male who had been admitted to the psychiatric unit with a diagnosis of agitated depression and unexplained recent weight loss. On examination, the patient was agitated, inattentive, and showed varying degrees of clouded consciousness. His T_3 and T_4 were found to be markedly elevated. With prompt treatment of his hyperthyroidism, his mental confusion, depression, and agitation all cleared within two weeks.

Hypothyroidism or myxedema can present in various ways; the most common being characterized by slowness, apathy, and poor performance on intellectual tasks. Other patients, however, do present with a full blown psychotic confusional state known as myxedema madness.[6]

Deficiencies as well as overactivity of the parathyroid or adrenal glands have also been implicated as causes of confusion and must be considered in the differential diagnosis.[12]

Vitamin deficiencies have long been known to cause various mental syndromes including the confusional states. Acute thiamine deficiency produces a confusional state known as Wernicke's encephalopathy (discussed more fully in Chap. 9). Nicotinic acid deficiency leading to pellagra, while not common, does occur in alcoholics and people with abnormal dietary habits. Pellagra can present with an acute confusional state even in the absence of the other clinical features of the disease (rash and diarrhea). B_{12} or folic acid deficiency can also be associated with mental confusion.[11,18] These patients often have a previous history of gastric surgery, although the condition can appear in isolation.

Abnormalities in copper metabolism are rare but of particular interest to the neurologist. Wilson's disease is a recessive genetic disease that has changes in mental function as one of its major symptoms. Although psychiatric or chronic mental deterioration are more typical presentations in this disease, acute episodes of confusional behavior can occur.

Another rare disease that frequently presents as acute confusion is acute intermittent porphyria. When patients develop a syndrome of confusion, inappropriate antidiuretic hormone secretion, repeated seizures, and a history of abdominal pain, this diagnosis should be considered.

ORGAN FAILURE

The decompensation of any major vital organ can often be accompanied by confusional behavior. Cardiac or pulmonary failure produce a relative anoxia which is poorly tolerated by the brain. Arrhythmias can also result in a significant decrease in cardiac output, thereby reducing cerebral oxygenation. Hepatic and renal failure cause a build-up of metabolic products that eventually act as toxins and cause cerebral dysfunction.

INFECTION

Any infectious disease, if sufficiently severe, can lead to an acute confusional state. There are several mechanisms by which infections produce confusional behavior. In encephalitis, the brain cells themselves are infected with viral particles. In meningitis, there is an inflammation of the cortical surface and edema, and a secondary vasculitis can develop in the vessels on the cortical surface, causing ischemia of patches of cortex. The most common infectious cause of a confusional state is the indirect effect on the brain seen in systemic sepsis. Although at one time it was felt that each specific agent produced a distinct type of confusional state, it is now recognized that the clinical picture of abnormal behavior is the same for any infective agent.[7]

OTHER NEUROLOGIC DISEASE

In several neurologic diseases, confusional behavior can be the only clinical manifestation. One is increased intracranial pressure which may be secondary to a tumor, infection, obstruction of cerebrospinal fluid flow, hypertensive crises, or benign intracranial hypertension (pseudotumor cerebri).

Seizure disorders (epilepsy) of various types can produce an acute confusional state. In grand mal epilepsy (generalized tonic-clonic seizures), the confusional behavior is most often seen after the seizure (postictal), although the prodrome or aura can also be characterized by a clouding of consciousness. In psychomotor or temporal lobe epilepsy (partial seizures with complex symptomatology) the seizure itself can simulate a confusional state. These patients often walk around aimlessly muttering to themselves for as long as an hour during a series of seizures.[37] The following case is an example of a patient in petit mal (absence) status epilepticus who presented in a confusional state.

A 55-year-old woman was brought to the office by the police. An officer stated that he had found the woman wandering around a bus stop mumbling incoherently. On neurologic examination she appeared to be completely out of contact with reality. She would try to talk but could only produce 4 or 5 slurred words and would then stop and begin to blink her eyes. She was agitated and restlessly pulled at her clothes and hair. Since many of her restless movements looked like psychomotor automatisms, she was taken to the electroencephalographic laboratory. Her EEG tracing showed almost continuous 3 cycle per second spike and wave bursts, compatible with petit mal (absence) status epilepticus. The patient was promptly treated with intravenous diazepam (Valium) and within 15 minutes was conversing normally.

Head trauma, particularly in the child and elderly adult, can lead to a behavioral change in the postconcussive period. Often the confusional state is present immediately after the injury as is seen in football players or boxers after a severe blow to the head. On some occasions, the onset is delayed by several days.

A 78-year-old man had been beaten up. Immediately after injury, he was clear mentally and required only stitching of his wounds and a cast on a broken arm. He returned home the same day. That night he did not sleep well because of pain and was given stronger analgesic medication. The second night he became quite restless and began to have rather florid paranoid ideation. On the following day, he was agitated and had great difficulty thinking and talking clearly. Neurologic evaluation did not reveal any focal findings, the brain scan and skull films were negative, but the EEG showed diffuse moderate slowing. The patient was treated conservatively with reassurance, thioridazine (Mellaril) and chloral hydrate for sleep. He made an uneventful recovery within several days and has not had any further difficulty.

This is the typical course of a post-traumatic confusional state, but occasionally the behavioral change is the first sign of a more serious condition.

A 76-year-old woman was recently admitted to the hospital in a confusional state after head trauma. Her neurologic examination was normal, but her level of consciousness steadily decreased over a 24 hour period. Evaluation including EEG, CT scan, and angiography revealed a large subdural hematoma. Surgery was immediately performed, but unfortunately she died postoperatively.

This case demonstrates the great importance of an agressive evaluation and close observation of the patient with behavioral change after head trauma.

VASCULAR DISEASE

Vascular disease is well-known for its ability to cause focal brain lesions with specific behavioral syndromes. There are, however, several vascular conditions that can produce an acute confusional state. The first results from subarachnoid hemorrhage. The mechanism by which the subarachnoid blood causes generalized disruption of brain function is uncertain, but several explanations are possible: (1) irritation of the cortex by blood or blood breakdown products, (2) vascular spasm, or (3) development of hydrocephalus from interference with cerebrospinal fluid circulation. The second vascular condition associated with confusional behavior is hypertensive encephalopathy. These patients are usually somewhat lethargic and complain of headache, but occasionally incoherent thought, clouding of consciousness, and bizarre behavior are the outstanding features. The third condition is cerebral vasculitis, particularly systemic lupus erythematosus. Although seizures are the most common cerebral manifestation of vasculitis, mental disorders occur in about one third of the cases.[21] The confusional state of delirious type is one of the most common of these mental disorders, while the remaining mimic psychiatric disorders. The fourth vascular etiology is occlusive cerebrovascular disease. It is common for patients to show a degree of confusion after any acute cerebral infarct. This confusion may be somewhat overshadowed by the more obvious neurologic deficits of hemiplegia and aphasia. Nevertheless, these patients frequently act inappropriately, display agitation, and have the typical clouding of consciousness seen in a confusional state. Usually this acute postinfarct confusion clears within 24 to 48 hours unless brain swelling is significant and intracranial pressure greatly increased.

However, some patients with focal infarcts do develop prolonged, significant confusional states. These cases are interesting because they raise the possibility that confusional behavior may be due in part to damage or dysfunction of specific brain areas. The first group of such patients described in the literature had occlusions of the anterior cerebral arteries or rupture of anterior communicating artery aneurysms.[38] These lesions resulted in infarction or destruction of the anterior cingulate gyri, orbital frontal cortex, and septal nuclei.[5] These patients usually had motor and reflex changes in their legs, but often the outstanding feature of their illness was the acute onset of confusion with lethargy or agitation. More recently an "agitated delirium" has been reported with occlusion of the posterior cerebral arteries and infarction of the occipital lobes plus the fusiform, lingual, and hippocampal gyri. The most dramatic cases had bilateral lesions, but the syndrome can be produced by a unilateral lesion.[19,27]

Some patients develop a transient confusional state with a very prominent memory disturbance. This state has been called a transient global amnesia and is felt to be secondary to vascular insufficiency in the distribution of the posterior cerebral arteries. This condition will be more fully discussed in Chapter 7.

Recently there has been a series of reports of cases in which patients with right middle cerebral artery occlusions presented with the features of a classic confusional state.[28] These patients did not have abnormalities on routine neurologic examination and were initially diagnosed as "confusional state secondary to metabolic inbalance." Only after a brain scan revealed the cortical lesion was it realized that these confusional states were secondary to focal lesions.

A final type of occlusive vascular lesion that can produce confusional behavior is that seen with severe bilateral extracranial carotid artery disease. In these patients, marked stenosis or occlusion of the carotid arteries significantly reduces the blood flow to the cerebral hemispheres. Any sudden change in hemodynamics can cause transient cerebral ischemia and confusion. Usually there are other transient neurologic symptoms and signs that suggest a vascular etiology, but on occasion confusional behavior is the only clinical manifestation.

SURGERY

The postoperative period is a common clinical setting for confusional behavior. As with all etiologies, the elderly are the most vulnerable. The abnormal behavior pattern frequently appears on the third or fourth postoperative night, but it can arise any time during the first two weeks. Many factors contribute to the development of confusional behavior in the patient after surgery, and the surgeon must carefully review the entire history, operative period, and postoperative course to determine the etiology of the confusion. Table 4-2 lists etiologic factors.

Anoxia during the operative procedure is a major factor and a review of the anesthesia record can help to uncover prolonged periods of hypotension, difficulty with adequate air exchange, or significant cardiac arrhythmia. The anesthetic agents themselves do not seem to be a problem; rather it is an inadequate oxygen supply to brain tissue that causes the cerebral dysfunction. If significant anoxia has been present during surgery, the patient will show confusion upon awaking from anesthesia. This is quite different from the patient who develops confusional behavior in the third or fourth postoperative day due to electrolyte imbalances that have arisen subsequent to surgery.

TABLE 4–2. Factors Leading to the Postoperative Development of an Acute Confusional State

1. Anoxia during surgery
2. Sepsis
3. Electrolyte imbalance
4. Abnormal reaction to sedatives and analgesics
5. Atelectasis with decreased oxygen pressure
6. Loss of sleep
7. Pain
8. Fear and stress
9. Cerebral emboli, particularly microemboli in cardiac surgery
10. Drug or alcohol withdrawal
11. Any combination of the above

Cardiac surgery is one type of surgery in which postoperative confusion and delirium have been a common and significant problem. Patients undergoing valve replacement frequently develop not only a confusional state but also scattered abnormal neurologic signs in the postoperative period.[34] Pathologic study of fatal cases has revealed multiple microemboli and evidence of anoxic damage to neurons in the hippocampus. It had been postulated that the microemboli came from the bypass pump and caused both microinfarcts and decreased cerebral oxygenation.[9] The introduction of a small pore filter into the pump-oxygenator has considerably decreased the incidence of postoperative brain damage and dysfunction.[17] Confusional behavior, however, continues to be a problem. In a study reported in 1979, 38 percent of 48 patients receiving single valve replacements demonstrated postoperative delirium.[16] In this series, cardiac output was carefully monitored, and it was apparent that a significant drop in output was a major factor in the production of the delirium. Patients undergoing valve replacement surgery have a higher incidence of confusional behavior than those having coronary bypass operations. Accordingly, intracardiac surgery appears to involve higher risk.

The actual surgery is not the only factor, however, since cardiac patients, like most other postoperative patients, tend to develop confusional states two to five days after surgery. The cardiac surgery patient has a somewhat different postoperative course because he remains in a special intensive care unit for several days before being returned to his regular hospital room. Nursing routines and general activity in such units give the patients virtually no sustained periods of sleep.[20] In one study, it was shown that the patients were disturbed an average of 47 times during each of the first three nights after surgery.[35] Such units are very sterile appearing and, in general, the environment is monotonous, nonstimulating, and disrupting. This sleep and sensory deprivation coupled with pain, uncertainty about prognosis, and the general stress of the illness combine to produce what has become known as "the intensive care unit psychosis" or "I.C.U. psychosis." That this is the origin of the psychosis is supported by the fact that patients usually demonstrate a rapid clearing of their confusion upon return to their own rooms.[23] Although first appreciated in postsurgery patients, this syndrome is also common in other patients restricted to coronary or medical intensive care units.

The physician must also be very attentive to the problems of electrolyte imbalance, adverse effect of analgesics, and fever. Electrolyte balance is particularly important in those patients requiring intravenous infusion for an extended period of time. One surgical procedure that is known to cause an immediate electrolyte imbalance and confusional behavior is the transurethral prostatectomy. During this sur-

108

gery, copious amounts of water are used to irrigate the operative field and some patients absorb large quantities of pure water and develop a dramatic water intoxication syndrome. This is easily recognized by the urologist and the patient's water intake is restricted. The use of hypertonic saline is dangerous because the patients are usually elderly and are already hypervolemic. The addition of salt will exacerbate the hypervolemia and often cause cardiac decompensation.

The postsurgical confusional state is an excellent example of how a combination of factors can produce a confusional syndrome. Advancing age with the additional possibility of early dementia; the adverse effects of strong analgesics, pain, fear, loss of sleep, and relative sensory deprivation; and the effects of sepsis and metabolic imbalance all may be present to some degree in the same patient. Though each may seem insignificant in isolation, their combined presence may exceed the patient's individual threshold and confusional behavior can ensue.

LABORATORY EVALUATION

After completing the history, physical examination, and considering the differential diagnosis, the medical basis of the patient's problem may be obvious and the laboratory need only be consulted for confirmatory evidence. However, as is all too frequently the case, the etiology may be elusive. At this point there is a series of tests that should be used to screen for the major causes of the confusional state. These are listed below:

General Testing Procedures

Test	*Clinical Implication*
1. White blood count and differential	Infection
2. Sedimentation rate	Infection or vasculitis (lupus)
3. Urine examination and toxicology tests	
Sugar and acetone	Diabetes
Leukocytes	Infection
Barbiturates and other toxic substances	
Albumin	Renal failure
Porphyria screen	
4. Serum tests	
Blood urea nitrogen and creatine	Renal failure
Sugar	Diabetes, hypoglycemia

T_3, T_4	Thyroid disease
Electrolytes	Evaluation for imbalance including Na^+, K^+, Ca^{++}, Cl^-, $PO_4^{\equiv}$; parathyroid induced change in calcium and phosphorus
Mg^{++}, Br^+	If available. Bromides are still present in some common drugs and overuse can inadvertently lead to toxicity.
Alcohol	
Specific drug levels	Barbiturates, etc.
5. X-rays, routine	
Chest	Infection, heart failure
Skull	Evidence of increased intracranial pressure, fractures

Special Neurodiagnostic Tests

ELECTROENCEPHALOGRAM (EEG)

The EEG can be very useful in evaluating patients diagnosed as or suspected of having an acute organic confusional state. Most patients who have clouding of consciousness and are confusional will have a diffusely slow EEG.[14] This fact can be very useful in separating the organic from a functional, purely psychiatric psychosis. Schizophrenics, while showing occasional EEG slowing, will show neither the degree nor magnitude of slowing seen in the confusional patient. In patients with delirium tremens the EEG usually shows slowing.[2] The EEG is also useful in determining if the confusional state represents an ictal (seizure) or postictal phenomenon. If the patient is actually in status epilepticus (a seizure state in which repeated seizures do not allow mental clearing between seizures), the EEG is highly diagnostic. If the patient is postictal, epileptiform activity may have been surpressed and replaced by slow activity. Accordingly, the absence of epileptiform discharges does not rule out seizures as the cause of the confusional state.

NUCLEOTIDE BRAIN SCAN OR COMPUTERIZED AXIAL TOMOGRAPHY (CT SCAN)

In cases in which the diagnosis is uncertain, the standard brain scan can help to rule out the presence of a brain tumor or subdural hematoma. Far more useful, but not available in every community, is the computerized tomography scan that provides the additional valuable information of ventricular size and the presence or absence of hemorrhage. Ventricular size will be normal in the majority of patients with confusional states of metabolic or toxic etiology unless the patient has preexisting dementia. Increased ventricular size without cortical atrophy is indicative of obstructed cerebrospinal fluid flow, a condition (hydrocephalus) that can present with increased pressure and confusional behavior.

SPINAL FLUID EXAMINATION

A spinal puncture is frequently advised, particularly when the etiology is uncertain. Viral meningoencephalitis, unsuspected subarachnoid hemorrhage, and the chronic meningitides (tuberculosis, cryptococcal and fungal infections) are not rare and are readily diagnosed with examination of the cerebrospinal fluid. Pressure measurements, cell count, protein, sugar, and extensive culture and staining procedures should be carried out.

INVASIVE NEURORADIOLOGIC PROCEDURES

Cerebral angiography or pneumoencephalography should be performed only in special cases where a tumor, specific vascular lesion, or hydrocephalus is suspected.

CONSULTATIONS

If a specific brain lesion such as a tumor or stroke is suspected, it is wise to consult the neurologist or neurosurgeon to assist in the evaluation. This is particularly important before undertaking any invasive neurodiagnostic procedures (i.e., angiography or pneumoencephalography).

Both neurologists and psychiatrists can be of assistance in the diagnostic evaluation and psychiatrists can also often be very helpful in the management of the case as will be discussed in the section to follow.

PATIENT MANAGEMENT

Two important avenues of treatment must be followed in the management of an acute confusional state: (1) the identification and correction of the underlying medical problem and (2) the control of the abnormal and often disruptive behavior. Hopefully, the primary physician can recognize the behavioral pattern as being an acute organically based behavioral change and will initiate medical management. If, however, he is unsure of the diagnosis he should consult a psychiatrist or neurologist. It is the primary physician's responsibility to review the patients's medical status and take steps to reverse any physiologic imbalance. With specific medical treatment, the behavior will eventually revert to the premorbid level. Unfortunately, this can sometimes take several days or even weeks. Accordingly, control of behavior must be an integral part of the overall treatment plan. If the physician is uncomfortable with this aspect of the treatment, he should consult a psychiatric colleague to assist him. The psychiatrist is accustomed to managing psychotic behavior and he can also serve as a valuable resource in supporting and reassuring the family and nursing staff.

Environmental Structuring

Effective control of the psychotic behavior is best achieved by a combination of the judicious use of tranquilizing medications and the rearrangement of the patient's immediate environment. If possible, the patient should be moved to a private room so that he can get adequate sleep and will not disturb other patients. Private duty nurses or family members should be with the patient at all times, particularly at night. This is very important for a number of reasons. The delirious patient may climb out of bed or pull out intravenous needles if not carefully watched, and regular nursing personnel cannot possibly be in the room constantly to prevent falls and other accidents. An attendant within the room reassures the patient that someone is there and that he is being taken care of properly. This reassurance is especially helpful at night when the effects of sensory deprivation are the greatest. The nurse or family member can also greatly reduce disorientation by talking frequently to the patient and actively trying to reorient him. Whenever the patient awakens or becomes agitated, a simple statement like, "John, it's me, Mary. Remember you are in the Memorial Hospital. It's Sunday and the doctor says that you are doing very well," can be very effective in calming and reorienting the patient. This type of environmental input is very helpful in both treating the confusional patient and preventing confusion in patients at risk. The incidence of confusional behavior after surgery can be greatly reduced if the nurses or family members will reorient patients at frequent intervals during the day.[10] We cannot stress too much the value of a constant attendant (which may be a family member) in handling the confusional patient.

The use of restraints is a question that frequently arises when dealing with the delirious patient and must always be discussed with the nursing staff. In general, restraints tend to agitate patients so they should be used only when absolutely necessary to prevent accidents or disruption of life support apparatus. With most patients, restraints can be used intermittently and should be removed promptly during periods of relative calm.

The room should be well lighted, but without bright lights aimed at the patient's face. At night, a light should be left on so that the patient can reorient himself quickly to his environment if he should awaken. It is good to have a clock, calendar, pictures, and perhaps a television

112

in the room to insure adequate sensory stimulation. Nightime interruptions should be kept to an absolute minimum so that the patient can get adequate sleep. If the patient can be moved from the bed, it is often helpful to let him sit up during part of the day. Occasionally several warm tub baths during the day can have a definite calming effect, and this is a useful adjunct in dealing with the agitated patient.

Medication

These specific environmental manipulations create an atmosphere that maximizes the effects of medical management. Usually, however, there is a need for sedation and tranquilization. We prefer the use of the major tranquilizers, chlorpromazine (Thorazine), haloperidol (Haldol) and thioridazine (Mellaril). The choice of dosage and route of administration will depend upon the degree of the patient's agitation. A dosage of 50 mg. of chlorpromazine, 25 mg. of thioridazine or 0.5 mg. of haloperidol three to four times daily is usually effective in ameliorating the agitation and other abnormal behavior. Haloperidol has the advantage of being administrable intramuscularly in severe cases. The initial intramuscular dose of haloperidol should be 2 to 5 mg. t.i.d. or q.i.d., although doses as high as 5 mg./hr. have been suggested.[29] The oral form should supplant the injectable as soon as is practical. Chlorpromazine given intravenously will cause a severe drop in blood pressure and should not be used. Paraldehyde is probably the safest drug to use (5 to 15 ml. orally, rectally, or intramuscularly 4 or 5 times daily), but the odor is often offensive to those caring for the patient. Other minor tranquilizers such as chlordiazepoxide (Librium) and diazepam (Valium) can be used, but these can sometimes excite the elderly patient and increase the agitation. Chlordiazepoxide, however, is very effective in treating delirium tremens, with doses of 100 to 400 mg. per day required.

Since sleep deprivation and disruption are a major contributory factor in production of the acute confusional states, it is best to sedate the patient at night until the confusion clears. Often all that is needed is an extra measure of tranquilizer at the hour of sleep, but at times the addition of a soporific is necessary. Chloral hydrate, 500 mg. to 1 gm., is usually sufficient. Barbiturates should be avoided in the elderly because of their occasional paradoxical effect.

Recovery

When the above steps of primary medical management, environmental structuring, and sedation/tranquilization are followed, the uncomplicated confusional state should gradually reverse and the patient's behavior return to its premorbid level. The period of recovery is quite variable. In some cases, confusion can clear in a matter of hours; this is most dramatically seen in patients who become confusional after cataract surgery. This confusion clears almost immediately after the removal of the eye patches. In such cases, the confusional state was caused primarily by sensory deprivation and reinstatement of normal sensory input reoriented the patients. In other cases of acute confusional state, the confusion will take several days to clear. Frequently there is a lag between the return to normal of serum chemistry levels and the reestablishment of normal cellular function. The return of normal synaptic membrane function may also be slow and in some cases the total recovery process may take 3 to 4 weeks.

The degree of recovery varies and is predicated to a great extent upon the type and severity of the underlying cause and the patient's age and general medical condition. Patients who experience a confusional state secondary to a drug reaction or postoperative electrolyte imbalance can usually expect a full recovery; while the patient who has sustained a period of anoxia with microembolism during cardiac surgery may suffer residual neurologic and cognitive impairment.

In many patients, the early signs of dementia or senility go unrecognized until they develop a confusional state secondary to a superimposed minor illness or after elective surgery. On initial examination it is usually impossible to discern whether a preexisting dementia has been present. This determination must await either an accurate history from the family or evaluation after the acute confusion has completely cleared. The superimposition of an acute organic behavioral change upon a chronic organic deterioration of mental function has been called "beclouded dementia," a convenient term that accurately describes this common clinical situation.[2] Although some families steadfastly claim that the patient's mental functioning was flawless prior to the illness, often careful questioning of the family elicits a history of failing memory or difficulty with work predating the acute illness or surgery by a number of months or even years. It is uncertain whether the physiologic disruption experienced during a confusional episode can actually exacerbate an early dementia or whether the family, patient, and physician are now able to see more clearly the early cognitive impairment. The following case history exemplifies this problem.

A 62-year-old marble cutter was working in his shop late one evening when he was hit on the head from behind by a prowler. The blow was not sufficient to render the man unconscious but merely frightened him. When the assailant left the building, the patient called a family member to take him to the hospital. Upon arrival at the hospital, he was anxious, somewhat lethargic, and restless. His conversation was some-

what disjointed and contained paranoid ideation. Following admission, he was inattentive and his level of consciousness fluctuated throughout the next day. This initial confusional period cleared in several days and his neurodiagnostic evaluation revealed only a slightly slow EEG. The patient was discharged and returned to work. He then found that he was unable to concentrate and that he could not keep the accustomed work details in proper order. He complained of memory difficulties and had become extremely anxious. He insisted that his mental functioning had been completely normal before the trauma, but mental status testing showed severe memory disturbance, retrograde amnesia for a period of several years, impaired abstract ability, and constructional impairment.

It was obvious on this exam and subsequent psychologic testing that this man had a substantial congnitive deficit which was consistent with a diagnosis of a degenerative dementia (Alzheimer's disease). At this point we questioned his wife more closely and she admitted reluctantly that his memory had, in fact, been getting worse over the last 1 to 2 years and that the head injury had only seemed to exacerbate it. A CT scan showed enlarged cerebral ventricles and generalized cortical atrophy.

This case could have been considered merely a posttraumatic encephalopathy had not additional investigation been undertaken. Although no pathology is available, we are quite certain that the trauma with its attendant confusional state served only to unmask a significant preexisting organic disorder.

PATHOLOGY AND DISCUSSION

Acute confusional behavior is characteristically the result of a physiologic disruption of the brain's entire neuronal population. Arousal, emotion, and intellectual processes are all disturbed. Whereas it is not possible to localize this behavioral pattern to involvement of any specific region of the brain, it is of theoretical interest to point out the possible contributions made by dysfunction of various anatomic structures.

Clouding of consciousness, the central symptom of the confusional states, implies an alteration both in the level of alertness and in the content of conscious processes. As discussed in Chapter 2, the level of alertness is largely determined by a balance between the ascending activating and inhibiting systems. Therefore, it is probable that these systems are dysfunctional in the confusional state. It can be postulated that patients with quiet or lethargic manifestations have suppression of the activating portion of the system and/or stimulation or release of the inhibiting portion. Conversely, the agitated or delirious type of patient may have the activating component stimulated and the inhibitory one suppressed. It has been shown that damage to the cerebral cortex can also cause a decrease in the level of consciousness.[3] Accordingly, it is probable that there are cortical as well as subcortical systems involved in the regulation of alertness. The clouding of mental processes reflected in incoherent thinking, disorientation, misperception, and the disruption of specific cognitive functions is the result of widespread cortical dysfunction.

The alterations in mood and emotions such as anxiety, paranoia, depression, and irritability do not seem to be primary personality reactions to illness but rather are the direct effect of organic limbic dysfunction or release.

Inattention and distractibility are often other characteristic features of the confusional syndrome and may reflect dysfunction of specific anatomic structures. Attention requires cortical and limbic input to focus the basic arousal energy. In the confusional patient, alterations in function are present at all three levels: ascending activation system, limbic system, and cortex. It is not surprising that the ability to selectively attend to some stimuli in the environment and to exclude other irrelevant stimulation is impaired in these patients. Although in most cases, inattention is the result of widespread dysfunction, there recently have been some cases of confusional behavior with gross alterations in attention described in patients with focal brain infarcts.[19,28] These infarctions have involved either the right inferior frontal lobe, the right inferior parietal lobule, the inferomedial temporal lobes, or the medial and deep frontal lobes. These areas are the convergence points for environmental stimuli and are necessary for continual monitoring of all incoming environmental input. The attention and confusional behavior that results from damage to these areas seems to result from the individual's inability to maintain a coherent sampling of ongoing thoughts or events.[28] If this hypothesis is correct, the previous theory that attention is a product of the brain's total function would have to be revised.

One aspect of the confusional state that cannot be well explained on anatomic grounds is the curious fact that some individuals develop a delirium from the same basic metabolic disturbance that produces lethargy in another. It is possible that individual differences in anatomy and membrane function result in these different reactions, but it is equally possible that each type of clinical presentation is determined by a unique combination of factors, with the most obvious cause of the illness being only one.

Although the anatomy and pathophysiology of the acute confusional state is not yet established, the clinical picture is well defined and may be readily recognized. The patient presenting in an acute confusional state should be considered to have a serious medical problem and a prompt and extensive evaluation is mandatory. With appropriate treatment, most cases will respond favorably with little, if any, residual. Without efficient evaluation and treatment, these patients may develop devastating neurologic sequelae or even die.

REFERENCES

1. Abruzzi, W.: Drug induced psychosis. . . . or schizophrenia? Am. J. Psychoanal. 35:329, 1975.
2. Adams, R.D., and Victor, M.: Delirium and other confusional states, in Wintrobe, M.M., Thorn, G.W., Adams, R.D., Braunwald, E., Isselbacher, K.J., and Petersdorf, R.G. (eds.): Principles of Internal Medicine. McGraw-Hill, New York, 1974, pp. 149–156.
3. Albert, M.L., Silverberg, R., Reches, A., and Berman, M.: Cerebral dominance for consciousness. Arch. Neurol. 33:453, 1976.
4. American Psychiatric Association: Diagnostic and Statistical Manual of Mental Disorders (DSM I, II, and III). American Psychiatric Association, Washington, 1952, 1968, 1980.
5. Amyes, E.W., and Nielsen, J.M.: Clinicopathologic study of vascular lesions of the anterior cingulate region. Bull Los Angeles Neurol. Soc. 20:112, 1955.
6. Asher, R.: Myxoedematous madness. Brit. Med. J. 2:555, 1949.
7. Bleuler, M.: Acute mental concomitants of physical disease, in Benson, D.F., and Blumer, D. (eds.): Psychiatric Aspects of Neurologic Disease. Grune and Stratton, New York, 1975, pp. 37–61.
8. Bleuler, M., Willi, J., and Buehler, H.R.: Akute psychische Begleiterscheinungen Koerperlicher Krankheiten. Thieme, Stuttgart, 1966.
9. Brennan, R.W., Patterson, R.H., and Kessler, J.: Cerebral blood flow and metabolism during cardiopulmonary bypass: evidence of microembolic encephalopathy. Neurology 21:665, 1971.
10. Budd, S., and Brown, W.: Effect of a reorientation technique on postcardiotomy delirium. Nurs. Res. 23:341, 1974.
11. Camp, C.D.: Pernicious anemia causing spinal cord changes and a mental state resembling paresis. Med. Rec. (New York) 81:156, 1912.
12. Cohen, S.: The toxic psychoses and allied states. Am. J. Med. 15:813, 1953.
13. Ebaugh, F.G., Barnacle, C.H., and Ewalt, J.P.: Delirious episodes associated with artificial fever: a study of 200 cases. Am. J. Psychiatry 23:191, 1936.
14. Engel, A.L., and Romano, J.: Delirium, a syndrome of cerebral insufficiency. J. Chron. Dis. 9:260, 1959.
15. Furlong, F.W.: Possible psychiatric significance of excessive coffee consumption. Can. Psychiatr. Assoc. J. 20:577, 1975.
16. Heller, S.S., Kornfeld, D.S., Frank, K.A., and Hoar, P.F.: Postcardiotomy delirium and cardiac output. Am. J. Psychiatry 136:337, 1979.
17. Hill, J.D., Osborn, J.J., Swank, R.L., Aguilar, M.J., deLaneralle, P., and Gerbode, F.: Experience using a new Dacron wool filter during extracorporeal circulation. Arch. Surg. 101:649, 1970.
18. Holmes, J.M.: Cerebral manifestations of vitamin B_{12} deficiency. Brit. Med. J. 2:1394, 1956.
19. Horenstein, S., Chamberlain, W., and Conomy, J.: Infarction of the fusi-

117

form and calcerine regions: agitated delirium and hemianopia. Trans. Am. Neurol. Assoc. 92:85, 1967.

20. Johns, M.W., Large, A.A., Masterton, J.P., and Dudley, H.A.F.: Sleep and delirium after open heart surgery. Brit. J. Surg. 61:377, 1974.

21. Johnson, R.T., and Richardson, E.P.: The neurological manifestations of systemic lupus erythematosus. Med. 47:337, 1968.

22. Knox, S.J.: Severe psychiatric disturbances in the post-operative period—a five year survey of Belfast hospitals. J. Ment. Sci. 107:1078, 1961.

23. Kornfeld, D.S., Zimberg, S., and Malm, J.R.: Psychiatric complications of open-heart surgery. New Engl. J. Med. 273:287, 1965.

24. Kounis, N.C.: Atropine eye-drops delirium. Can. Med. Assoc. J. 110:750, 1974.

25. Lipowski, Z.J.: Delirium, clouding of consciousness and confusion. J. Nerv. Ment. Dis. 145:227, 1967.

26. Lipowski, Z.J.: Delirium: Acute Brain Failure in Man. Charles C Thomas, Springfield, Illinois, 1979.

27. Medina, J.L., Rubino, F.A., and Ross, A.: Agitated delirium caused by infarction of the hippocampal formation and fusiform and lingual gyri: a case report. Neurology 24:1181, 1974.

28. Mesulam, M.M., Waxman, S.G., Geschwind, N., and Sabin, T.D.: Acute confusional states with right middle cerebral artery infarctions. J. Neurol. Neurosurg. Psychiatry 39:84, 1976.

29. Moore, D.P.: Rapid treatment of delirium in critically ill patients. Am. J. Psychiatry 134:1431, 1977.

30. Morris, G.O., and Singer, M.T.: Sleep deprivation: the context of consciousness. J. Nerv. Ment. Dis. 143:291, 1966.

31. Solomon, P., Mendelson, J.H., Kubzansky, P.E., Trumbull, R., Leiderman, P.H., and Wexler, D. (eds.): Sensory deprivation: A symposium held at Harvard Medical School. Harvard University Press, Cambridge, Massachusetts, 1961.

32. Stengel, E.: The organic confusional state and the organic dementias. Brit. J. Hosp. Med. 2:719, 1969.

33. Stone, M.H.: Drug related schizophrenic syndrome. Int. J. Psychiatry 11:391, 1973.

34. Tufo, H.M., Ostfeld, A.M., and Shekelle, R.: Central nervous system dysfunction following open-heart surgery. JAMA 212:1333, 1970.

35. Woods, N.F.: Patterns of sleep in postcardiotomy patients. Nurs. Res. 21:347, 1972.

36. Bond, T.C.: Recognition of acute delirious mania. Arch. Gen. Psychiatry 37:553, 1980.

37. Mayeux, R., Alexander, M.P., Benson, D.F., Brandt, J., Rosen, J.: Poriomania. Neurology 29:1616, 1979.

38. Okawa, M., Maeda, S., Nukui, H., Kawafuchi, J.: Psychiatric symptoms in ruptured anterior communicating aneurysms: social prognosis. Acta Psychiatr. Scand. 61:306, 1980.

5

ALZHEIMER'S/SENILE DEMENTIA

Mrs. R. B. is a 55-year-old poetess. In 1975, when her family initially brought her to the neurology clinic, her husband gave the history that the patient had been experiencing a gradual loss of memory and mental capacity for about one year. Six months previously, she had been fired from a job as a real estate agent because of frequent errors and personality clashes with other employees. Her ability to keep her personal calendar of upcoming events had declined and thus she frequently missed scheduled commitments. She forgot household details as well and seemed oblivious to the date and season. She had always been a very verbal person who spoke frequently in metaphore, but in the few months preceding her hospitalization her family noted that her speech had become rambling, tangential, and often quite empty of meaning. Though her personality had not changed substantially, her eccentric traits had become more dramatic. She had also become quite euphoric and indifferent until stressed, at which time she became irritable, argumentative, and often paranoid.

On initial medical and neurologic examination, the abnormalities were confined to the mental status examination. She was awake, hyperalert (any stray stimulus in the environment attracted her attention), and very inattentive to the examiner's specific questions. She denied any illness and staunchly held to the belief that she was in the hospital to see about a shoulder that had been bruised during a minor bus accident some months before. She demonstrated a remarkable press of speech and her conversation was loosely organized, perseverative, and almost completely tangential. Although quite agitated and occasionally paranoid, she seemed content to remain in the hospital and to be examined for short sessions.

She demonstrated no aphasia in running speech. Comprehension was impaired for complex material but not for routine conversation. She had some difficulty in naming objects and occasionally produced frank paraphasic errors. Her orientation and ability to learn were markedly impaired as was her recall of recent events. Her remote memory, however, was quite intact. Her drawings were relatively good, but block construction was impaired. Her thinking was very concrete and despite many years of using metaphorical language in her speech and poetry, she was unable to give an abstract interpretation to even the simplest of proverbs.

Neuropsychologic testing showed a Verbal IQ (WAIS) of 90, with very low scores on Comprehension and Similarities, and a Performance IQ of 76. Full Scale IQ was 83, a remarkable drop for a college graduate with additional graduate level work in journalism. Her Memory Quotient was only 52, considerably less adequate than her depressed IQ scores.

The only abnormal laboratory tests were an EEG which showed mild generalized slowing and a computerized tomography scan that demonstrated generalized cerebral atrophy (Fig. 5-1). A tentative diagnosis of Alzheimer's disease was made.

Over the past five years, the patient's mental capacity has steadily decreased, and she is currently (1980) totally incapacitated and confined to a state psychiatric hospital for custodial care.

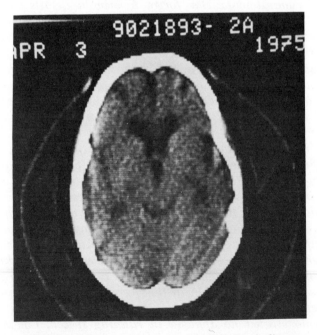

FIGURE 5–1.   CT scan of patient with Alzheimer's disease.

This case history exemplifies one of today's major mental health problems—dementia. This problem affects those under 65 years of age as well as the elderly, and it has been estimated that the dementias alone account for a staggering 70,000 to 110,000 deaths in the United States each year.[27,64] As life expectancy increases, the percentage of elderly in our society will increase proportionally. With age, unfortunately, comes the increasing probability of developing some type of dementing illness. In a sample of 80 year olds, for instance, a clinical picture of significant dementia was present in approximately 20 percent.[28] Organic brain syndromes in general account for 75 percent of all first admissions to mental hospitals in the 65 to 74-year-old age group. This percentage reaches 90 for those over the age of 75.[28] These figures are impressive and will certainly not reverse in the foreseeable future.

Dementia is a descriptive term which is usually used to denote a group of brain diseases in which the patients have suffered a slowly progressive deterioration in intellectual and adaptive functions. The process is not necessarily irreversible nor is there usually a uniform or generalized decline of *all* cognitive and social functions, two points that are at variance with many standard notions concerning dementia. The actual clinical picture of dementia can develop acutely after head injury, encephalitis, anoxia, and other conditions. Traditionally these entities have borne the pathologic label of encephalopathies, but in regard to the clinical feature of reduced mental capacity, they are often included under the rubric of dementia. In a given patient, a dementia must be distinguished from a primary amentia or mental retardation, a situation in which mental development was defective from birth or early life.

Dementia is a common clinical syndrome that has both varied etiology and clinical presentation. Although the dementias known as Alzheimer's disease, Pick's disease, and multi-infarct dementia have fairly characteristic modes of presentation, there is considerable variation within each group. In general, however, the demented patient demonstrates changes in several areas of functioning: usually memory, intellect, judgement, and affect or personality. These symptoms develop slowly in an unrelenting fashion over a period of months to years in the average case.

In this first chapter on the dementias, we will describe the general clinical features, the neurologic and laboratory evaluations, and the general principles of patient management. Because of its frequency, we have chosen to use Alzheimer's/senile dementia as the prototype for our discussion. Although traditionally Alzheimer's disease and senile dementia have been considered distinct entities, it is now apparent that they have more similarities than differences. Their clinical picture and pathologic findings are identical and the only substantial difference seems to lie in the arbitrary assignment of one label to those patients under 65 years of age (i.e., Alzheimer's presenile dementia) and another to those in the senium (i.e., senile dementia).[16,26]

Presenile Alzheimer's disease was thought to be a devastating dementia with extensive neuropathologic abnormalities, while the senile form was more indolent, less dramatic, and had similar, yet less intense, pathologic changes. Whether there are, in fact, two different conditions has not yet been proven. The incisive suggestion has been made that the disease itself is the same in both conditions, yet the neuropathologic and clinical response differs at different ages.[76] As immunologic systems and host responses change with age, diseases often also change in their clinical expression; this is certainly true of lymphomas, hepatitis, and tuberculosis. Accordingly, a similar variation in host response may be responsible for the differences within the Alzheimer spectrum. Since the concept of separating this condition into two groups has not withstood close scrutiny, we feel justified in discussing all patients with this type of degenerative dementia under the term Alzheimer's disease.

DESCRIPTION OF THE CLINICAL SYNDROME

Alzheimer's disease can occur at almost any age, the youngest recorded case being a child only 6 years old,[3] but 96 percent of the cases present after the age of 40.[58] There is a very consistent preponderance of female cases with a female/male ratio of 2:1 at all ages of onset.[58] The incidence of the disease increases with age, as does the prevalence; it is estimated that approximately 10 percent of the population over the age of 65 are affected to some degree.[26] The disease usually occurs sporadically, although there is a 5 percent familial incidence; a few of these familial cases have a dominant inheritance pattern, but most are polygenic.[3,58] Although the vast majority of the cases are classified as sporadic, the appearance of a case of Alzheimer's disease in a family increases the probability considerably above chance that a second case will be present in a parent or sibling.[58] This fact certainly suggests some hereditary tendency of polygenic type.

Initial Stage

Clinically the initial symptoms and signs of Alzheimer's disease fall into several categories: emotional, social, or intellectual (cognitive). In most cases the symptoms gradually become apparent, but in some instances the dementia can be abruptly manifested during a period of stress due either to an upheaval in the patient's environment (e.g., the death of a spouse) or an intercurrent illness or injury. As was mentioned in the previous chapter, a superimposed confusional state often unmasks a latent unsuspected dementia. Although usually slowly progressive, there have been several cases reported in which the disease ran a very malignant course with death occurring within six weeks from the time of onset of symptoms.[12]

The full-blown dementia, be it of Alzheimer type or another, is usually not difficult to recognize, rather it is the subtle early signs that the clinician must train himself to recognize if he is to help his patients avoid the social disaster of trying to "keep up the pace" of life when they cannot. Emotional changes can often be the first clue. These include a loss of interest in work, family, and vocation or increased irritability. A recent patient described himself by saying, "I just don't find work interesting anymore. I go and do my work, but it isn't any fun. Little things get on my nerves." Many patients try to find a physical explanation for their feeling that "something is wrong." They come to the physician's office with increasing frequency, complaining of minor aches and pains that do not seem to have a physical basis. This hypochondriasis in a previously healthy middle-aged or elderly patient should always raise the suspicion of dementia. Other patients, however, steadfastly deny any problem at all with their health and euphorically state that they have never felt better when, in fact, they are showing definite signs of intellectual deterioration.

Depression and anxiety can also constitute early features of the illness; this may represent not only the primary effects of neuronal degeneration in the frontal lobes and limbic system but also the patient's emotional reactions to his declining mental acuity. Restlessness, feelings of fatigue, and lack of accustomed initiative are frequent subtle emotional changes experienced by the Alzheimer patient in the first stage of his illness. Activity level tends to be high and the patients often wander incessantly.[61] These behavioral symptoms are usually better appreciated by the patient's family and coworkers than by the physician, so it is important to listen carefully and ask the appropriate questions of relatives if these early symptoms are to be recognized.

The social behavior and personality of the patient during the initial phases of his illness most often show an accentuation of previous personality traits superimposed upon a background of apathy or euphoria.[53] R.B.'s son-in-law remarked on one occasion, "My mother-in-law always acted a little strange, but now she seems *really* crazy." In some patients, where the degeneration of the frontal lobe is extensive (particularly in Pick's disease, Huntington's chorea, and general paresis), the patients develop a full blown frontal lobe syndrome with inappropriate behavior that is quite uncharacteristic of their previous personalities. This is less likely in the early Alzheimer's patient but can occur.

Cognitive changes occur early and are frequently the presenting complaint of the patient or his family. Memory disturbance is by far the most common and is manifested by a significant difficulty in forming new memories (i.e., new learning ability or recent memory). For example, an inspector at a local shipbuilding yard described his problem graphically, "When I go out on an inspection tour in the morning, there are a lot of different places that I have to check because the work is in different phases in various parts of the yard. I find now that I get out to the first station all right, but after that I can't remember where I am supposed to go next. I have to carry a schedule around with me to make sure I don't miss any stops on my rounds." This type of problem with work details plus misplacing things around the house and forgetting names are usually the most common complaints. Remote, well established memories, on the other hand, are usually quite well retained. It is not uncommon for a sympathetic relative to remark, "Now, his memory is better than all of ours. He can remember things about our childhood that I had long forgotten."

Though it is common, memory difficulty is not the only intellectual dysfunction noticed by the patient with Alzheimer's disease. General problem solving ability wanes; this is particularly evident when the patient attempts to solve complex novel problems in which he cannot rely upon well established routinized skills and strategies. We saw a real estate accountant who was showing signs of personality change but could still do the routine bookkeeping for his firm. The company tolerated his gradually progressing inappropriate social behavior because the books always balanced. One day, however, the company took over the establishment and management of a very different type of business, and the patient was asked to carry out a financial prospectus on the venture; he did so with great effort, frustration, and error. The business failed, and the firm finally realized that the patient was totally incompetent outside of the most routine bookkeeping matters. When we tested the man, he was not even able to accurately carry out written compound multiplication problems. He rejoined that he "always used a calculator and I've become rusty with arithmetic."

Comprehension and expression of complex ideas, thinking in an abstract fashion, and making critical judgements are all dulled in the patient with early Alzheimer's disease. Along with these higher level cognitive deficits, there is a definite loss of basic visual-motor integrative ability (constructional ability). Most patients will not complain of this problem unless they are architects or engineers, but it is easily demonstrated on mental status testing by having the patients copy some simple line drawings.

During this first stage of memory difficulty, subtle high level intellectual failing, and constructional deficits, the routine neurologic examination remains normal. The diagnosis, therefore, depends entirely upon the clinician's ability to carry out a careful mental status examination and recognize these early behavioral signs.

Although frequently appearing as described above, there is considerable variation in the presentation and course of the disease; in some cases the emotional change is more dramatic than the intellectual, while in others the reverse is true. In most patients, memory failure will be the first complaint, but we saw one patient whose initial symptom was a disturbance in writing and calculating.[63] The most important clinical point is that these patients are experiencing a change in behavior, and it is that change that the clinician must learn to search for and recognize.

Second Stage

As the disease progresses to a second stage, there is an accentuation of the emotional, social, and cognitive changes discussed above. The patients are less able to manage their personal and business affairs because of failing memory, increasing lack of initiative, and decreased ability to meet the challenges of any demand.

Language, which earlier had been normal, now becomes very concrete, tangential, circumlocutory, and perseverative. Mrs R.B., for instance, when asked why she was in the hospital would start by saying that she had some trouble with the arm which she needed to write and did we know that she was putting together a group of her poems for a new publication. Within moments we had been told about her name appearing in *Who's Who in American Poetry* and then about her graduate school experience at Cornell. This general string of conversation was produced with clockwork regularity after almost every inquiry. These changes in language are primarily a reflection of a dissolution of intellectual processing, but true aphasic errors also appear. Speech remains fluent at first but contains paraphasias, word-finding pauses, circumlocutions, and a surprising lack of substantive words (nouns and action verbs). For instance, a hospitalized patient upon being asked what kind of place she was in answered, "Oh, it's a sort of place where people are, and it is a resting area, a sort of clinic but not really for sick people."

Patients in this second stage may become quite upset at night and tend to wander about the house and neighborhood. They become quite restless and their hands are frequently found to be picking at imaginary bits of lint on their clothes (corphologia) or constantly manipulating objects in their hands. A napkin or handkerchief is commonly folded and refolded as the patient sits in a chair.

During the first two stages of the dementing process, the patients often retain sufficient insight into their condition to develop secondary anxiety and depression. It is very important to recognize these reactive emotional states because they cause the dementia to appear more severe than it is, and specific treatment of these states can produce a remarkable improvement in the patient's overall functioning.

Third Stage

With further progression, the patients enter a more distinctly aphasic, apractic, and agnosic stage. Not only have their general intellectual capacities deteriorated, but they begin producing unmistakable aphasic speech. Spontaneous speech decreases. They tend to echo what is said to them (echolalia), their comprehension is greatly reduced, and they have significant anomia (inability to name objects to confrontation or to come up with the names of people or things in running speech). However, they often have remarkably preserved repetition.

Their anomia is interesting because the difficulty with naming objects is more than a simple linguistic problem in which the word is unavailable. They actually seem not to recognize previously familiar objects. For instance, one patient was shown a pen and asked what it was. He picked it up as though he had never seen such an implement before, toyed with it for a moment, and then handed it back without verbal response. This type of failure of recognition is called a visual agnosia and is one of the typical features of advancing Alzheimer's disease.

Difficulty in the execution of previously learned skilled movements (apraxia) also becomes prominent during this stage. The apraxia becomes more than mere difficulty with individual limb movements such as hammering a nail, flipping a coin, or combing the hair (ideomotor praxis). These patients experience total disruption in the ability to carry out a serial act such as taking a match from a box and lighting a cigarette (ideational praxis). We watched one woman carefully unwrap a lump of sugar for her coffee only to be completely baffled about what to do thereafter. She had the sugar in one hand, wrapper in the other, and after painful deliberation, she put the paper in the coffee and threw away the sugar. Another woman of 53, who was moderately demented, found it almost impossible to turn down the sheet and get into the hospital bed. We watched her as she regarded the bed, put her hand on it, turned around, touched it again, then finally looked at us sheepishly and said, "I just can't get in." This combined apraxia and agnosia (occasionally called apractagnosia) is a prominent feature of moderately advanced Alzheimer's disease in many patients. R.B.'s husband called frantically one day saying that she had almost set the house on fire. She was working in the kitchen when one of the dish

126

towels became very wet, and she decided to dry it in the oven. She then forgot about the towel only to be led back to the kitchen some minutes later by the smell and billows of smoke. Such disasters are the fate of the patient at this point in their disease and frequently precipitate the patient's admission to the hospital.

Inattention and distractibility also become very common at this stage. Personality changes are accentuated and insight becomes very tenuous. At times patients seem painfully aware of what is happening and at other times they seem totally oblivious of their plight. Crying spells develop and at times appear related to the patient's realization of the loss they are suffering, while at other times the emotions seem involuntary and manifestations of a developing pseudobulbar state. In this third stage, the primitive or infantile reflexes such as the snout, root, grasp, and palmomental begin to show themselves. Individual patients rarely show all of these reflexes but rather demonstrate one or two.[47,48] The snout reflex is the most common, seen in more than half of demented patients, whereas the grasp reflex is the least frequent, appearing in less than 20 percent.[47] The palmomental reflex is seen in over 50 percent of all people over the age of 65, thus it cannot be used alone to suggest the presence of dementia.[46,80] The limbs begin to resist passive motion (gagenhalten or paratonia), and the naive examiner often thinks that the patient either has parkinsonism or is intentionally uncooperative. In fact, this inability to relax the limbs to passive motion is the result of both a loss of the patient's ability to inhibit his natural reflexes (a cortical, probably frontal, phenomenon) and actual cell loss in the basal ganglia producing a genuine cogwheel rigidity.[58] The resistance to movement is less consistent than is seen in the parkinson patient but does have a certain flavor of cogwheeling.

Carphologia (lint picking) is quite prominent in many patients and frequently is accompanied by chewing movements. Urinary and fecal incontinence also begin during this stage. Occasional emotional outbursts coupled with periods of agitation and shouting also may occur. One additional curious behavioral aberration that has been described in these advanced Alzheimer patients is sitting in front of a mirror and talking to themselves.[58,61] This "mirror sign," although often used by Hollywood to denote "craziness," is probably more common in the organically psychotic patient than the schizophrenic. When the demented person begins to display this and other bizarre behavior and is obviously becoming quite out of touch with reality, his dementia has reached the point of organic psychosis.

Muscle stretch reflexes may be somewhat increased and scattered other pathologic reflexes occasionally appear (e.g., Babinski toe signs); but in other respects, the routine neurologic examination remains remarkably normal. Another feature that is typical of Alzheimer's disease is that during the early stages, the patients appear very alert. Although often disinterested in carrying out any sustained activity, their ability to quickly shift attention to any novel stimulus in the environment characteristically makes them appear much brighter than they actually are.[37] An outstanding example of this was a 53-year-old violinist who had become extremely demented intellectually but retained a pleasant, yet formal, demeanor. He still enjoyed music and frequently went with his wife to the symphony. One of us (R.L.S.) saw him there one night and introduced him and his wife to my wife. The patient nodded formally then walked on. This apparent aloofness prompted my wife to comment, "Is that one of your snooty professors from the medical school?"

Final Stages

In the final stages of the disease, the patients become very noncommunicative, uttering only short phrases or undirected babbling. They often show evidence of pseudobulbar effect (i.e., involuntary emotional expression, either crying or laughing), aimless wandering, and little meaningful social interaction. They become peevish if bothered, delusional, and finally completely apathetic and withdrawn. The patients develop a masked facies (facial diparesis) and 22 percent will have generalized seizures during their last year of life.[58] At this point they often take on the features of the Klüver-Bucy syndrome with its attendant memory loss, constant mouthing, sexual inappropriateness, and emotional outbursts. If patients remain in bed for any length of time, either because of apathy or intercurrent illness, they begin to experience flexion of the lower extremities. At first they are noted to sleep in a fetal position, but with time their legs draw up during the waking hours as well and pelvicrural contractures develop.[77] Once this process starts, it is almost impossible to reverse the trend and the patients remain in this fetal position, muttering and taking only small amounts of food. Death usually results from pneumonia, aspiration, or urinary infection and sepsis. In this final stage of virtual decortication, Alzheimer's disease is clinically indistinguishable from any other dementia. In the earlier stages, however, Alzheimer's disease has some specific features that help differentiate it clinically. These features will be emphasized in the discussion of the differential diagnosis.

COURSE

The course of the illness is variable, with the average life span from time of diagnosis to death being slightly over seven years.[58] Twenty-five to 30 percent of the patients, however, live over 10 years, and some live for as long as 20 years.[4] The longevity ranges from a few months to 25 years, accordingly it is very difficult to advise a family concerning the prognosis until a period of observation indicates the rate of progression. However, several factors, have been found to have predictive value in respect to mortality and these merit special mention. In general, the degree of functional impairment of the patient is of more value in predicting longevity than is structural change (atrophy) demonstrated on the CT scan.[25] Patients with poor memory scores and decreased expressive language function appear to have the least favorable prognosis irrespective of the degree of cortical atrophy.[25] When the disease has progressed to the point where hospitalization is required, life expectancy is quite limited. Eighty-two percent of patients will die within two years of their hospitalization.[51] The fact remains that Alzheimer's disease is a long and emotionally painful illness for both the patient and his family. The diagnosis should not be made lightly, for a false positive diagnosis of Alzheimer's disease may take years to correct and cause considerable unnecessary anguish.

HISTORY AND EVALUATION

The diagnosis of dementia relies upon a comprehensive history and appropriate physical examination. Below we have provided an outline of the essential elements in the routine history and examination that will help the physician to identify patients with a dementing illness. We have emphasized both the specific symptoms that should alert the physician that his patient may be developing a dementia and also, once suspicion has arisen, those additional symptoms and signs that will verify or negate the initial diagnostic impression.

The diagnosis of dementia in general can often be made on historical information alone; but, unlike most medical conditions, the patients themselves are all too frequently unable to provide accurate information concerning the evolution of their illness. For this reason, it is extremely important for the physician to verify and augment the patient's history by consulting family members, friends, or co-workers. This second history is best taken in the patient's absence, so that the informant will feel free to discuss the problem openly without fear of upsetting or embarrassing the patient.

First and most importantly the sequence of events that resulted in the patient's presenting problem (i.e., a history of the present illness) must be established. Most dementing illness has a slow and relentless course, and it is important to inquire at what time the patient was felt to be completely normal and how long his problem has been noticeable. With a typical dementia, particularly Alzheimer's disease, the history spans months to years rather than the days to weeks seen in confusional states. In taking the history there are many specific symptoms that should be conscientiously explored. Many of these will be spontaneously offered by the patient as specific complaints, while others may have to be specifically elicited. The important areas of symptomatology are outlined below:

1. Change in behavior: In general, is the patient's present behavior different than his previous behavior? If so, how?
2. Was the change gradual and steady or have there been sudden stepwise alterations? This latter pattern is typical of the vascular dementia that develops after multiple small cerebral infarctions. Gradual diminution in function is characteristic of degenerative diseases such as Alzheimer's disease.
3. Changes in emotion:
   a. Is there evidence of depression?
   b. Are anxiety and agitation developing?
   c. Does the patient sense that things are not right? Is there insight that something is amiss?
   d. Is there a general lack of interest in work, family, and hobbies or avocations?
   e. Is paranoia, grandiosity, or confabulation present?
   f. Does it seem that previous personality traits have been exaggerated?
   g. Has the patient developed multiple physical complaints that do not have an organic basis?
4. Social behavioral change: Patients with dementia primarily involving the frontal lobes such as Pick's disease frequently display very inappropriate social behavior early in their illness while these exaggerated changes are less typical of Alzheimer's disease.
   a. Has the patient become embarrassingly loud and jocular?
   b. Has sexual interest and action changed? Has it escaped the bounds of social propriety?
   c. Has the patient become short-tempered, irritable, or aggressive?
   d. Is social judgment impaired?
5. Changes in intellectual behavior:
   a. Is memory affected? Memory disturbance is both the most frequent and earliest symptom in many dementias but particularly in Alzheimer's disease. Ask about the patient's ability to remember recent events. The maintenance of old, remote memories is generally spared in the early stages of Alzheimer's disease, whereas the ability to learn new facts is impaired. It is, therefore, important to stress recent memory or new learning ability in questioning the patient and family.

b. Is the patient having difficulty doing his or her work? Is the ability to solve difficult or unfamiliar problems and keep track of complicated work details intact? Since abstract reasoning and conceptualization are often affected early, patients with demanding occupations will notice difficulty earlier than those individuals with menial jobs.

c. Does the patient become disoriented in new environments or does he become lost when driving and walking to other than routine places? Does the patient actually get lost even in familiar places? Spatial and geographic orientation are frequently affected in Alzheimer's disease, though rarely are they the only initial symptom.

d. Does the patient have difficulty and make mistakes when carrying out complex skilled motor tasks (apraxia)?

e. Is the patient's language normal? Does his speech ramble and wander from the point (tangential)? Does he talk around a point without ever clearly stating what he means (circumlocution)? Does he have difficulty comprehending complex or extensive amounts of material? Does he have trouble remembering names of people and objects (anomia)? Difficulty in writing (agraphia) often is manifest early in dementia and is an important sign when elicited.

6. Is there a fluctuation in the patient's level of consciousness? Such fluctuations are not characteristic of Alzheimer's disease, and their presence should suggest either a different disease or a superimposed confusional state.

The above areas of inquiry were specifically chosen because they represent specific symptoms of dementia and are not usually included in the routine medical history. Complete medical history taking is well covered in standard physical diagnosis texts and will not be covered here. There are, however, specific medical and neurologic conditions which must be considered when taking the history of an apparently demented patient:

1. Cerebral vascular disease: Transient ischemic attacks, hypertension, diabetes, previous strokes.

2. Seizures: Can be the symptom of brain tumors, old cerebral infarctions, late events in the course of the degenerative dementias, particularly Alzheimer's disease, or central nervous system infection.

3. Unilateral weakness: Could be due to vascular or neoplastic disease.

4. Headaches: Can be associated with tumors, infections of central nervous system, hydrocephalus, depression.
5. Abnormal movements: Choreiform movements look like fidgetiness and often go unnoticed; therefore, careful observation of the patient at rest is important. Huntington's chorea is a common disorder and must be considered in the differential diagnosis of dementia.
6. Imbalance: Parkinsonism and progressive supranuclear palsy give both dementia and balance problems. A curious imbalance of gait is also seen in hydrocephalus.
7. Thyroid surgery or symptoms of hypothyroidism: Myxedema can present as dementia.
8. Stomach surgery: Vitamin B_{12} deficiency can develop after gastrectomy and this may produce dementia.
9. Old subarachnoid hemorrhage: Can lead to hydrocephalus.
10. Old or recent head trauma: Brain damage or subdural hematoma may produce a dementia.
11. History of veneral disease: Syphilis is often unrecognized and undertreated in patients with gonorrhea or other veneral infection.
12. Cancer, particularly reticuloendothelial: The remote effects as well as direct metastases can mimic dementia.
13. Medication use or abuse: Chronic overuse of barbiturates, antidepressant medications, and combinations of psychotropic drugs can cause mental changes.
14. Use of illicit drugs.
15. Heavy use of alcohol.

This review of current symptoms and past medical history provides most of the historical data necessary in the differential diagnosis of dementia. In some cases, additional family history can be very helpful. This is particularly true in the diagnosis of Huntington's chorea, a dominantly inherited dementia. Since there are some familial cases of Alzheimer's disease, it is always important to inquire if any other relatives are or were demented. Pick's disease has a stronger familial tendency but is much less common.

MENTAL STATUS EXAMINATION

The neurobehavioral or mental status examination is most easily done directly after the history taking as the patient is usually seated in a chair or on the edge of the bed, as yet unruffled by the process of physical and neurologic examination. When dementia is suspected from the history, the mental examination provides the definitive data for the diagnosis.[62] Throughout the history, the clinician should be making mental note of the patient's behavior and mental functioning. He should also assess the patient's ability to give an accurate history, remember details, and comprehend complicated or lengthy questions. His ability to communicate at a level commensurate with his education should also be evaluated. Personal cleanliness, appropriateness of attire, general mood, and emotional status must also be noted. This conscientious observation of the patient's behavior during the entire session is an important part of a good mental status examination. The second aspect of the examination is a systematic evaluation of a large number of cognitive factors, particularly those known to be affected in early dementia. Below is summarized a complete examination with brief discussions of the abnormalities seen in a typical case of Alzheimer's disease:

Level of Consciousness

The patient with Alzheimer's disease is usually bright and alert early in the course of his illness. Several exceptions to this bear mentioning:

1. Superimposed confusional state.
2. Concomitant depression: While not actually decreasing the level of consciousness, per se, depression causes the patient to become sleepy, withdrawn, and adynamic.
3. Extensive frontal lobe atrophy: This is not the usual pattern in Alzheimer's disease, but some cases will have marked frontal lobe involvement which results in apathy and lack of spontaneity disproportionate to the intellectual changes.

In the late stages of the disease, these patients become very apathetic, unable to interact, and seem to have a true decreased level of arousal.

Behavioral Observations

APPEARANCE

The patient with Alzheimer's disease usually shows no changes in his dress and appearance in the early stages of his illness. The exception to this are those patients with marked frontal atrophy who, early in their course, will demonstrate slovenliness in personal hygiene. As the disease progresses, most patients lose interest in their physical appearance and must be coaxed to bathe, cut their nails, and comb their hair.

133

ORGANIC BEHAVIORAL CHANGES

Apathy, euphoria, lack of insight, irritability, fatuousness, and inappropriate social interactions are often seen. These changes are not as prominent in the early stages of Alzheimer's disease as they are in Pick's disease. Restlessness and overactivity are, however, typical behavioral patterns in patients with Alzheimer's disease.

SECONDARY DEPRESSION OR AGITATION

Personality reactions to the primary organic condition such as depression or agitation should be noted as they can often be successfully treated psychotropically.

Attention

In the very early stage, the demented patient is usually attentive, but with time, concentration powers fail. The patient can no longer accurately perform the "A" test and frequently digit repetition also becomes faulty. Clinically, the patients exhibit two rather interesting alterations in attention: (1) they can be easily distracted by any extraneous stimulus in the environment and (2) they will sometimes rivet their attention on one thing in the environment and be unable to shift to other stimuli. This can be well demonstrated when asking a patient to follow your finger when testing extraocular eye movements. Frequently, the patient stares only into the examiner's face and will not follow the moving finger.

Language

The patient with Alzheimer's disease should have careful language testing because this function begins to show changes early in the disease. Initially there is a decrease in the amount of language output; this can best be demonstrated by having the patient produce lists of words under the pressure of time. The patient with Alzheimer's disease can usually produce less animal names, words beginning with a specific letter, and so forth, within one minute than normal individuals. This deficiency in generating word lists precedes other language changes and is one of the earlier cognitive changes noted. As the disease progresses spontaneous speech tends to become circumlocutory, repetitive, concrete, tangential, and exhibits word finding pauses yet remains fluent.[41] Comprehension of complex material decreases, naming begins to show errors, but repetition ability is usually spared until quite late. In the later stages, aphasia becomes more obvious with increased comprehension difficulty, word finding pauses, anomia, echolalia, and a general emptiness of discourse. Spontaneous speech may eventually deteriorate to the point of stereotyped utterances. Writing skills decrease along with spoken language but at a more rapid rate. It is often helpful to ask the patient to write a short paragraph about his job or the weather in hopes of demonstrating language errors if none are apparent in spoken language.

Memory

Memory testing is the most important aspect of the mental status examination in dementia. Memory problems develop in many of the dementias, but in Alzheimer's disease failure of recent memory is the outstanding early feature. Remote memories are relatively resistant until the disease is quite advanced. It is quite common for a patient with Alzheimer's disease to carry on endlessly about events in the past but be unable to keep track of the date and what he is supposed to do that day.

Memory testing should include orientation, recent historical events, ability to remember four unrelated words, and visual memory. The dementing patient typically will remember only one or two of the words and hidden objects, will know a recent president (often not the current one), but will not remember the date. Patients with memory trouble tend to confabulate or try to lead the examiner away from memory questions, so the examiner must often be persistent. One patient, when asked the date, looked with disgust at the examiner and said, "What, do you think I'm crazy? What do you mean asking me a silly question like that?" Undaunted, the examiner finally coaxed the patient to divulge the fact that it was 1946 when it was actually 1980.

Constructional Ability

Every patient with suspected organic mental disease should be asked to draw and copy a series of line drawings. Abnormalities in these constructional tasks are seen in most cases of early Alzheimer's disease and as the disease progresses, drawing ability deteriorates dramatically.[58] Figure 5-2, B shows examples of drawings executed by patients with early Alzheimer's disease. Compare these with the ones made by a patient with hydrocephalus (Fig. 5-2, A) in which the cortex is distorted but not severely damaged.

Because of their sensitivity in identifying early cerebral atrophy, construction tasks often give the best objective evidence of brain disease.

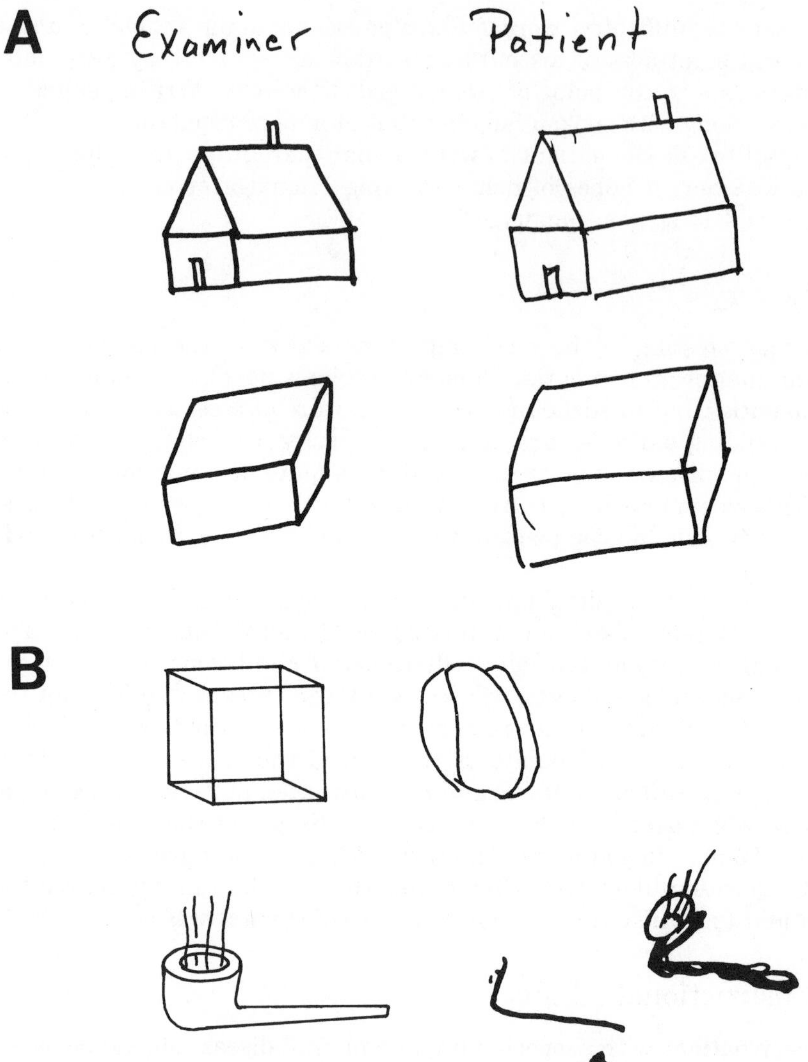

FIGURE 5–2. A, Drawings executed by a hydrocephalus patient and B, by a patient with Alzheimer's disease.

Higher Cortical Function

ARITHMETIC

Arithmetic errors are common early in the course of Alzheimer's disease, particularly when the task is complicated and requires carrying, borrowing, and multiple steps as in complex multiplication. Errors may occur in basic arithmetic concepts, memory of rote tables, and also in number alignment in compound written problems.

PROVERB INTERPRETATION

Interpretation of proverbs or maxims, such as, "People in glass houses shouldn't throw stones," is an exercise in abstract verbal reasoning that is frequently disturbed in the early stages of Alzheimer's disease. Patients become very concrete in their approach to such sayings and often answer quite glibly, "Well, if you throw stones you will break the glass. That's clear enough." Despite attempts to cajole these patients into adopting a metaphorical stance, they steadfastly hold to their concrete interpretations.

SIMILARITIES

Recognition of similarities is an abstract verbal reasoning task that, like proverb interpretation, is often taken literally by the demented patient. The question "What is the similarity between an apple and a banana?" often brings the concrete response, "Why, they aren't alike at all. One is round and one is long." We find recognition of similarities somewhat more sensitive to the effects of cortical atrophy then interpretation of proverbs in many cases. In some patients' lives proverbs have been so overused that the meaning no longer requires much abstract thinking and is more of an exercise in remote memory than a true interpretation. The concept of similarities is a bit less familiar than proverbs to most patients, but this may change with succeeding generations because of the great emphasis on similarities in standardized testing, on children's television, and in the schools.

With a complete history, physical, neurologic examination, and a screening mental status evaluation, a positive diagnosis of dementia can be established in most cases. In many instances, it is also possible to make a presumptive diagnosis of Alzheimer's disease, but as confident as we may feel at times about the diagnosis, it is essential to consider a wide range of possibilities in our differential diagnosis of any patient with a picture of dementia.

MEDICAL EVALUATION

The physical examination should be complete and concentrate on the factors suggested by the outline provided in the history: hypertension, cerebral vascular disease, hypothroidism, infections, systemic cancer,

137

chronic alcoholism, and pernicious anemia. In Alzheimer's disease, particularly in the presenile patient, the examination is usually normal.

The neurologic examination should be complete with particular emphasis on the following features:

1. Cranial nerves
    a. Optic fundus examination: Evidence of acute or chronic increased intracranial pressure and vascular changes should be looked for.
    b. Pupil: Irregular pupils that react to accommodation but not light (Argyll Robertson pupil) are seen in central nervous system syphilis.
    c. Extraocular rotations: Weakness of outward gaze (abduction) with diplopia may indicate increased intracranial pressure.
    d. Downward gaze: Parkinsonism patients often have gaze paralysis, but specific downward gaze difficulty is a typical early sign in progressive supranuclear palsy.
2. Nucal rigidity: Chronic meningitis, particularly cryptococcal, will cause dementia.
3. Motor examination
    a. Strength: Unilateral weakness suggests a unilateral cerebral lesion.
    b. Gait: Imbalance is seen in hydrocephalus, parkinsonism, and progressive supranuclear palsy (PSP), while retropulsion is quite typical of PSP and parkinsonism. "Stickiness" of gait (small steps with feet seemingly stuck to the floor) is seen with frontal lesions as well as hydrocephalus.
    c. Reflexes (muscle stretch): Asymmetries suggest unilateral central nervous system lesions. Increased leg reflexes (bilateral) can be seen in frontal or parasagittal tumors and hydrocephalus.
    d. Primitive reflexes (snout, grasp, root, and palmomental): These are usually the only abnormal neurologic findings in Alzheimer's disease until the later stages. These signs are also present in patients with other frontal lesions.
4. Sensory examination (particularly the integrative functions of stereognosis and graphesthesia): Abnormalities of these cortical sensations will occur on the side opposite a parietal lesion. In the later stages of Alzheimer's disease, patients fail to recognize shapes or numbers traced on the hand. This results from a variety of reasons, one being atrophy of parietal sensory tissue, another being a basic language deficit (i.e., the patient is unable to name the object).

As mentioned, in the early stages of Alzheimer's disease, the routine neurologic examination is usually normal except for the primitive reflexes. If prominent abnormalities are found in cranial nerve function, motor control, or elementary sensation, it is important to carry out a very comprehensive neurodiagnostic evaluation in search of a cause for the dementia other than Alzheimer's disease. Consultation with a neurologist or neurosurgeon is suggested in such cases.

DIFFERENTIAL DIAGNOSIS

There are many causes of the clinical syndrome of dementia. Since some of these are treatable, it is most important for the clinician to undertake a comprehensive evaluation to determine the exact etiology of an individual patient's dementia. Some of these conditions mimic Alzheimer's disease in its gradual onset of subtle emotional changes, memory difficulty, drawing problems, and slowness in abstract reasoning; but many others have somewhat distinctive clinical features that should cause the clinician to suspect an alternate diagnosis. Understanding these subtle differences in symptomatology of the dementias allows the clinician to reject that long held idea that all dementia presents a unitary clinical picture. Since Chapter 6 is devoted to an extensive discussion of dementias other than those caused by Alzheimer's disease, only a brief outline is included here as a differential diagnosis.

Aging

A number of elderly patients complain of symptoms that superficially resemble Alzheimer's disease, yet they do not show the typical history of progressive deterioration. They continue to be able to care for themselves and live an independent life until their death from unrelated causes. This group of patients represents part of the normal aging population; who, for the various reasons discussed below, give a superficial appearance of senility but never actually become demented. The clinician must determine which of these patients with complaints of apathy, failing memory, and difficulty at work actually have Alzheimer's disease and which are part of the normal aging population.

Before discussing this differential process, it is important to review the present knowledge on aging as it applies to mental functioning. Although it had been traditionally felt that the intellect begins to fade rather perceptibly after age 60[73] in the normal individual, recent studies have not supported this view.[30]

The Wechsler Adult Intelligence Scale (WAIS), for instance, awards a 30-year-old patient an IQ of 101 with a raw score of 100 points;

whereas the 75 year old receives an IQ of 119 for the same raw score.[72] The difference is not great, but built into this "old age credit" is the implication that a loss of intellectual abilities is the natural course of aging. More careful analysis of the older population reveals many unsuspected reasons why the overall population of elderly citizens performs less adequately on standard tests than their younger counterparts: (1) Many older persons have medical diseases such as hypertension, atherosclerotic disease, or diabetes which may not cause a major stroke but often cause intellectual decline through the occurrence of multiple small areas of cortical infarction. (2) Emotional problems, such as depression, are common in the elderly, particularly in those persons who are retired, live alone, or have medical illnesses which limit their activities. (3) Physical illness alone often reduces the patient's ability or motivation to perform at his level of competence either in life or formal testing situations. (4) Educational level and life experience are very different for the general population of 70 to 80 year olds (born at the turn of the century) and the 25 to 35 year olds who have had all their education in the post World War II era. All of these factors affect performance but are not a direct effect of aging brain cells. The question then arises, is there any actual alteration in the functioning of the brains of those elderly who have escaped the effects of the problems mentioned above? Is there such a thing as "normal" or expected changes in behavior that result from the aging process itself? The answer is probably yes, but the changes are more subtle than previously appreciated. For instance, complex problem-solving tasks that do not rely upon familiar routine strategies (fluid intelligence) are more difficult for the older person. Many factors, such as the older person's lack of competitiveness or motivation can certainly be important in reducing performance; but, beyond this, there seems to be genuine decline in the ability to carry out high level abstract thinking.[30] In contrast, tests that assess vocabulary, general information, and comprehension (crystallized intelligence) do not show this decline with age.[24]

There are certain elderly persons who complain primarily of forgetting specific dates and people's names, yet, unlike the patient with Alzheimer's disease, accurately keep track of ongoing events. The memory deficit is inconsistent and names forgotten one day may be recalled with ease on the following day. An additional feature of interest is that the information forgotten is frequently from remote rather than from recent memory stores. This type of memory disturbance is exactly the opposite of that found in Alzheimer's disease. This condition, often called benign senescent forgetfulness, shows only mild deficits on formal memory testing. Whereas the memory problem may

140

progress slightly with the passing years, these patients do not develop other cognitive deterioration and they live a normal life span.[31]

It would be most surprising not to find some changes in behavior accompanying aging, since nerve cell changes are seen on pathologic study of brains of elderly people. The changes are similar to those seen in Alzheimer's disease, but they are much less numerous and widespread.[4,68,69] These observations suggest that Alzheimer's disease may represent an acceleration of the aging process, but this position remains unproved at present. These normal changes of aging do not interfere with the social adaptive skills of most individuals; so, in the absence of any complicating factors, it does not appear that aging per se compromises intelligence to a significant degree.

If the clinician accepts this view of aging and understands the factors that complicate a valid assessment of the elderly patient with memory or other similar complaints, he should be able to separate most normal patients from those with Alzheimer's disease. The following steps must be taken in the differential diagnosis:

1. Assess the patient's social situation, previous education, and personality to see if there is any obvious reason for the problem.
2. Examine the patient closely for evidence of depression and anxiety.
3. Do a careful mental status examination; the normal patient will not have genuine new learning problems, will not show evidence of aphasia, will be able to complete the constructional drawings and, if encouraged, will be able to interpret proverbs satisfactorily. The dementing patient, on the other hand, will usually show evidence of errors in several areas of mental status testing.

Depressive Pseudodementia

Depression can often masquerade as dementia and failure to realize this can lead to a very unfortunate diagnostic error.[29,43] Depressed patients frequently complain of memory difficulty and problems with concentration. These complaints, coupled with the depressed patient's apathy and lack of interest in the environment, often suggest the diagnosis of Alzheimer's disease or other dementia. The memory, concentration, and problem-solving complaints, however, are a function of the patient's lack of motivation and not a true cognitive deficit. To learn new material or to keep track of ongoing work details, dates, or plans requires effort. Some memories are stored in a rather passive fashion such as remembering if one had breakfast; but most memory storage is an active process that requires continual rehearsal and concentration on the details (the truth of this should be quite obvious to any student who has had to prepare for an examination).[42] The depressed patient simply cannot muster the mental energy for this type of sustained mental work.

If the clinician is aware of the possible confusion between depression and dementia, it will usually be possible to differentiate between the two. Some important differential points are listed below:

1. The patient with depressive illness often has a significant early life history of cyclic emotional problems.
2. Acute psychotic depression or other reactive depression usually has an antecedent precipitating cause.
3. In depression, the emotional change (apathy) precedes the cognitive (memory) change by many months; whereas, the reverse is usually true in dementia, where memory and intellectual changes are noticed first.[51]
4. The depressed patient frequently demonstrates sleep disturbance, crying spells, self-deprecating feelings, deep sighing respiration; while the demented patient is usually merely apathetic.
5. Mental status testing of the depressed patient reveals no aphasia, good drawings, and with encouragement, evidence of adequate new learning ability and proverb interpretation capacity.
6. Neuropsychologic testing in depression reveals normal nonverbal skills and errors mostly in memory, reasoning, and tasks requiring speed and sustained attention.[43]

Utilizing the above observations, most patients can be correctly diagnosed. There are many patients in whom depression accompanies dementia; there are also many chronically depressed patients who ultimately become demented. Accordingly, the clinical picture can be confusing. It has been estimated that 25 to 30 percent of all demented patients suffer from depression at some point in their illness and for many of them, it is the presenting symptom.[33,35] Since the depression is treatable, it is of more than passing importance for the clinician to be able to separate depression from the dementia in each patient's case.

Character disorders such as hysterical personality disorder, hysterical neurosis with conversion reactions, and more serious psychiatric conditions are also known to present with a spurious dementia.[75] Such patients may have the features of a depressive affect but do not present a full picture of depression. This group of patients tends to be more vehement about their symptoms, quite unlike the demented patient. Their stated memory loss is quite inconsistent with the detailed discussion of their history that they recount. They tend to have scattered remote as well as recent memory loss, a feature not seen in most dementia. The pure depressive pseudodementia patient tends to produce less information than these patients. He usually merely claims that he just does not remember. In contrast, the hysterical individual when asked a specific question concerning his or her life will often emphatically state, "I don't remember. You see, doc, that's the kind of thing that happens all the time. Things that I used to know I just can't remember." These nondepressive pseudodementia patients, like the depressive patients, frequently have previous psychiatric history and at the time of examination have many current emotional symptoms such as anxiety, depressive mood, and psychophysiologic symptoms (e.g., headaches, gait abnormalities).

Brain Tumor

Although characteristically presenting with focal neurologic symptoms or seizures, occasionally brain tumors will present with a dementia-like picture.

Arteriosclerosis (Multi-infarct) Dementia

It is common for elderly patients, whether demented or not, to have several small areas of cerebral softening.[68,69] As the number of these small infarcts increases and if some occur in strategic locations, such as the speech area or hippocampi, mental changes begin to occur. Although the clinical picture of gradual steady deterioration is not usually the same as that seen in Alzheimer's disease, multi-infarct dementia is an important condition to consider in differential diagnosis (see Chap. 6). Patients with Alzheimer's disease also are frequently found to have scattered small cerebral infarcts. At times these lesions are sufficiently extensive to add to the clinical dementia,[69] and it has been estimated that approximately 20 percent of all dementia is caused by a combination of Alzheimer's disease and multiple small infarctions.[67,69]

Confusional State

Although most confusional states are not mistaken for dementia, on occasion confusional behavior can be present for weeks or months and initially be misdiagnosed as dementia. Usually the alteration and fluctuation in level of consciousness and the other features of the confusional state are sufficiently obvious to allow the differentiation from early Alzheimer's disease. However, if the patient with Alzheimer's disease has a superimposed physiologic disturbance, the features of both illnesses will be present and the clinical picture will be that of a beclouded dementia.

Hydrocephalus

This condition usually presents with other neurologic signs such as incontinence and gait disturbance before mental changes are very obvious. The first mental changes are frequently those suggesting frontal lobe pathology (e.g., apathy, social inappropriateness, irritability, and sloppiness) rather than the problems with memory, drawing, and abstractions that are seen in Alzheimer's disease. However, we have seen several patients in which memory loss was the first sign of mental change in hydrocephalus.

Chronic Drug Use

Most patients with alterations in mental and adaptive capacities from the excessive intake of sedatives or combinations of psychotropic medications display alterations in consciousness and intermittent confusional behavior, although there are some patients whose clinical picture is more typical of a dementia than a confusional state. This is particularly true for chronic barbiturate use[15] and possibly with tricyclic antidepressant use.

Thyroid Disease

Hypothyroidism is a condition well-known for its ability to present as dementia. The patients, however, are usually less alert and active than the patients with Alzheimer's disease.

Pernicious Anemia

Dementia appearing in a patient with a history of stomach disease or previous stomach surgery should always suggest the possibility of vitamin B_{12} deficiency.

Pick's Disease

Pick's disease usually presents with substantial changes in personality before there is loss of memory and parietal lobe functions. Late in the disease, Alzheimer's and Pick's may look similar, but in the early stages there is usually a striking difference. The patient with Pick's disease is slovenly, socially inappropriate, flip, and unconcerned yet intellectually he is relatively intact. On the other hand, the patient with Alzheimer's disease is clean, neat, socially quite appropriate yet he suffers from devastating intellectual decay.

Huntington's Chorea

While the chorea is usually obvious before the dementia presents, there are some patients with Huntington's chorea in whom mental changes appear first. As with Pick's disease, the changes are usually emotional in the initial stages: inappropriate social behavior, emotional instability, and often a history of suicide attempts.

General Paresis

Although not common today, cases of parenchymatous neurosyphilis of the brain are still with us. General paresis usually presents with frontal lobe damage much the same as Pick's disease or Huntington's chorea. Differentiation from Alzheimer's disease should not be difficult, particularly with a review of the history and a careful neurologic examination.

Subdural Hematomas

Chronic subdural hematomas are always found in a small percentage of patients dying in mental hospitals. Since an antecedent history of head trauma is present in less than half of the older patients with subdural clots, the absence of trauma in the history is of little significance when entertaining this diagnosis. The clinical picture of a subdural collection is usually one of focal neurologic or neurobehavioral signs rather than dementia, but occasionally, particularly with bilateral lesions, a picture of dementia may be seen.

LABORATORY EVALUATION

Since the differential diagnosis of Alzheimer's disease in particular and dementia in general includes many potentially reversible conditions, it behooves the physician to carry out an extensive evaluation when the initial diagnosis is made or suspected. To diagnose Alzheimer's disease in a patient is tantamount to saying, "You have ahead of you 5 to 10 years of progressive enfeeblement. Go forth and put your affairs in order." Such a pronouncement should be made (hopefully in more gentle terms) only after the diagnosis has been firmly established. The few hundred dollars spent on the initial evaluation is nothing compared to the years of unnecessary mental anguish suffered by the family and patient in whom later (hopefully not too late) the diagnosis of myxedema or benign brain tumor is made.

With the idea of doing a complete screening evaluation, we recommend the following standard laboratory tests, all of which are readily available in most communities.

Blood Tests

Test	Result	Implication in Relation to Dementia
Hemoglobin and hematocrit	High	Polycythemia
	Low	Pernicious anemia
White blood cell count	High	Chronic infection
	Low	Systemic lupus erythematosus
VDRL	High	Syphilis
Erythrocyte sedimentation	High	Collagen disease Metastatic cancer to brain Chronic infection
Calcium	High	Hyperparathyroidism
	Low	Hypoparathyroidism
Liver function studies	Abnormal	Hepatocerebral degenerations
Bromide, barbiturate	High	Chronic toxicity
Cholesterol	High	Myxedema
T_3, T_4	High	Thyrotoxicosis
	Low	Hypothyroidism/ myxedema
Lipid profile	High	Cerebral vascular disease Rare hyperlipidemic dementia[21]
Vitamin B_{12}, folate (not always necessary but useful, serum must often be sent to a central lab)	Low	Pernicious anemia

Plain X-rays

There are no specific plain x-rays that can diagnose Alzheimer's disease. The typical patient with Alzheimer's disease has normal routine studies. However, many other conditions present with dementia and abnormal skull x-ray (e.g., brain tumor); therefore, a routine chest x-ray and skull series are advisable.

X-ray	Finding	Relation to Dementia
Chest x-ray	Cancer	Metastatic disease to brain
		Progressive multifocal leukoencephalopathy
		Carcinomatous meningitis with hydrocephalus
	Enlarged heart	Failure with chronic anoxia (the resulting chronic confusional state can occasionally resemble dementia)
		Hypertensive disease with multi-infarction
kull x-ray	Enlargement of sella turcica	Increased pressure from tumor or hydrocephalus
		Pituitary tumor with frontal lobe extension
	Focal hyperostosis or focally enlarged meningeal vessels	Meningioma
	Calcium in basal ganglia	Familial intracranial calcinosis Parathyroid disease
	Shift of the gland	Tumor Subdural hematoma

Electroencephalogram

The electroencephalogram (EEG), like the skull x-rays, is much more helpful in ruling out other causes of dementia such as tumor, metabolic disturbance, subdural hematoma, or the rare case of Creutzfeldt-Jakob disease, than it is in making the positive diagnosis of Alzheimer's disease. For this reason the EEG is very useful in diagnosing the treatable forms of mental deterioration and is a vital part of the laboratory evaluation.

One of the problems in utilizing the EEG to diagnose Alzheimer's disease is that not only is the EEG normal in many early cases, but subtle abnormalities in the EEG occur with increasing frequency in the normal elderly population.[2,32] In many older patients, the EEG shows a decrease in the percentage and frequency of the background alpha as well as the appearance of scattered slowing (unilateral temporal or bilateral frontoparietal).[44] Unfortunately, the identical changes can also be seen in early Alzheimer's disease.[20] In a large sample, patients with Alzheimer's disease will show a greater percentage of EEG abnormalities than normal patients, but the EEG alone cannot be the deciding factor in an individual case.

There is, however, a direct relationship between the degree of dementia and the slowness of the EEG.[74] Therefore, as the dementia progresses, more consistent and extensive slowing usually emerges. The slowing is usually diffuse or scattered and can contain both theta and delta activity.[56] Low voltage fast records, which are common in the normal elderly, are uncommon in patients with Alzheimer's disease.[56]

Radioisotope Brain Scanning

The routine brain scan is normal in patients with Alzheimer's disease. However, traditionally this scan has been the most accurate method of identifying the presence and location of focal brain lesions such as tumors, subdural hematomas, and abscesses, all important differentials in the diagnosis of dementia. The advent of the more comprehensive computerized axial tomography scan (CT) has made the regular radioisotope scan less useful. The expense of obtaining both scans seems unjustified in most cases, although, in occasional cases, the radioisotope scan will identify a subdural hematoma that is not seen on the CT scan.

Studies for Visualization of Cerebral Ventricles and Cortical Sulci

To properly evaluate any demented patient, the physician *must* obtain a test that can demonstrate if the patient has enlargement of his cerebral ventricles and/or cortical atrophy. In Alzheimer's disease there is widespread atrophy of the cerebral cortex which is reflected pathologically and radiologically as narrowing of cortical gyri and widening of the intergyral sulci (Fig. 5-3). There is also enlargement of the cerebral ventricles, principally due to the loss of the fiber tracts from degenerated cortical neurons. This hydrocephalus ex vocuo is mild to

148

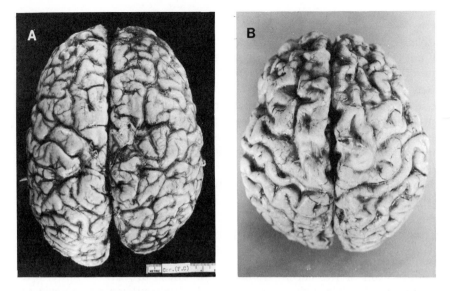

FIGURE 5–3. A, Normal brain. B, Brain from patient with Alzheimer's disease.

moderate and usually not as extensive as the hydrocephalus seen in obstructive conditions.

The test of choice for the evaluation of cortical atrophy and ventricular enlargement is the computerized axial tomography (CT) scan.[22] This procedure allows not only the evaluation of the ventricles and subarachnoid spaces but also can identify the presence of tumor, abscess, infarction, and hemorrhage. The development of this technique has made the radiologic evaluation of dementia much safer and easier than was previously the case when pneumoencephalography and arteriography were the only tests available. At present, CT scanners are available in most large communities. If necessary, the patient should travel to a nearby city where the scan can be obtained. The evaluation for dementia is rarely, if ever, an emergency and the patient can usually have the scan done electively as an outpatient. If a CT scanner is truly inaccessible, a pneumoencephalogram should be performed. The physician should be very cautious about diagnosing any nontreatable disease such as Alzheimer's disease unless cortical atrophy has been clearly demonstrated.

However, there are limitations to any laboratory test which must be fully appreciated and incorporated into the diagnostic evaluation of all individual cases. The correlation of dementia with cortical atrophy is high, though not 100 percent. Several investigators have noted that 15 to 30 percent of normal elderly individuals demonstrate mild cerebral atrophy.[10,34,68] This atrophy is seen on CT scanning and has been verified by autopsy studies of patients with normal mental status who died of unrelated medical illnesses.[68] Thus, the demonstration of atrophy on a scan in a patient with migraine headaches, for example, is not adequate justification for suggesting that a patient is also dementing. Conversely, some patients who have died of Alzheimer's dementia have shown all the microscopic features of the disease but no evidence of gross atrophy.[69] The degree of dementia, therefore, correlates more strongly with the microscopic evidence of senile plaques and neurofibrillary tangles than it does with cortical atrophy. These exceptions to the rule that Alzheimer's disease has atrophy and that atrophy indicates dementia serve to caution the physician to use these radiologic tests as an aid to diagnosis and not as the absolute arbiter.

Cerebrospinal Fluid Examination

Several diseases which produce dementia can be diagnosed only by examination of the cerebrospinal fluid. These are late syphilis and chronic meningitis such as cryptococcosis, tuberculosis, sarcoidosis, or fungal infection. Though these conditions are rare, a spinal puncture should be done as part of the complete diagnostic evaluation for dementia.

CONSULTATIONS

Neurologist

In conjunction with the laboratory investigation, the physician will often wish to ask the assistance of a consultant in evaluating and managing an individual patient. Since many of the treatable conditions are primary neurologic diseases (e.g., tumors, hydrocephalus, or chronic meningitis), a neurologist should see the patient and supervise the evaluation whenever possible. If necessary he will order more extensive neuroradiologic studies and consult a neurosurgeon.

Psychologist

Whenever possible a psychologist should also evaluate the patient. The psychologist's value is greatest in the early stages of the condition when the diagnosis may be in doubt or emotional factors have clouded the clinical picture. When a patient is severely demented with aphasia, amnesia, apraxia, and gross atrophy on the CT scan, the psychologist's services are not usually necessary for diagnosis but may be needed for management or placement suggestions. In the early phase of Alzheimer's disease, psychologic testing can supply a tremendous amount of important information: (1) Testing can determine if dementia is actually present. (2) The extent of cognitive deficits and residual strengths can be objectively assessed; this information can help to determine the patient's capability of meeting his vocational demands and also his general mental and legal competence. (3) A complete test battery can also evaluate if the patient has significant concommitant emotional difficulty which is influencing his overall adaptive and cognitive functioning.

The patient with Alzheimer's disease often shows a rather characteristic neuropsychologic test profile in the early stage:

1. Performance on objective tests of memory is less adequate than overall intellectual performance, with the lowest scores typically found on the logical memory paragraphs, paired associate words, and visual memory subtests.
2. Performance Scale IQ will usually be lower than the Verbal Scale IQ due to impairments of speed and accuracy.
3. Verbal IQ is more resistant to deterioration, with the exception of performance on the comprehension subtest which requires higher level abstract interpretation and judgement (fluid intelligence). Subtests of such areas as vocabulary, digit repetition, and information rely primarily on previously well learned material and results usually remain relatively intact (crystallized intelligence).
4. Overall IQ declines. As well as a significant verbal/performance discrepancy, there is usually an appreciable variation (scatter) of subtest scores.
5. Bender Gestalt drawing will be more defective than expected from intellectual level.
6. Halstead category test will show marked impairment.
7. Trail-Making Test performance will be within the organic range, particularly on Form B (alternating number and letter sequences).

Comparison of the psychologic test profile with estimates of premorbid intellectual functioning usually establishes the presence or absence of organic dementia and often definitely suggests the diagnosis of Alzheimer's disease.[45]

Psychiatrist

A third consultant who is helpful in the evaluation and management of these patients is the psychiatrist. The psychiatrist can evaluate the possible emotional features of the patient's condition and is thoroughly familiar with the medications used for controlling the behavioral aberrations. Psychiatrists are also familiar with and have access to inpatient psychiatric units and institutions. This type of in-hospital care is usually not necessary in the early stages of the illness; but often the patient is initially brought to the physician in a crisis situation and temporary hospitalization in a psychiatric facility may be necessary for a complete and satisfactory evaluation.

All of these referral sources are not available in every community and the primary physician who desires assistance with a complicated evaluation may wish to send his patient to a neighboring city to obtain these services. The physician may then utilize his consultant's suggestions to more effectively manage the long term care of his patient.

PATIENT MANAGEMENT

Social and Environmental Aspects

A diagnosis of Alzheimer's/senile dementia or any of the other irreversible dementias requires that the management of the case shift from specific disease treatment to minimizing the adverse effects of the condition and planning for the social future of the patient and his family. The physician can be of invaluable continuing assistance and should not feel that his job is complete after the diagnosis of an untreatable disease has been made. A sympathetic physician who understands the many problems of dementia can help the patient to avoid personal and social disaster while giving the family much needed support and direction.

There are two major areas of difficulty for the demented patient (1) the insidious intellectual decline and (2) the significant organic and reactive emotional changes that accompany the disease. The demented patient reacts negatively, both to the basic realization of his failing mental ability and also to stress in general. Whenever demands are made that cannot be met or the environment changes so that familiarity is lost, the patient responds with exaggerated anxiety that sometimes completely overwhelms him and produces full-blown confusional behavior.

The physician must be prepared to effectively deal with all of these psychologic and psychosocial problems. The precise details of management depend on the stage of the patient's disease. Accordingly, the problems arising at each stage and their appropriate management are outlined below.

The initial step must be to discuss as fully as possible with the patient and his family the nature of the patient's problem. Point out that the

152

initial complaints, such as of memory trouble, are in fact real and that the patient is having genuine difficulty with tasks that had previously been easy for him. We usually suggest that he is having the type of problems that many older persons have. Such comments are much less offensive than allusions to a "shrinking brain" or "early senility." Advising them that the condition probably will not improve but is usually very slowly progressive with a longevity of many years is not overly comforting but at least allows everyone involved to realize that plans can be formulated and the family's emotional adjustments to the situation arrived at gradually. The need for logical planning and the physician's willingness to help cannot be over emphasized; families caring for a dementing patient need a great deal of emotional support for extended periods of time.

In terms of practical management, the first consideration should be to determine the extent of the patient's intellectual loss and how this loss affects his work and social life. The following decisions must be made: (1) Is the patient able to continue his work? (2) Is he competent to carry on his personal business (i.e., pay bills and manage his own money)? (3) Is he legally competent to enter into legal contracts and to make a will (testamentary capacity)? (4) Does he need supervision for such activities as cooking or smoking? (5) Can the patient continue to drive a motor vehicle safely? None of these questions can be easily answered during the early stages of the illness. For instance, we have one patient who owns and runs a dry goods store who, when his memory began to fail, carried a notebook with him and constantly wrote down various things that he had to remember. As his memory worsened, his wife worked with him so that she could attend to many of the details that he could not. This patient could continue working without any great liability to either himself or his business. The same degree of memory failure in a judge, physician, accountant, or a building engineer would probably be sufficiently serious to prevent him from adequately performing his duties. If we feel that a patient's disease is sufficiently severe, we encourage early retirement. Although it is impossible to force a patient to stop working, we feel justified in trying to convince the patient and his family that he should not continue to work in his present state. This issue of fitness for work among older persons is a difficult problem. Unfortunately, there is no satisfactory mechanism for evaluating independent citizens with highly responsible positions such as government officials, lawyers, accountants, and physicians in the hope of avoiding embarrassing and possibly very serious errors.

The question of when a dementing patient should turn over his monetary affairs to a responsible relative or agent is too often asked too late. The following vignette illustrates this point.

A 65-year-old widow was referred because she was extremely agitated and according to the family had become very suspicious and "scatter-brained." Upon examination, the patient was obviously paranoid, anxious, and almost frantic. Her memory, drawings, object naming, and proverb interpretation were all faulty and it was quite apparent that she was in fact demented. After we gained her confidence, she told us that the precipitating event for all of her problems was that she had made many errors in paying her rent and that she was threatened with immediate eviction. When she tried to correct her errors, they only increased and she sank into a veritable financial morass. She became anxious and paranoid and when her well-meaning lawyer son-in-law said that he would manage her affairs, she felt that he was only after her money.

In this case, the situation had deteriorated to such a point that legal interdiction was necessary and a conservator was appointed. It is far better for the patient and family to realize the seriousness of the situation early and to have a lawyer help them with the responsibility of everyday financial affairs then to wait until the issue is forced and ill will created within the family.

Early in the course of the illness a will should be written; this must be done at a time when the patient understands what is contained within his estate and clearly knows what relatives should share this estate. If the patient's memory is poor and he does not remember what he owns or is irrational concerning financial affairs, it is best to have a legal declaration that the patient is incompetent to make a will.[17] In such cases, the court appoints a conservator and approves the will.

Supervision at home is usually not a major problem during the early stages of Alzheimer's disease. Most of these patients can fairly well attend to their personal affairs and function within a familiar environment. As the disease progresses, however, patients tend to wander and become lost, their memory for the details of cooking is faulty, and apraxia can develop to the point where simply preparing a cup of coffee or lighting a cigarette becomes impossible. It is obvious that the patient at this point needs constant supervision.

Driving is another difficult situation in which there are no absolute guidelines. We, quite frankly, are not too enthusiastic about having our demented patients drive (particularly in our neighborhoods!). Their spatial orientation is not good, judgement is failing, and they tend to become very upset whenever anything out of the ordinary occurs. These factors plus their poor memories make us feel it prudent to gently urge them to give up driving for their own safety and protection.

Most of the above suggestions are aimed at manipulating the patient's environment so that stressful situations are avoided. Stress leads to anxiety, feelings of failure, depression, and occasionally confusional behavior. These are best avoided by simplifying the patient's environment and life. Make life as routine as possible. Nothing is more upsetting to a dementing patient than moving him from place to place. That trip to Europe or across the country might sound like "just what grandpa needs to relax," but by the fifth day, in the fourth hotel, and the third country, grandpa is so confused and agitated that he has to be sent home under heavy sedation. The need for order and structure is not as acute in the beginning of the disease process but becomes increasingly important as adaptive capacities dwindle.

At some point in the progression of the disease the patient becomes largely dependent upon others to meet all of his daily needs. This is a crisis point for many families; they simply do not have anyone in the family who has the amount of time necessary to care for the patient. The crisis is frequently precipitated by an episode of incontinence, a nocturnal wander about the neighborhood, or a particularly boisterous series of verbal or social outbursts during a trip to the grocery store. At this time a sensible long-term care plan must be made. A professional social worker will now be the physician's best ally. We encourage our patients' families to establish contact with the social worker before the crisis arises, but this suggestion is often not very enthusiastically received until the obvious need is at hand. Regardless of the timing, the social worker can help assess the patient's and the family's needs and is then able to advise the family of the resources available in the community to meet those needs. Visiting nurses, aides, or sitters are one solution. Day care centers for the elderly will occasionally accommodate some demented patients in the earlier stages of their illness, or nursing home or institutional placement may be required. Unfortunately, all of these services are expensive. For the wealthy patient, the easiest and most satisfactory solution is to have help in the house constantly. In this way the patient does not undergo the upsetting experience of being moved; he is in his own home and family members can help when they are available. Expensive, elaborate nursing or residential facilities are also available to give very comfortable care to those who can afford it. The poor often have a variety of services available through welfare programs, although they are usually not as satisfactory as the services for those with financial means. The middle-class, fixed income families who own their own homes are the most hard pressed to provide the necessary care as they do not have the available finances to buy adequate help and do not qualify for public assistance programs. This is a genuine social problem in our country. Many of our patients' families have had to make considerable personal and financial sacrifices to care for the patient as he slowly becomes more and more incapacitated.

155

Medical Management

In addition to social and environmental aspects of management, there are avenues of medical management the physician must follow in treating the demented patient. Some of these are similar to those discussed in the chapter on the confusional states. Good, conscientious medical care will prevent confusional behavior and greatly simplify the patient's overall care. Judicious use of non-barbiturate sleeping medication (e.g., Benadryl, chloral hydrate, or a phenothiazine drug) when sleep has been interrupted on several consecutive nights is advisable.

A major area in which the physician may be of assistance is in the treatment of concomitant depression or anxiety. As mentioned earlier, these emotional manifestations or reactions in patients with dementia can adversely affect the intellectual and adaptive functioning of the patient; it is thus important to treat these problems promptly. For depression we most commonly use the tricyclic antidepressants amitriptyline HCl (Elavil), imipramine HCl (Tofranil), or amitriptyline HCl combined with perphenazine (Triavil). To control anxiety and agitation in the earlier stages of the illness, we use chlordiazepoxide (Librium), diazepam (Valium), and occasionally meprobamate (Equanil or Miltown). In the later stages when agitation is more of a problem than minor anxiety, a major tranquilizer is more appropriate (e.g., chlorpromazine [Thorazine], haloperidol [Haldol], or thioridazine [Mellaril]). Some physicians successfully treat agitation with barbiturates, but we find the risk of additional agitation plus the frequent rather substantial sedative effect undesirable. It is advisable initially to use small doses of any medication since the demented patient is often very sensitive to these psychotropic drugs. When used, antidepressant medications must be taken daily, but we feel that tranquilizing drugs should be used only when necessary and not on a regular basis except when absolutely required, since these medications can precipitate an acute confusional state. The physician may wish to consult a psychiatric colleague before prescribing any psychotropic medication.

The use of medications that are advertised as improving the patient's mental status by increasing blood flow or cerebral oxygen uptake (e.g., Deapril or Hydergine) is controversial. Alzheimer's is a disease of degenerating nerve cells and as yet the metabolic error that causes this to occur has not been discovered. It is generally felt that these medications have not been shown to significantly help the patient with Alzheimer's disease, therefore, we do not prescribe them.[9,78]

Another treatment, and one that has been popularized in the lay press, is the use of hyperbaric oxygen.[36] Claims have been made that 90 minutes in 100 percent oxygen at 2.5 atmospheric pressure, twice daily for 15 days can have a remarkable restorative effect on patients with atrophic brain disease.[36] All investigators do not agree, and this treatment has failed to gain general acceptance.[66]

The most recent medical treatment has been the use of choline or its precursor lecithin. The rationale for this treatment is that it is the cholinergic neurons that seem to be the first and primary neurons to deteriorate in Alzheimer's disease (see following section for discussion). Using the same reasoning employed in treating parkinsonism with dopamine, many investigators are attempting to reduce memory and intellectual deficits in Alzheimer's disease by supplying exogenous acetylcholine precursors[13,57,60] or inhibiting cholinesterase activity.[8,50,59]

The use of the precursors alone has not produced successful results; however, utilizing parenteral physostigmine with or without oral lecithin, significant, albeit transient, memory improvement has been reported.[8,50]

PATHOLOGY AND ETIOLOGY

The gross and microscopic features of Alzheimer's disease have been well known since their initial description in 1906 by Alois Alzheimer.[39] It is only very recently, however, that researchers have begun to understand the pathophysiology of this curious condition.[79] Unfortunately, its etiology still eludes the investigators.

Present evidence, very convincingly suggests that Alzheimer's disease is primarily a disease affecting the cholinergic neurons.[1,7,49,76] In several studies, biochemical analysis of cells in the regions of most intense pathologic change have shown a marked decrease in choline acetyltransferase, an enzyme intimately associated with cholinergic transmitter function. Other transmitter systems, principally GABA appear to be intact.[7] It is not yet known why these cells, in a fashion similar to the dopamine cells in Parkinson's disease, are unable to sustain their metabolic subsystems but undergo premature degeneration.

A genetic predisposition has been proposed, since it has been noted that there is an increased incidence of the disease in the relatives of patients with Alzheimer's disease.[58] There is also a small percentage of cases with a definite dominant inheritance pattern.[3] Many interesting observations have recently been made in these familial cases. Neither the significance of these findings nor their applicability to Alzheimer's disease in general is known.

The most unusual reports on familial Alzheimer's disease were made in 1977 by Gajdusek and his associates.[14,70] They innoculated brain tissue from a large number of sporadically occurring cases of Alzheimer's disease and from 12 familial cases into the brains of monkeys. Within two and a half years, two of the monkeys had developed a dementia similar to Creutzfeldt-Jakob disease. This immediately

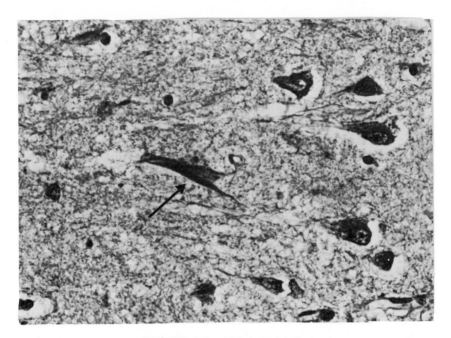

FIGURE 5–4. Alzheimer tangle.

caused the speculation that Alzheimer's disease might be caused by a slow transmissible virus. Many factors do not support this view, however. Transfer occurred in only two of the 12 familial cases and in none of the sporadic cases. Also, the disease did not transfer as Alzheimer's disease, but as a spongiform encephalopathy. While the findings are interesting, at this point it would seem prudent to suggest that the patient with familial Alzheimer's disease is more susceptible to latent virus infection, rather than to propose a viral etiology to this disease.[5]

Another feature recently described in familial cases is a chromosomal abnormality. Lymphocytes have been shown to have an increased incidence of aneuploidy (abnormal numbers of chromosomes).[3] The aneuploidy is caused by an abnormality in microfilament function during mitosis. It is the microfilamentous and microtubular structures within the cells that become abnormal in Alzheimer's disease. From these observations it is speculated that Alzheimer's disease may be a generalized abnormality in tubulofilamentous physiology.[3] A high level of aluminum has been found in the brains of some patients suggesting that in those cases the disease might be triggered by the toxic effect of this metallic ion.[6] This finding has not been reproduced by all investigators, however, and the consensus is that the basic defect is primarily metabolic and not toxic.

Microscopically, the first pathological changes are the degeneration

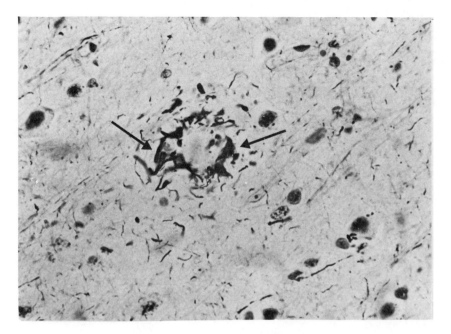

FIGURE 5-5. Senile plaque of Marinesco.

of the presynaptic terminals and loss of the horizontal dendrites that allow intercommunication between cortical cells.[28,40,54,64,65] After sufficient degeneration of the cell processes, tubular processes within the axon begin to twist and clump to form the characteristic finding of this disease—the neurofibrillary tangle of Alzheimer[71] (Fig. 5-4). This tangle of tubular elements impedes axoplasmic flow and further aids in the degeneration of the cells. When the cells degenerate, they leave argentophilic cellular detritus in a stereotyped pattern which becomes the senile plaque of Marinesco (Fig. 5-5), the second characteristic microscopic feature of Alzheimer's disease. Some cells also become packed with lipofuscin and undergo granuovacuolar degeneration (Fig. 5-6), but the significance of this pathologic change is uncertain. Amyloid deposition, both in the center of old senile plaques and in the walls of blood vessels is an additional typical finding whose significance is also yet to be explained.

These microscopic findings are localized in the cholinergic system, which is most strongly represented in the hippocampi and in the association areas of the parietal and frontal lobes.[11] This localization correlates well with both the gross pathologic findings and the clinical features of the disease. The first area to show pathologic change is the hippocampus. Regional cerebral blood flow studies support this by showing a decrease in flow initially in the temporal leads.[18,19,23]

159

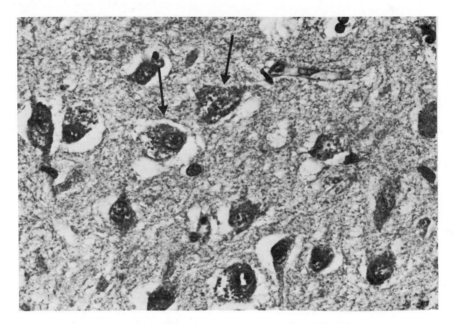

FIGURE 5-6. Cells demonstrating granulovacuolar change.

These findings correlate directly with the clinical observation that recent memory, a function intimately associated with hippocampal activity, is usually the first cognitive area to be disrupted in Alzheimer's disease. The areas that next demonstrate atrophy and decrease in regional blood flow are the parieto-occipital areas. This finding correlates well with the early appearance of failure on drawings and the later development of aphasias, apraxias, and agnosias. The frontal areas where, with the limbic structures, the emotional and personality aberrations are felt to originate also show decrease in flow early in the disease.[23]

Atrophic cells are also found in the subcortical regions, particularly in the substantia nigra, cerebellum, and motor cortex.[54,58] This is felt to be the reason that these patients frequently show the extrapyramidal findings of cogwheel rigidity and bradykinesia.

The gross brain usually shows rather significant atrophy, with increased sulcal width and ventricular dilatation. As was mentioned previously, the degree of dementia often correlates more directly with the intensity of the microscopic changes than with gross atrophy. This observation does not, however, negate the fact that extensive cortical atrophy is the usual gross pathologic picture of this condition (Fig. 5-6).

The brain of the patient with Alzheimer's disease also frequently shows areas of cerebral softening from small infarctions. In some cases there can be enough of these to contribute to production of the dementia, whereas in others the number is small and clinically unimportant.[69]

The uncanny pathologic similarity of this disease to the normal aging process raises an unanswered question. All the pathologic features described above are noted in the brains of so-called normal old persons. The intensity and extent of the changes are not as great, but the process appears to be identical.[68] Senile plaques can be quite widespread in the normal old brain and tangles are also seen in the elderly, albeit restricted to the hippocampi. The question as to whether Alzheimer's disease is merely an accelerated aging process or a discrete disease entity awaits future investigation.

REFERENCES

1. Bowen, D.M., and Davison, A.N.: Changes in brain lysosomal activity, neurotransmitter-related enzymes, and other proteins in senile dementia, in Katzman, R., Terry, R.D., and Bick, K.L.: Alzheimer's Disease: Senile Dementia and Related Disorders, Vol. 7 of Aging. Raven Press, New York, 1978, pp. 421–426.
2. Busse, E.W., Barnes, R.H., Friedman, E.L., and Kelty, E.J.: Psychological functioning of aged individuals with normal and abnormal electroencephalograms. I. A study of non-hospitalized community volunteers. J. Nerv. Ment. Dis. 124:135, 1956.
3. Cook, R.H., Ward, B.E., and Austin, J.H.: Studies in aging of the brain: IV. Familial Alzheimer disease: Relation to transmissible dementia, aneuploidy, and microtubular defects. Neurology (Minneap.) 29:1402, 1979.
4. Corsellis, J.A.N.: Aging and dementia, in Blackwood, W., and Corsellis, J.A.N. (eds.): Greenfield's Neuropathology. Arnold, London, 1976, pp. 796–848.
5. Corsellis, J.A.N.: On the transmission of dementia. Br. J. Psychiatry 134: 553, 1979.
6. Crapper, D.R., Krishnan, S.S., and Quittkan, S.: Aluminum, neurofibrillary degeneration and Alzheimer's disease. Brain 99:67, 1976.
7. Davies, P., and Maloney, A.J.F.: Selective loss of central cholinergic neurons in Alzheimer's disease. Lancet 2:1403, 1976.
8. Davis, K.L., Mohs, R.C., and Tinklenberg, J.R.: Enhancement of memory by physostigmine. Lancet 2:946, 1979.
9. Drugs for dementia. Drug. Ther. Bull. 13:25, 1975.
10. Earnest, M.P., Heaton, R.K., Wilkinson, W.E., and Manke, W.F.: Cortical atrophy, ventricular enlargement, and intellectual impairment in the aged. Neurology 29:1138, 1979.
11. Editorial: Cholinergic involvement in senile dementia. Lancet 1:408, 1977.
12. Ehle, A.L., and Johnson, P.C.: Rapidly evolving EEG changes in a case of Alzheimer's disease. Ann. Neurol. 1:593, 1977.
13. Etienne, P., Gauthier, S., Johnson, G., Collier, B., Mendis, T., Dastoor, D., Cole, M., and Muller, H.F.: Clinical effects of choline in Alzheimer's disease. Lancet 1:508, 1978.
14. Gajdusek, D.C.: Unconventional viruses and the origin and disappearance of kuru. Science 197:943, 1977.
15. Geschwind, N.: Personal communication, 1977.

16. Grufferman, S.: Alzheimer's disease and senile dementia: one disease or two? in Katzmann, R., Terry, R.D., and Bick, K.L. (eds.): Alzheimer's Disease: Senile Dementia and Related Disorders, Vol. 7 of Aging. Raven Press, New York, 1978, pp. 35–41.
17. Gunn, A.E.: Mental impairment in the elderly: Medical-legal assessment. J. Am. Geriat. Soc. 25:193, 1977.
18. Gustafson, L., and Risberg, J.: Regional cerebral blood flow related to psychiatric symptoms in dementia with onset in the presenile period. Acta Psychiat. Scand. 50:516, 1974.
19. Hagberg, B., and Ingvar, D.H.: Cognitive reduction in presenile dementia related to regional abnormalities of the cerebral blood flow. Br. J. Psychiatry 128:209, 1976.
20. Harner, R.N.: EEG evaluation of the patient with dementia, in Benson, D.F., and Blumer, D. (eds.): Psychiatric Aspects of Neurologic Disease. Grune & Stratton, New York, 1975, pp. 63–82.
21. Heilman, K.M., and Fisher, W.R.: Hyperlipidemic dementia. Arch. Neurol. 31:67, 1974.
22. Huckman, M.S., Fox, J., and Topel, J.: The validity of criteria for the evaluation of cerebral atrophy by computerized tomography. Radiology 116:85, 1975.
23. Ingvar, D.H., Risberg, J., and Schwartz, M.S.: Evidence of subnormal function of association cortex in presenile dementia. Neurology 25:964, 1975.
24. Jarvick, L.F., Eisdorfer, C., and Blum, J.E. (eds.): Intellectual Functioning in Adults. Springer Publishing Co., New York, 1973.
25. Kaszniak, A.W., Fox, J., Gandell, D.L., Garron, D.C., Huckman, M.S., Ramsey, R.G.: Predictors of mortality in presenile and senile dementia. Ann. Neurol. 3:246, 1978.
26. Katzman, R.: The prevalence and malignancy of Alzheimer disease. Arch. Neurol. 33:217, 1976.
27. Katzman, R., and Karasu, T.B.: Differential diagnosis of dementia in Fields, W.S. (ed.): Neurological and Sensory Disorders in the Elderly. Stratton Intercontinental Medical Book Corp., New York, 1974, pp. 103–134.
28. Kay, D.W.K.: Epidemiological aspects of organic brain disease in the aged, in Gaitz, C.M. (ed.): Aging and the Brain. Plenum Press, New York, 1972, p. 15–27.
29. Kiloh, L.G.: Pseudodementia. Acta Psychiatr. Scand. 37,336, 1961.
30. Kinsbourne, M.: Cognitive decline with advancing age: an interpretation, in Smith, W.L., and Kinsbourn, M. (eds.): Aging and Dementia. Spectrum Publications, New York, 1977, pp. 217–235.
31. Kral, V.A.: Benign senescent forgetfulness in Katzmann, R., Terry, R.D., and Bick, K.L. (eds).: Alzheimer's Disease: Senile Dementia and Related Disorders, Vol. 7 in Aging. Raven Press, New York, 1978, pp. 47–52.
32. Levy, R.: The neurophysiology of dementia. Br. J. Psychiatry, Special no.9, 1975, pp. 119–123.
33. Liston, E.H.: Occult presenile dementia. J. Nerv. Ment. Dis. 164:263, 1977.
34. Mann, A.H.: Cortical atrophy and air encephalography: a clinical and radiological study. Psychol. Med. 3:374, 1973.
35. Marsden, C.D., and Harrison, M.J.G.: Outcome of investigation of patients with presenile dementia. Br. Med. J. 2:249, 1972.
36. Martin, P.: Hyperbaric oxygen and you. The Lion, October, 1978, pp. 24–29.

37. Mayer-Gross, W.: Discussion on the presenile dementias: symptomatology, pathology and differential diagnosis. Proc. R. Soc. Med. 31:1443, 1938.
38. McDermott, J.R., Smith, A.I., Iqbal, K., and Wisniewski, H.M.: Brain aluminum in aging and Alzheimer disease. Neurology 29:809, 1979.
39. McMenemey, W.H.: Alois Alzheimer and his disease, in Wolstenholme, G.E.W., and O'Connor, M. (eds.): Alzheimer's disease and related conditions. Churchill, London, 1970, pp. 5–10.
40. Mehraein, P., Yamada, M., and Tarnowska-Dziduszko, E.: Quantitative study on dendrites and dendritic spines in Alzheimer's disease and senile dementia, in Kreutzberg, G.W. (ed.): Advances in Neurology, Vol. 12. Raven Press, New York, 1975, pp. 453–458.
41. Miller, E., and Hague, F.: Some characteristics of verbal behavior in presenile dementia. Psychol. Med. 5:255, 1975.
42. Neisser, U.: Cognitive Psychology. Appleton-Century-Crofts, New York, 1967, pp. 219–242.
43. Nott, P.N., and Fleminger, J.J.: Presenile dementia: the difficulties of early diagnosis. Acta Psychiatr. Scand. 51:210, 1975.
44. Obrist, W.D.: The electroencephalogram in normal aged adults. Electroencephalogr. Clin. Neurophysiol. 6:235, 1954.
45. Orme, J.E.: Non-verbal and verbal performance in normal old age, senile dementia, and elderly depression. J. Gerontol. 12:408, 1957.
46. Otomo, E.: The palmomental reflex in the aged. Geriatrics 20:901, 1965.
47. Paulson, G.: The neurological examination in dementia, in Wells, C.E. (ed.): Dementia. F.A. Davis Co., Philadelphia, 1971, pp. 169–188.
48. Paulson, G., and Gottlieb, G.: Development reflexes: the reappearance of foetal and neonatal reflexes in aged patients. Brain 91:37, 1968.
49. Perry, E.K., Perry, R.H., Blessed, G., and Tomlinson, B.E.: Necropsy evidence of central cholinergic deficit in senile dementia. Lancet 1:189, 1977.
50. Peters, B.H., and Levin, H.S.: Effects of physostigmine and lecithin on memory in Alzheimer disease. Ann. Neurol. 6:219, 1979.
51. Post, F.: Dementia, depression and pseudodementia, in Benson, D.F. and Blumer, D. (eds.): Psychiatric Aspects of Neurologic Disease. Grune and Stratton, New York, 1975, pp. 99–120.
52. Roth, M.: The natural history of mental disorder in old age. J. Ment. Sci. 101:281, 1955.
53. Roth, M., and Myers, D.H.: The diagnosis of dementia. Br. J. Psychiatry. Special no. 9, 1975, pp. 87–99.
54. Scheibel, A.B.: Structural aspects of the aging brain: Spine systems and dendritic arbor, in Katzman, R., Terry, R.D., and Bick, K.L. (eds.): Alzheimer's Disease: Senile Dementia and Related Disorders, Vol. 7 in Aging. Ravens Press, New York, 1978, pp. 353–373.
55. Scheibel, M.E., Lindsay, R.D., Tomiyasu, U., and Scheibel, A.B.: Progressive dendritic changes in the aging human limbic system. Exp. Neurol. 53:420, 1976.
56. Short, M.J., and Wilson, W.P.: The electroencephalogram in dementia, in Wells, C.E. (ed.): Dementia. F.A. Davis Co., Philadelphia, 1971, pp. 81–97.
57. Signoret, J.L., Whiteley, A., and Lhermitte, F.: Influence of choline on amnesia in early Alzheimer's disease. Lancet 2:837, 1978.
58. Sjögren, T., Sjögren, H., and Lindgren, A.G.H.: Morbus Alzheimer and Morbus Pick; genetic, clinical and pathoanatomic study. Acta Psychiatr. Scand. Suppl. 82: 1, 1952.

59. Smith, C.M., and Swash, M.: Physostigmine in Alzheimer's disease. Lancet 1:42, 1979.
60. Smith, C.M., Swash, M., Exton-Smith, A.N., Phillips, M.J., Overstall, P.W., Piper, M.E., and Bailey, M.R.: Choline therapy in Alzheimer's disease. Lancet 2:318, 1978.
61. Stengle, E.: A study on the symptomatology and differential diagnosis of Alzheimer's disease and Pick's disease. J. Ment. Sci. 89:1, 1943.
62. Strub, R.L., and Black, F.W.: The Mental Status Examination in Neurology. F.A. Davis Co., Philadelphia, 1977.
63. Strub, R.L., and Geschwind, N.: Gerstmann syndrome without aphasia. Cortex 10:378, 1974.
64. Terry, R.: Editorial. Arch. Neurol. 33:1, 1976.
65. Terry, R.D., and Wisniewski, H.M.: Ultrastructure of senile dementia and of experimental analogs, in Gaitz, C.M. (ed.): Aging and the Brain. Plenum Press, New York, 1972, pp. 89–116.
66. Thompson, L.W., Davis, G.C., Obrist, W.D., and Heyman, A.: Effects of hyperbaric oxygen on behavioral and physiological measures in elderly demented patients. J. Gerontol. 31:23, 1976.
67. Todorov, A.B., Constantinidis, J., Go, R.C.P., and Elston, R.C.: Specificity of the clinical diagnosis of dementia. J. Neurol. Sci. 26:81, 1975.
68. Tomlinson, B.E., Blessed, G., and Roth, M.: Observations on the brains of non-demented old people. J. Neurol. Sci. 7:331, 1968.
69. Tomlinson, B.E., Blessed, G., and Roth, M.: Observations on the brains of demented old people. J. Neurol. Sci. 11:205, 1970.
70. Traub, R., Gajdusek, D.C., and Gibbs, C.J.: Transmissible virus dementia: The relation of transmissible spongiform encephalopathy to Creutz-feldt-Jacob disease, in Smith, W.L., and Kinsbourne, M. (eds.): Aging and Dementia. Spectrum Publications, New York, 1977, pp. 91–146.
71. Van Doorm, J.M., and Hemker, H.C.: Aluminium and Alzheimer's disease. Lancet 2:708, 1977.
72. Wechsler, D.: Manual for the Wechsler Adult Intelligence Scale. The Psychological Corporation, New York, 1955.
73. Wechsler, D.: The Measurement and Appraisal of Adult Intelligence. Williams and Wilkins Co., Baltimore, 1958.
74. Weiner, H., and Schuster, D.B.: The electroencephalogram in dementia—some preliminary observations and correlations. Electroencephalogr. Clin. Neurophysiol. 8:479, 1956.
75. Wells, C.E.: Pseudodementia. Am. J. Psychiatry 136:895, 1979.
76. White, P., Goodhardt, M.J., Keet, J.P., Hiley, C.R., Carrasco, L.H., Williams, I.E.I., and Bowen, D.M.: Neocortical cholinergic neurons in elderly people. Lancet 1:668, 1977.
77. Yakovlev, P.I.: Paraplegia in flexion of cerebral origin. J. Neuropathol. Exp. Neurol. 13:267, 1954.
78. Yesavage, J.A., Tinklenberg, J.R., Hollister, L.E., and Berger, P.A.: Vasodilators in senile dementia. Arch. Gen. Psychiatry 36:220, 1979.
79. Strub, R.L.: Alzheimer's disease-current perspectives. J. Clin. Psychiat. 41:110, 1980.
80. Jacobs, L., and Gossman, M.D.: Three primitive reflexes in normal adults. Neurology 30:184, 1980.

6

OTHER DEMENTIAS

S.G. is a 57-year-old businessman referred for neurologic evaluation because of a 6 year history of increasing forgetfulness. The patient dated the onset of his difficulty from a bout of supposed encephalitis. At the time we saw him, the patient required assistance in remembering the everyday details of his work. Fortunately, he supervised a family business and relatives were available to assist him. As a memory aid, he also carried a little book in which to jot down important details and appointments. His only other complaint was an occasional feeling of gait unsteadiness. According to his wife, his geographic orientation was failing, and he had great difficulty orienting himself in new environments. In addition, his wife reported a general increase in irritability and diminished ability to cope with normal day-to-day stress.

On examination he appeared very anxious, but was alert and cooperative. Mental status testing showed good attention, with a digit span (forward) of 7. His language was intact as was his constructional ability (Fig. 6-1) and proverb interpretation, but his memory was definitely faulty. He could recall only one of four words after a five minute delay and his knowledge of recent political events was very sketchy. Routine neurologic examination demonstrated brisk reflexes bilaterally but no abnormalities of gait or motor control.

Intelligence testing showed a Verbal IQ of 137 and a Performance IQ of 116 (Full Scale IQ of 129). His Memory Quotient, however, was only 94. Verbal abstraction, using a test of complex verbal reasoning (Shipley-Hartford) was compromised, with the conceptual quotient being only 80.

Brain scan, skull x-rays, EEG, and routine serum studies were negative. Pneumoencephalography was attempted, but ventricular filling was not attained. Questionable cortical atrophy was noted in the sylvian cisterns. Following the test, the patient had a severe headache and

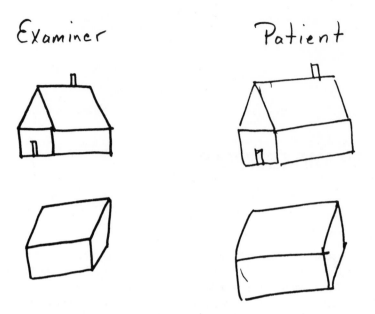

Examiner

Patient

FIGURE 6–1.

refused a repeat study. A presumptive diagnosis of Alzheimer's disease was made; however, the history of mild gait difficulty and the absence of constructional impairment were worrisome features.

Over the next two years, the patient did quite well. His memory actually improved with the use of mild tranquilizers to ameliorate his marked anxiety, but his gait had become quite broad-based and unstable. He also had experienced several confusional episodes and began to notice urinary urgency. At neuropsychologic reevaluation, his measured IQ remained at previous levels and the Memory Quotient had actually increased to 122. Since a CT scanner had recently been installed in the city, it was suggested that this test would be a much better alternative than a repeated attempt at pneumoencephalography. The study showed obstructive hydrocephalus (Fig. 6-2). At this point the patient was hospitalized, a pneumoencephalogram revealed aqueductal stenosis and a ventriculoperitoneal shunt was placed in the right lateral ventricle.

Since surgery (1976) the patient has done very well. The lateral ventricles have decreased in size (Fig. 6-3), his Memory Quotient is now 130, and general activities have returned almost completely to normal. The only significant residual of the hydrocephalus is a Conceptual Quotient which remains impaired relative to his other cognitive performance (C.Q.=93).

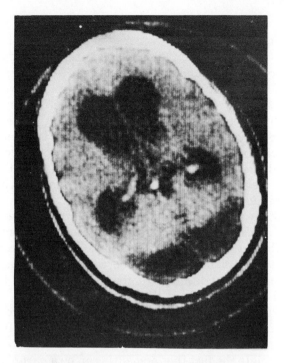

FIGURE 6–2.　Preoperative CT scan.

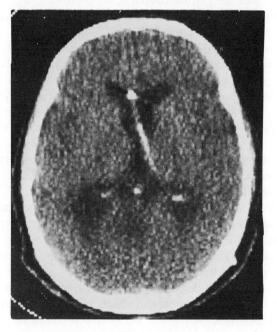

FIGURE 6–3.　Postoperative CT scan.

The above case exemplifies the vagaries of dementia. Other than the disturbing lack of constructional impairment, this patient's initial history of memory difficulty and anxiety certainly were compatible with a diagnosis of Alzheimer's disease. One year later, however, after his memory had actually improved and his gait had become more impaired, his clinical picture was more typical of a patient with hydrocephalus. Such cases emphasize the necessity of carrying out a full evaluation including visualization of the cerebral ventricles and cortical sulci in all cases of suspected dementia. This patient could have been correctly diagnosed a year earlier if a CT scanner had been available in the community.

In this chapter we will discuss many of the different diseases in which dementia is the principal or at least a prominent symptom. It is obviously impossible to discuss all of the rare and obscure conditions in which an associated dementia has been described. Extensive lists of these less common conditions are found in Wells,[186] Pearce and Miller,[132] and Slaby and Wyatt.[165]

In many of the dementias, other neurologic or systemic features of the illness typically manifest before mental deterioration. In such cases the differential diagnosis is not difficult, but it is important that the clinician appreciate the fact that dementia can be a part of that particular illness so that he can be prepared to cope with that eventuality should it arise. This is true for parkinsonism, pernicious anemia, pituitary disease, and many other conditions.

We will stress two primary clinical points in this chapter: (1) many of the dementias are treatable and (2) there are often subtle differences in clinical presentation in the various dementias that allow the clinician to make the specific diagnosis from physical and mental status findings alone. It was long thought that dementia was a nonreversible condition regardless of its type. However, several recent studies have shown this to be untrue. In one investigation of 106 patients with a presumptive diagnosis of dementia, 22 actually had psychiatric or other diagnoses, and 13 of the remaining 84 cases had treatable, albeit not always curable, lesions.[106]

Table 6-1 is a compilation of data from several investigations of the etiology of dementia in different samples. It is apparent from this table that most patients with dementia have untreatable diseases such as Alzheimer's disease or arteriosclerosis of the brain. The reversible dementias, such as those seen with myxedema and pernicious anemia are decidedly rare, but are extremely important to diagnose because of their reversibility. Hydrocephalus, which is certainly potentially reversible in many cases, represents between 5 to 10 percent of all cases of dementia and further points out the need for careful evaluation of the demented patient. The outlook for the demented patient is still not

TABLE 6–1. Etiologies of Dementia Expressed in Percentages

Diagnosis	Marsden and Harrison[106]	Harrison and Marsden[71]	Freeman[55]	Pearce and Miller[132]	Sourander and Sjögren[167]	Tomilson and Blessed[179]	Malamud[103]	Todorov[178]	Seltzer and Sherwin[161]
Atrophy									21
Alzheimer's disease	57	39	44	92	51	50	42	40	
Pick's disease							3		
Arteriosclerotic dementia	10	10	8		28	18	29	29	1
Mixed atrophy/ arteriosclerotic dementia						18	23	24	
Mass lesion	10	4	3	3					
Hydrocephalus	6	6	12						
Alcoholic dementia	7	8	7			2			10
Huntington's chorea	3.5		7						
Creutzfeldt-Jakob disease	3.5						3		
Chronic drug toxicity		4	8						
Post-trauma	1.5					2			3
Post-subarachnoid hemorrhage	1								
Encephalitis	1.5								2
Syphilis			2	1					
Subclinical hematoma				1					
Hypothyroidism			2	1					
Other	29	29	7		21	10		7	7
Total number of patients	84	49	59	63	258	50	1225	675	44

169

overly hopeful in general; but, compared to the futile view of the past, the diagnostic and treatment possibilities available today offer hope to many patients.

TREATABLE DEMENTIAS THAT ARE REVERSIBLE OR POTENTIALLY REVERSIBLE

Hydrocephalus

Hydrocephalus is a general term which denotes an enlargement of the cerebral ventricles. In Alzheimer's disease or other degenerative dementias, the ventricles expand as the underlying brain tissue atrophies. This process is called hydrocephalus ex vacuo and is a secondary rather than a primary hydrocephalus. The type of hydrocephalus to be discussed in this section is that which occurs with obstruction to cerebrospinal fluid (CSF) flow. The obstruction can be in the area of the cerebral aqueduct (most common in children), at the outlets of the fourth ventricle, around the base of the brain, over the convexities of the hemipheres from arachnoid adhesions, or in the arachnoid granulations themselves. Hydrocephalus secondary to aqueductal stenosis is called noncommunicating hydrocephalus, whereas ventricular dilatation due to circulation obstruction or absorptive failure in the subarachnoid spaces is called communicating hydrocephalus.

Although communicating hydrocephalus has been recognized for many years, interest in this condition has been renewed following reports of an idiopathic variety of communicating hydrocephalus with normal CSF pressure.[3,69,114] The reasons for the tremendous attention given these reports were: (1) the lumbar CSF pressure was within normal limits, (2) the patients were demented, and (3) the dementia reversed after a ventricular shunt procedure was carried out. There has been considerable controversy surrounding the evaluation and management of patients with normal pressure (noncommunicating) hydrocephalus. Several review articles[31,33,88] have appeared recently and current thinking is summarized below.

CLINICAL PICTURE

The clinical picture of communicating and noncommunicating hydrocephalus is quite similar. The patients usually initially develop a gait disturbance which can have various features with imbalance being the most characteristic. The first behavioral changes seen are those commonly associated with frontal lobe disease: apathy, euphoria, irritability, and disinhibited social behavior.[128] Intermittent episodes of lethargy and confusion are also frequently present. Increased reflexes,

170

particularly in the legs, with Babinski's signs are found in many cases. Urinary urgency or frequency may also be seen. Cognitive changes are usually minimal during the early stage of the hydrocephalus. Mild forgetfulness, dullness in thinking, and some slowness in carrying out work assignments may be the patients' only behavioral complaints. Occasionally, severe memory deficits are seen, but this is the exception. In general, the cognitive and emotional changes seen in early hydrocephalus are much less dramatic than the gait and reflex abnormalities. This is an important feature in the differential between hydrocephalus and Alzheimer's disease. In the latter, cognitive and emotional changes are usually pronounced before there is any suggestion of primary motor difficulty.

The clinical picture in hydrocephalus can remain stable but usually progresses over a period of weeks to months. Balance becomes worse and the patients have increasing difficulty in initiating gait. They take small steps and appear almost rooted to the floor. Active toe grasping is often seen and the patients will easily fall if lightly pushed. This type of prehensile gait with marked imbalance is the typical finding of a severe frontal gait disturbance, called by some a gait apraxia.[39] Emotionally, the patients become progressively abulic (without animation) and eventually are totally mute. Some cases of dramatic psychiatric problems including paranoia, depression, and attempted suicide have been described, but these are unusual.[137,141] During these later stages the dementia continues to progress, incontinence becomes pronounced, and primitive reflexes (e.g., snout, grasp) appear.

By and large the clinical signs are the result of the expansion of the anterior horns of the lateral ventricles. The behavioral changes are typical of frontal lobe damage and the gait, reflex, and bladder changes are also secondary to expansion of the frontal horns. As the frontal horns expand, fiber tracts from the frontal vertex (e.g., motor fibers to legs and autonomic fibers) are stretched and rendered nonfunctional. This produces the leg spasticity, imbalance, and incontinence that is so characteristic of the syndrome.[191] The paucity of early cognitive signs is due to the gradual distortion of the cortex rather than to its distruction.

LABORATORY EVALUATION

The laboratory evaluation of these patients has included many studies: EEG, CT scan, pneumoencephalography, RISA cisternography, subarachnoid saline infusion, and intracranial pressure monitoring. The EEG has not been a particularly useful tool in diagnosing hydrocephalus because it is normal in as many as 50 percent of all cases.[21] When considering the diagnosis of hydrocephalus, the most efficacious initial test is the CT brain scan. This safe, rapid test will correctly diagnose the presence or absence of hydrocephalus, often demonstrate whether the hydrocephalus is communicating, and will also show cortical atrophy if present.[82] Demonstration of significant cortical atrophy usually rules out the possibility of shunting, even though an occasional patient with significant hydrocephalus plus atrophy has been shown to improve with shunting.[82] It is the presence of a prominent gait abnormality that should suggest shunting.

In cases of noncommunicating hydrocephalus, the patients are referred for neurosurgical evaluation and shunting. Cases of communicating hydrocephalus require additional evaluation to determine which patients will benefit from shunting. Since the CT scan gives only a static picture of the ventricular system, additional studies to measure spinal fluid pressure, CSF flow dynamics and saline absorption have been advocated.[51,57,64,88,116] We have not yet had sufficient experience with the saline infusion technique, accordingly our procedure includes a measurement of spinal fluid pressure and RISA cisternography (injection of radioactive iodinated serum albumin [RISA] into the subarachnoid space) with brain scans taken at 6, 24, and 48 hours to assess cerebrospinal fluid circulation and absorption). An abnormal cisternogram is one in which the RISA (1) fills the ventricles within 6 hours, (2) fails to circulate out of the ventricle in 24 hours, and (3) is still in the cisterns and over the convexity at 48 hours.[14,110,116]

A final procedure that can be carried out if other tests strongly favor the diagnosis, is the monitoring of intracranial pressure for at least 48 hours.[27,36] In patients with communicating hydrocephalus, there are often waves of sustained increased intracranial pressure (B waves). If such waves are present for at least 2 hours during the 2 day period of monitoring, this suggests that the patient's hydrocephalus has not stabilized and that shunting may reverse the neurologic picture.

CRITERIA FOR SHUNTING

One of the great problems in evaluating these patients has been to determine what findings on which tests will not only diagnose the disease but also predict those patients which will benefit from a shunt procedure. Many tests and factors have been considered, but there is still no infallible formula for making these important decisions.[14] The currently accepted criteria for shunting include many factors. The first and most important is the clinical picture. Patients with significant gait difficulty yet little or mild dementia are unequivocally the best candidates for surgery.[51,81,162] In a recent study of 30 cases involving surgery, 12 of 16 patients having successful outcomes initially had gait symptoms with little dementia, whereas 9 of the 11 treatment failures had appreciable dementia as the initial and most prominent feature.[51] The remaining 3 cases could not maintain a functional shunt. Patients with dementia and no motor signs typically do not respond favorably.[81] A second important prognostic factor is etiology. If the patient has a well documented history of an antecedent neurologic illness, particularly subarachnoid hemorrhage, meningitis, or head trauma, he has a 65 percent chance of improvement with surgery. Patients with ideopathic hydrocephalus have only a 41 percent success rate.[88]

Laboratory criteria for the selection of patients for shunt surgery are less certain. The CT scan or pneumoencephalogram should not show cortical atrophy and actually should not show sulcal markings at all. In the typical case of hydrocephalus, the sulci have been obliterated completely. On CT scan, there is frequently evidence of low density areas capping the anterior horns of the lateral ventricles due to the transependymal absorption of spinal fluid. The width across the frontal horns of the lateral ventricles should be greater than 53 mm.[52] and the temporal horns should be very prominent. The lumbar spinal fluid pressure should not be below 110 mm. of water,[51] and intracranial pressure monitoring, if done, should demonstrate sustained increased pressure waves for a total of 2 hours during the 48 hour monitoring period. Although we still obtain a RISA cisternogram on our patients, the correlation of results with successful shunt outcome is not perfect. One problem in the interpretation of the cisternogram is that many patients with Alzheimer's disease also show abnormal CSF flow dynamics.[31,166] One very useful procedure is a therapeutic spinal puncture in which 20 to 25 ml. of spinal fluid are removed and the patient's clinical response is observed for a few days or weeks before surgery.[52] In many cases that are destined to improve with shunting, a temporary improvement can often be seen. Such improvement has been reported to last up to 4 months in some cases and leads some clinicians to treat their patients with periodic lumbar punctures rather than shunting.[52] It is difficult to understand why this treatment might work since the small amount of CSF removed would ordinarily be replaced in a few hours, but it is possible that the period of lowered pressure after the tap alters some critical membrane function and allows normal reabsorption to be reestablished during the period of clinical improvement.

If patients are carefully selected (as they should be since shunt complications such as subdural hematoma and infection are common), at least 50 percent of patients undergoing shunting should show significant improvement. Dramatic improvement can be seen in the first few days after surgery, but usually a course of gradual amelioration is experienced during the first postoperative month. However, the degree of improvement is inversely proportional to the total duration of the patients symptoms. This makes early detection and intervention essential.[81]

ETIOLOGY AND PATHOPHYSIOLOGY

The etiology and pathophysiology of communicating hydrocephalus, especially that with normal CSF pressure, has been actively discussed since 1964. The basic mechanism involves some interference of CSF flow or absorption. In many cases, the history of subarachnoid hemorrhage, meningeal inflammation, trauma, or tumor, easily leads to the conclusion that subarachnoid adhesions have been formed blocking CSF flow. In some cases, fibrosis of the arachnoid granulations has been demonstrated at autopsy.[38] In many cases even detailed microscopic examination has not revealed the cause of the obstruction. Some patients with either Alzheimer's disease or multi-infarct disease develop an associated meningeal thickening and hydrocephalus; these patients have the combined features of the two diseases but seldom benefit from shunting.[27,31,43,88,93]

One puzzling feature of the cases in which normal CSF pressure has been recorded is the mechanism of ventricular expansion in the presence of the normal pressure. One situation must obtain if the ventricles are to expand: the pressure in the ventricles must be sufficient to overcome the tensile strength of the ventricular walls and surrounding brain parenchyma. In some cases of Alzheimer's disease or multi-infarct disease, the tensile strength of the ventricle may weaken and allow normal intraventricular pressure to stretch the walls.[60] In other cases, the basal obstruction may create low pressure in the subarachnoid spaces over the convexity because of the negative hydrostatic pressure in the dural sinus. Such a pressure differential between ventricle and subarachnoid space could allow the ventricles to expand while maintaining essentially normal intraventricular pressure.[117]

Although there may be many mechanisms at work, it seems most probable that the subarachnoid or arachnoid granulation block initially causes increased pressure that expands the ventricles. As the ventricles expand, the ependymal lining stretches and CSF enters the surrounding parenchyma. Over time the ependyma and brain tissue absorb the CSF and a new production-absorption balance is established. On many occasions the CSF pressure is in the normal range, but from intracranial pressure monitoring, we know that the pressure frequently is increased for short periods of time.[27,36,73] These intermittent pressure waves seem to be the dynamic feature causing progression of the hydrocephalus.

Brain Tumors

The behavioral manifestations associated with brain tumors are usually either those of a confusional state secondary to increased intracranial pressure or specific behavioral deficits secondary to focal pathology.[94,172] Tumors involving the temporal and frontal lobes, however, are well-known for their propensity to produce a variety of mental changes of which dementia is only one.[66] This is particularly true of tumors arising in the frontal lobes in which the earliest and most characteristic clinical signs are mental dullness, amnesia, and confusion.[76] Often personality changes such as apathy, euphoria, irritability, and inappropriate social intrusiveness are common. In one large series of patients with temporal lobe tumors, 8 percent of patients experienced memory difficulty and 20 percent intellectual decline as the initial symptoms.[90] Eighty percent of these patients, however, developed sensorium changes by the time of definitive diagnosis. In general, it is unlikely that a brain tumor would produce a dementia simulating Alzheimer's disease without producing either concomitant neurologic abnormalities or a clouding of consciousness. A careful neurologic examination will identify many of the tumor cases, but a CT or isotope scan should always be obtained on all patients suspected of having a brain tumor. Tumors of the posterior fossa or those obstructing spinal fluid flow will create hydrocephalus and demonstrate the findings outlined in the previous section.

Subdural Hematoma

Chronic subdural hematoma can occur at any age but is particularly common in older patients. The elderly individual's brain has often undergone slight atrophy, a process that stretches the fine subdural veins. These delicate bridging veins are thus quite susceptible to tearing from minor head trauma—trauma often so insignificant that it is unappreciated by the patient and not reported. At least 50 percent of all elderly patients with verified subdural hematomas do not recall a specific incident of head trauma. As the hematoma enlarges from blood leaking into the subdural space, focal neurologic findings or alterations in level of consciousness are usually present. Occasionally, however, a picture of dementia is all that is evident clinically. In one series of 75 elderly patients who were treated for subdural hematoma, a majority (94%) had altered levels of consciousness or other neurologic findings, while 12 (16%) were hospitalized with only mental or personality changes.[173] In our experience, several patients with dominant hemisphere subdural hematomas have presented with subtle aphasia which was unrecognized and initially misdiagnosed as toxic delirium. Although the patient with a subdural hematoma does not typically present with a clinical picture of dementia, subdural hematoma must be ruled out in the differential diagnosis of any patient presenting with significant cognitive or behavioral changes.

Cerebral arteriography is definitive in evaluation of subdural hematoma and should be obtained if this lesion is even remotely suspected. We recently saw a 53-year-old woman with a large subdural hematoma in which the CT scan was negative and only our persistence in obtaining an arteriogram allowed us to make the diagnosis.

Surgery with removal of the hematoma is, of course, the treatment of choice and prompt restitution of mental function usually occurs if the dementia has been of short duration. Conversely, if the dementia has been present for many months or years, a less favorable response to surgery is to be expected.

Vasculitis (Systemic Lupus Erythematosus)

Systemic lupus erythematosus (SLE) is probably the most common of the collagen vascular diseases and is certainly the one with the most prominent central nervous system manifestations. A variety of neurologic symptoms have been reported, with mental symptoms being among the most frequently recorded findings.[84] It has been reported that 10 to 50 percent of patients with SLE display some mental change during the course of their illness.[30,126] The most common mental symptoms are psychiatric or emotional (usually acute confusional behavior or rapid psychiatric change[12]) rather than cognitive and will be discussed more fully in Chapter 12, Cerebrovascular Disease. Cases have been described, however, in which symptoms of dementia, including difficulty in work performance, failing memory, and problems with concentration were the patient's initial symptoms.[29,101] In most cases, the diagnosis of SLE has been firmly established from the other systemic signs and symptoms before the appearance of dementia[153] and therefore, the dementia seen in SLE rarely presents as a differential diagnostic problem.

An important point in differentiating SLE from Alzheimer's dementia is that lupus is characteristically a disease of young females. The average age of onset is the midthirties, at least two decades before the usual onset of Alzheimer's disease.[75] This age differential, the difference in quality of the mental symptoms, and the presence of other systemic signs should greatly increase the suspicion of systemic lupus in any female under the age of 40 who presents with a picture of apparent dementia.

Lupus can now be readily diagnosed with the aid of standard laboratory tests, particularly of the erythrocyte sedimentation rate, antinuclear factor, serum electrophoresis, and complement fractionation. Prompt diagnosis and treatment with steroids has been known to reverse many of the acute mental symptoms and on occasion can also improve a longstanding dementia.[29] The degree of improvement depends upon the extent of the pathologic changes in each case. The neuropathologic change seen in lupus consists of multiple areas of cerebral infarction. Because the SLE patient with longstanding dementia does have infarcted brain tissue, improvement will be limited to reversal of those mental changes due to the superimposed acute immune or inflammatory vasculitis.[47,126]

Metabolic Disorders and Deficiency States

Most metabolic imbalances or vitamin deficiencies will eventually result in a form of dementia if they are unrecognized and allowed to run their natural course. However, in most of these conditions, characteristic systemic signs are present which allow identification of the disease before the cognitive features become prominent. In the exceptional case, the mental changes of dementia may precede the other manifestations of the disease. Thus the physician should include these metabolic and deficiency states in a comprehensive differential diagnosis of dementia.

In most of these conditions, emotional or psychiatric mental changes are more frequent than primary cognitive changes. Depression, agitation, and paranoid feelings with delusions of grandeur are quite typical of the early mental symptoms. The cognitive changes, when they do occur early, are characteristically a dullness of intellect, slow thinking, memory problems, and occasional difficulty with abstract thinking. Whether the memory problem is a genuine memory deficit or merely a reflection of depression and lethargy has never been adequately established.

If these conditions remain untreated, a clinically significant dementia will almost invariably develop. The longer that the dementia is present, the less likely it is that the intellectual changes can be reversed by treating the primary disease.

In general, these dementias are not difficult to separate clinically from Alzheimer's disease. The patients are usually younger, have the appearance of lethargy and dullness, typically show other signs of the primary disease, and most frequently present with confusional behavior or psychiatric symptoms. Some of the more common of these conditions are described below.

THYROID DISEASE

Hyperthyroidism can have associated behavioral abnormalities which are usually characterized by either confusional behavior or psychiatric symptoms (more specifically, anxiety or agitated depression). Hypothyroidism or myxedema, to the contrary, can present with the symptoms of gradual intellectual failure typical of dementia.[151]

The mental changes of myxedema were well recognized in the 19th century.[32] However, these observations fell into relative obscurity until 1949 when Asher drew attention to the condition he called myxo-edematous madness.[10]

As is true with all of the diseases discussed in this section, the other clinical features of the primary metabolic disease usually precede or accompany the mental changes. Well-documented cases of a pure dementia syndrome as the initial manifestation of myxedema are distinctly uncommon.[97]

It has been reported that approximately one-third of all patients with myxedema have psychiatric changes and that 30 percent will also show memory changes.[83,125] Many of the cases of hypothyroidism that have mental changes, display emotional symptoms of psychotic proportions. Paranoia and depression are the most common features, but hypomania, agitation, explosiveness, and schizophreniform psychosis have been described.[10] Of the dementia symptoms, mental dullness, slow thinking, decreased memory, and difficulty in abstract reasoning are the most common. Full-blown confusional states are also seen at times, with active hallucinations reported in 50 percent of these cases.[32]

Although the clinical diagnosis is usually not difficult to make because of the overall clinical picture of myxedema (e.g., weight gain, husky voice, thin dry hair, loss of lateral eye brow hair, facial puffiness, cold intolerance, and hearing difficulty) we routinely screen all dementia patients for thyroid disease utilizing a serum T_3 and T_4.

Treatment can dramatically reverse all symptoms, but permanent intellectual change has been noted in about 10 percent of cases.[10,66,83,104] Infrequently, these patients' mental changes can actually worsen when they are placed on thyroid medication. In our experience, confusional and psychotic behavior, rather than worsening dementia, are more common adverse effects of treatment.

PITUITARY DISEASE

As with thyroid disease, mental changes, including dementia, can be seen with either hyperfunction or hypofunction of the pituitary gland. The hyperfunction which produces adrenal hyperplasia and Cushing's syndrome also commonly causes a mental state that can mimic the early signs of dementia. Easy fatigability, irritability, depression, mental dullness, and memory impairment are the most common symptoms. These are seen in moderate or greater degree in 40 percent of patients with Cushing's syndrome and to a milder degree in an additional 30 percent of the cases.[168,182] Such patients are typically young (25 to 50 years of age) and have weight gain and other physical signs of excessive steroid production by the time that mental changes are noticed. Because of the characteristic features, this condition can usually be easily

178

differentiated from the more common degenerative dementia described by Alzheimer. Diagnosis can readily be confirmed by a dexamethasone suppression test and urinary and serum 17-hydroxysteroid levels. Treatment of the primary disease will reverse the mental symptoms unless they are of long standing.

Hypopituitarism, though uncommon, can also present with slowly evolving mental changes that must be differentiated from degenerative disease. As with other metabolic conditions, mental slowness, memory loss, depression, and other emotional changes dominate the clinical picture. The disease usually occurs in young patients, with many cases occurring in the postpartal period secondary to hemorrhage into the pituitary gland (Sheehan's syndrome). Again, prompt treatment with replacement steroids will usually reverse the mental symptoms.

PARATHYROID DISEASE

Mental symptoms occur with both the elevation (hyperparathyroidism) or depression (hypoparathyroidism) of serum calcium levels seen in parathyroid disease. In hypercalcemia, the picture is more characteristic of a confusional state than of a dementia, although the chronic nature of the behavioral change can sometimes lead to diagnostic uncertainty. Two-thirds of the patients primarily have personality or emotional changes, whereas less than 20 percent demonstrate memory difficulty or other organic cognitive changes.[133] Loss of spontaneity and initiative are also common subjective complaints. The most common cause of hypercalcemia is a parathyroid adenoma. This lesion must be assiduously sought in every case. Removal of the tumor and restoration of normal serum calcium levels has been reported to rapidly reverse the mental changes in most cases, even when they had been of long standing.[133]

Low serum calcium, either due to hypoparathyroidism or pseudohypoparathyroidism will induce mental changes that can present as a dementia even in the absence of tetany.[45,145] More commonly, the patient demonstrates a confusional state accompanied by tetany.[163, 174] The type of mental picture is somewhat related to the rapidity of the fall of serum calcium. A gradual drop in calcium will result in less dramatic personality and memory changes, while a precipitous lowering will produce an acute agitated confusional state (delirium).

The condition is usually seen in middle-aged patients (40 to 50 years of age), but cases of idiopathic hypoparathyroidism have been reported in patients up to the age of 80.[45] Most cases are secondary to inadvertent removal of all parathyroid tissue during total thyroidectomy. Accordingly, any patient with a progressive mental syndrome who has had recent thyroid surgery must be screened for parathyroid dysfunction. Cataracts, features of parkinsonism, seizures, and increased intra-

179

cranial pressure are also seen in patients with hypoparathyroidism, and their presence can aid in establishing the diagnosis clinically. Laboratory investigation typically demonstrates a depressed serum calcium level and elevated phosphate level in the presence of normal renal function. Treatment with calcium has been known to reverse the mental picture quite dramatically, but frequently permanent intellectual loss is seen.

HEPATOCEREBRAL DEGENERATION

Wilson's Disease (Hepatolenticular Degeneration)

Wilson's disease is a somewhat rare recessively inherited condition in which an abnormality in copper metabolism causes deposition of the copper ion in the liver, various structures in the nervous system (primarily the putamen and globus pallidus), and other tissues.[188] The usual onset of the disease in its adult form is during the patient's 20s, although cases have been reported whose first symptoms were not noted until the middle and late 40s.[63,184]

Most of the cases first present with neurologic symptoms (tremor, involuntary grimacing, dystonic posturing, choreoathetosis, dysarthria, and rigidity), although at least 25 percent of the cases present initially with only behavioral abnormalities.[155,183,184,188] Patients with a behavioral manifestation as the initial sign of their disease tend to be those with late onset, making Wilson's disease one of the diseases that should be considered in the differential diagnosis of mental changes occurring in middle age. In most cases, the mental aberrations involve uninhibited social behavior. The patients tend to be explosive, immature, silly, impulsive, sexually promiscuous, unkempt, and emotionally labile. Many patients become delusional and despondent, and some attempt suicide.[80] In conjunction with these common psychiatric or behavioral changes, some patients demonstrate cognitive difficulties including memory failure, decreased judgement and academic performance, and lack of concentration. If the disease remains untreated, a progressive, severe dementia develops. By the time that a full picture of dementia is seen, the other neurologic manifestations of the disease are also present.

The diagnosis of Wilson's disease is made in most cases by laboratory studies showing low serum ceruloplasmin, low serum copper, and high urinary copper. A liver biopsy for copper content is more definitive but somewhat more risky than collecting a 24-hour-urine sample. Treatment with penicillamine can effect a remarkable improvement in behavioral as well as neurologic symptoms. In one group of 17 patients who had psychologic testing before and after treatment, the authors reported a significant improvement on the WAIS Verbal IQ and the memory score of the Wechsler Memory Test.[63] In a larger series of 49 patients in which 61 percent had significant psychiatric abnormalities, over half experienced demonstrable improvement in their moods and antisocial behavioral problems with treatment.[155] Though Wilson's disease is uncommon, the encouraging response to treatment in many cases makes us feel justified in mentioning Wilson's disease in this discussion of the mental changes occurring in middle life.

Acquired Hepatocerebral Degeneration

A small percentage of patients with liver disease of any cause will develop a general intellectual deterioration secondary to their hepatic disease. This dementia usually begins as a sequela of hepatic coma, but 15 percent of the cases present with cognitive symptoms before the diagnosis of liver disease is made.[2] Alcoholic cirrhosis and other liver diseases are sufficiently common that the physician should be aware of the possibility of hepatocerebral degeneration in the differential diagnosis of dementia.

VITAMIN DEFICIENCIES

Pellagra

Niacin deficiency will characteristically produce a mental syndrome of confusion, memory impairment, disorientation, apathy, irritability, and apprehension. This mental picture, which can often look superficially like an early degenerative dementia, is soon followed by the dermatitis, peripheral neuropathy, and diarrhea which constitute the full clinical syndrome of pellagra. The epidemic form of this condition is no longer seen in this country, rather it has become a sporadic disease in alcoholics, food fadists, and others with very abnormal eating habits.

Vitamin B_{12} and Folate Deficiency

In the search for treatable causes of psychiatric disease and dementia, vitamins B_{12} and folate have received considerable attention. Depletion of either substance can produce a mental syndrome that can be confused with early Alzheimer's disease.[59,77,147,152,158] Mild depression and anxiety, loss of sexual interest, irritability, memory impairment, and concentration difficulty constitute the typical clinical presentation. All of these findings can occur years before the onset of hematologic abnormalities.[142,157] The etiology of the symptoms does not seem, therefore, to be directly related to the anemia frequently associated with the vitamin deficiency but rather to vitamin deficiency itself. There is little doubt that B_{12} deficiency causes a neurologic syndrome

181

with prominent mental changes, but the actual relationship of B_{12} to folate and to mental symptoms is much debated. Some authors allege that there is a close relationship between the two vitamins in the production of dementia.[140] Others question the fact that folate itself is an important factor.[150,158]

Since efficient screening methods for determining B_{12} and folate levels are not available in every laboratory, the physician must be selective in requesting these tests. Certainly, any patient with a history of gastric surgery, malabsorption, or strict vegetarianism should be investigated.[61] Any case of dementia without cerebral atrophy for which no alternate explanation can be established should have serum levels of B_{12} and folate determined. Patients with well-documented abnormal levels of B_{12} (< 100 pg./ml.) and/or folate (< 2 ng./ml.) who also have dementia and/or mental symptoms, should be treated with both B_{12} (100 mgm. daily for 7 days, then 3 times weekly for 1 month, and then once weekly for 1 year) and folate (5 mg. daily). If the mental condition is of recent onset, the behavioral changes should reverse. If it is longstanding, however, demyelination will have occurred and the cognitive as well as psychiatric changes may be permanent.[4,87]

Chronic Meningitis

Tuberculosis, Cryptococcus, Coccidiodes, and various rarer fungal agents produce indolent infections that can result in a chronic meningitis, frequently without signs of the illness in other organs.[121] In such cases, mental symptoms are very prominent features. For example, mental changes have been reported in more than 50 percent of patients with cryptococcal meningitis.[154]

The typical clinical picture is of a middle-aged patient (many of whom have been on immunosuppressive drugs, steroids, or have lymphomas) who develops a chronic headache (almost 100% of patients) with memory difficulty, chronic confusion, clouding of consciousness, fever (almost 100% of patients), malaise, and often scattered neurologic signs such as ataxia, visual blurring, or seizures. The headache, fever, and mental confusion dominate the early clinical picture, whereas a decreased level of consciousness, nuchal rigidity, cerebellar dysfunction, and cranial nerve signs develop as the disease progresses.[96,112,149]

In the case of tuberculosis, the progression of symptoms is quite rapid, with death occurring in the undiagnosed patient within 4 to 6 weeks. These cases should not be confused with a degenerative dementia because of their characteristic rapid clinical course.

The patient with the more slowly developing infections as with Cryptococcus or one of the fungi can often have a history of 6 to as many as 24 months of gradual mental change—not an atypical history for Alzheimer's disease. Dementia due to these infections is uncommon, but as they are amenable to treatment, they should be considered in the differential diagnosis.

The diagnosis of such infectious processes is made most efficiently on spinal fluid examination. Spinal fluid protein and often pressure are elevated, sugar is depressed, and cells (mostly lymphocytes) are present. The infective agent can frequently be identified on microscopic examination or culture. However, the aptly named Cryptococcus is often quite difficult to find on a single microscopic examination (even with India ink) and repeated spinal punctures may be necessary.

Treatment is quite effective for all the chronic meningitides, although it is lengthy and many of the drugs have significant side effects. As with most of the diseases discussed in this section, the reversal of mental symptoms is best achieved with early treatment before the inflammatory reaction in the meninges causes extensive vasculitis in the basal vessels and widespread infarction.

General Paresis (parenchymatous neurosyphilis, general paralysis of the insane, dementia paralytica)

Neurosyphilis has long been known for its ability to produce an extremely wide variety of clinical syndromes. One of the most common of these is a form of dementia usually referred to as general paresis. Since the advent of penicillin, the later stages of syphilis are infrequently seen, but every physician should be acquainted with the clinical picture of this disease to complement his knowledge of dementia. Since the condition is much less common in this country today, one must look to foreign or older literature for comprehensive clinical descriptions.[28,118,187]

Although there are many different behavioral manifestations of general paresis, the most commonly recognized features are those relating to frontal lobe damage. In the early stage of paresis, the patient shows subtle changes in personality, which are frequently exaggerations of his premorbid personality traits. A lack of attention to personal appearance, poor judgement, aggressiveness, and abnormal or bizarre behavior are also often seen initially. In time, "peculiarities of conduct,"[187] irritability, mood swings, apathy, memory and concentration deficits, geographic disorientation with aimless wandering, and a deterioration in personal habits occurs.[28] Delusions are often present; these are very gradiose in 10 to 20 percent of the patients.[118] However, at least 45 percent of the patients present with only a simple dementia, with apathy being a major symptom.[28]

The literary picture of the paretic is that of a male with a napoleonic complex, strutting about like a megalomaniac, and claiming to have extraordinary powers, financial resources, or physical prowess. Such cases certainly do occur but are not as common as generally believed and less spectacular presentations predominate. With progression of the disease, the patients become more severely demented with marked memory failure, aphasia, apraxia, and agnosia.[187] The duration of symptoms before diagnosis varies, with 20 percent of the patients presenting in the first 4 weeks of their illness, 25 percent in 1 to 6 months, and a few after a year of behavioral change.[28]

The behavioral features of paresis can be the initial and, during the early stages of the illness, the only clinical findings in some patients. However, the physician should look for other neurologic signs as they are frequently seen in conjunction with the behavioral change. Argyll Robertson pupils (irregular, unreactive to light but reactive to accomodation), tremors of tongue and limbs, slurring dysarthria, and increased reflexes in the legs are those signs most commonly seen in the paretic patient.[118,187]

The diagnosis is easily made on spinal fluid examination. An increase in cells and protein is present in many cases, but the most accurate test is the VDRL (Venereal Disease Research Laboratory) test. Treatment with penicillin can have a very favorable influence on prognosis when used early in the course of the disease.[15,66,156] There is some question as to how much penicillin should be used, and for how long treatment is necessary, but it is consensually considered to be within the range of millions of units daily for several weeks.

The pathology of paresis has been well studied, and there is a good correlation with the clinical features. The frontal lobes have extensive atrophy with associated meningeal thickening. The infection enters the outer layers of cortex and causes neuronal loss and reactive gliosis. Vascular lesions may also be seen, these account for many of the focal neurologic signs seen in patients with advanced neurosyphilis.[118]

TREATABLE, NONREVERSIBLE DEMENTIAS

There are several conditions which cause dementia in which treatment of the underlying disease can slow or arrest further progression of the dementia, yet cannot reverse the damage already present. Many of the conditions discussed in the preceding section are nonreversible if the disease has been unrecognized for many years and permanent neuronal damage has occurred (e.g., vitamin deficiency, Wilson's disease, or chronic hydrocephalus). The two most important treatable but nonreversible dementias are those associated with arteriosclerotic and/or hypertensive cerebrovascular disease and the chronic abuse of alcohol.

Arteriosclerotic Dementia

There are still many physicians who loosely apply the term "arteriosclerotic dementia" to any elderly patient who shows signs of senility.

While it is true that "hardening of the arteries" (arteriosclerosis) and hypertension are very common in older patients, these diseases, per se, are implicated in the production of a clinical dementia in only a small number of patients. Table 6-1 summarizes the clinical and pathologic studies of demented patients which demonstrate that only 10 percent of the patients in the clinical studies had a dementia judged to be secondary to vascular disease, whereas approximately 20 to 25 percent of the autopsied demented patients demonstrated vascular disease judged by the neuropathologist to be sufficient to produce a dementia. The patients in these clinical series presented with a history of gradual deterioration in intellectual and adaptive processes without evidence of major vascular accidents. In the autopsy series, however, patients who had had multiple major strokes were often included in the arteriosclerotic dementia category, thereby exaggerating the incidence of dementia attributed to vascular disease. Although many demented patients have signs of arteriosclerotic disease, relatively few of them develop a gradually progressive dementia secondary to this disease process. Alzheimer's disease remains by far the most common cause of dementia in patients over the age of 50.

Within the group of patients in whom dementia is, in fact, due to arteriosclerotic disease, there is a variety of both proven and postulated mechanisms by which vascular disease can produce the chronic progressive mental changes.

MULTIPLE MAJOR STROKES

If a patient has sustained several significant vascular accidents destroying large areas of cortex in both cerebral hemispheres, he will characteristically show intellectual loss in association with his other obvious neurologic impairments. The reason for mentioning this encephalopathy in this section is not because this condition is likely to be confused with a degenerative dementia, but because many such patients are admitted to chronic care facilities with a subdiagnosis of dementia. Because of the subdiagnosis, any statistical or pathologic study of such patients will greatly increase the percentage of cases of dementia attributed to arteriosclerosis in the sample. This leaves the erroneous impression that a high percentage of the progressive dementias are due to arteriosclerosis.

MULTI-INFARCT DEMENTIA

The progressive dementia syndrome that is caused by arteriosclerotic or hypertensive cerebrovascular disease is secondary to multiple small cerebral infarctions.[49,67,72] Clinically, these patients are usually quite easily differentiated from those with Alzheimer's disease. The important features of the multi-infarct dementia are as follows:

1. Presence of hypertension and/or arteriosclerotic cerebrovascular disease (e.g., transient ischemic attacks, carotid bruits, etc.).
2. A history of step-wise decreasing mental and neurologic functions which may or may not be associated with a history of transient ischemic attacks.[49,180]
3. Neurologic signs which are more dramatic than the dementia: Asymmetric reflexes, abnormal reflexes, sensory abnormalities.
4. Presence of a pseudobulbar state, (found only in multi-infarct dementia and not in Alzheimer's disease).[49]
5. Memory which is much better than other cognitive functions, particularly speech (a feature uncharacteristic of Alzheimer's disease).[50]

These clinical features combined with a history of a previous stroke that cleared completely should result in a relatively sound diagnosis of multi-infarct dementia.

There are several mechanisms by which multi-infarction can occur and several well recognized pathologic entities have been described.

Lacunar State

This represents one of the end stages of hypertensive cerebrovascular disease in which multiple small infarctions have occurred in the subcortical regions of the brain leaving many small lacunae.[49]

Multiple Cortical and Subcortical Infarctions

In this type, diffuse multi-infarction results from microemboli from the heart or great vessels. This can also be seen with multiple, somewhat larger, infarctions in the distribution of the major cerebral arteries.

Subcortical Arteriosclerotic Encephalopathy of Binswanger

Binswanger's disease is fairly uncommon in its fulminant form, but the multiple white matter lesions that are its hallmark are frequently seen in the brains of hypertensive patients. Clinically the disease is a fairly typical multi-infarct dementia, except that it usually is seen in a slightly younger age group, with an onset between 50 and 60 years of age.[26,129] The patients usually are hypertensive and have extensive atheromatous change in their cerebral vessels.[23] The lesions are a combination of perivascular infarctions in the cerebral white matter and an unexplained secondary, often massive, demyelination of all but the corticocortical (u) fibers in the cerebral hemispheres.

Granular Atrophy

Granular atrophy consists of an extensive C shaped band of multiple microinfarctions in the border zones between anterior and middle cerebral arteries and middle and posterior cerebral arteries. (Fig. 6-4) This border zone infarction occurs primarily because of significant carotid artery disease which decreases the overall blood flow in the entire carotid system. Under such conditions, it is the border zones that suffer the most extensive ischemia and subsequent infarction.[49,146]

DEMENTIA SECONDARY TO CAROTID STENOSIS AND ANOXIA WITHOUT INFARCTION

A great controversy surrounds the very appealing concept that carotid stenosis decreases blood flow to the brain and therefore can, if chronically present, cause gradual atrophy of cortical neurons and an attendant dementia. Although seemingly logical,[48,131] evidence to support this contention is lacking.[49]

Carotid stenosis can produce transient cerebral ischemia; when this is localized, specific neurologic symptoms are produced, but when it is generalized, a confusional state results. What may occur is that some patients suffer repeated episodes of transient ischemia without actual infarction, but physiologic function fails to return to full capacity between attacks. Clinically such patients would present a picture of chronic, fluctuating confusion or focal neuropsychologic dysfunction, findings which could be called a dementia if they persisted over a period of months.

In this group of patients, carotid artery surgery which increases

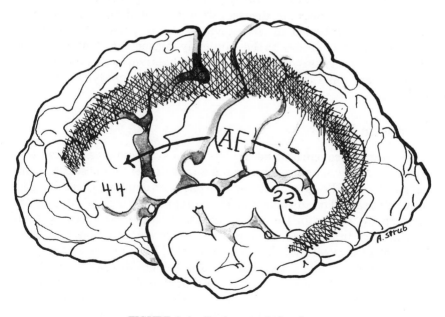

FIGURE 6–4. Border zone infarction.

187

blood flow can increase overall mental functioning and to an extent reverse the dementia-like symptoms. This situation is quite rare and in most of the cases reported, the patients have had some evidence of residual cerebral infarction and a clear history of focal transient cerebral ischemia.[41,46]

MIXED DEGENERATIVE AND ARTERIOSCLEROTIC DEMENTIA

When evaluating demented patients and attempting to classify the etiology in the individual patient, one must remember that some demented patients have both atrophic brain disease and significant numbers of small cerebral infarctions (Table 6-1). This mixed group is very confusing diagnostically because (1) the dementia seems too great for the paucity of neurologic signs necessary to diagnose a multi-infarct dementia, and (2) the presence of focal neurologic findings is inconsistent with the diagnosis of a typical Alzheimer's disease.

Evaluation of the patient suspected of having a vascular dementia should include evaluation of blood pressure, heart rhythm, and evidence of old myocardial infarction and a full evaluation of the cerebral vasculature, particularly the extracranial vessels. Treatment cannot reverse cerebral infarction but is guided toward preventing future additional strokes. Hypertension, cardiac arrhythmia and other cardiovascular disease should be treated. The patient should discontinue smoking. Anticoagulation therapy, carotid surgery, and other treatment of cerebrovascular disease should be undertaken where indicated. As mentioned in the previous chapter, we have not found the use of vasodilators to be clinically efficacious. Unfortunately, the overall prognosis is not good in vascular disease of the brain, nevertheless some cases can be helped, thereby justifying the effort expended.

Alcoholic Dementia

There are several chronic neurobehavioral syndromes associated with long term alcohol abuse. The first is a true dementia, most commonly seen in the middle-aged alcoholic who has been drinking excessively for 15 to 20 years. The initial signs are a progressive lack of interest and concern for events in the environment, carelessness about personal appearance, impairment of judgement, defective attention, and a general slowness in all thought processes.[42,74,79] Most of these abnormalities are those usually associated with frontal lobe disease and are quite similar to the changes seen in general paresis. The similarity was so striking to many of the earlier investigators that they called the condition an alcoholic pseudoparesis. However, the marked personality lability and grandiosity of the true paretic are not found in such prominence in alcoholic pseudoparesis.[74]

Intellectually such patients show difficulty with abstract reasoning, problems with new learning (recent memory), some mild aphasic symptoms, and perseveration.[79] In one study, 95 percent had some difficulty with recent memory, while a smaller percentage (61%) suffered disorientation in their environment. Only 10 percent of the patients had difficulty with drawings or constructional tasks, however.[79] The lack of constructional impairment is not usually seen in Alzheimer's disease and can be a helpful differential point. On formal neuropsychologic testing, the patients show deficits in the Full Scale IQ, memory testing, complex perceptual motor tasks (particularly those requiring rapid performance), and frontal lobe tests such as the card sorting test that requires shifting from one scheme of sorting to another (e.g., first by shape then by color or size).[20,91,176]

If the patients continue to drink, these symptoms and signs of dementia will continue; exacerbations are often brought on by bouts of delirium tremens. Improvement is slight and infrequent even if temperance is achieved. Pneumoencephalography or computerized tomography scanning shows ventricular dilation in as many as 70 percent of chronic alcoholics even though the dementia is not obvious. These findings verify the contention that alcohol can and often does do irreversible brain damage.[20,54]

The pathophysiology of alcoholic dementia is still not completely understood and in many patients seems to be a combination of factors. Firstly, alcohol itself appears to be toxic to brain cells and actually causes atrophy of cortical neurons. On the other hand, a significant percentage of alcoholics are known to experience episodes of delirium tremens, seizures, repeated head trauma, and the effects of chronic liver disease. The actual part played by each of these factors is not known and certainly differs in each case.

Pathologically the findings are quite characteristic. There is macroscopic cortical atrophy frontally, a finding which correlates well with the clinical picture; thinning of the cerebral cortex; and enlargement of the ventricular system. Microscopically, pigmentary atrophy and loss of cortical neurons is obvious, maximally in the frontal areas and primarily in the middle layers of the cortex. There is some glial proliferation (astrocytic) and in occasional patients an actual laminar necrosis of the third cortical layer is found.[35,120,123,185]

The other chronic mental syndromes associated with alcoholism are Marchiafava-Bignami disease and Korsakoff's syndrome. Marchiafava-Bignami's disease is a dementing illness but sufficiently rare that we do not think it merits specific discussion here. Korsakoff's syndrome is not a dementia as we define it, but it is rather a disease with a discretly

189

localized pathology and a restricted type of cognitive impairment. We will discuss this syndrome in the next chapter on focal brain lesions in the section on the organic amnesias.

UNTREATABLE DEMENTIAS
Degenerative Diseases

Many of the degenerative diseases have intellectual and social deterioration as a primary or associated manifestation of the illness. The most common of these is Alzheimer's disease, a condition which traditionally was considered synonymous with presenile dementia. Another of the classic degenerative dementias which should be differentiated from Alzheimer's disease is Pick's disease. Other conditions such as Huntington's chorea, parkinsonism, progressive supranuclear palsy and the spinocerebellar degenerations usually have dementia as a late component of the illness. In these cases, the dementia is an additional manifestation to be taken into account in managing the patient and his illness. Such cases do not typically present a diagnostic problem.

PICK'S DISEASE

Many textbooks disagree on the clinical separability of Pick's from Alzheimer's disease. Although it should be acknowledged that there is a clinical spectrum to each condition which makes differentiation impossible in every case, particularly during the later stages; the initial symptoms of the two conditions are usually quite distinct and recognizable.[86,89,105,144,164,165,170]

Pick's disease characteristically presents with a change in personality and social behavior rather than a primary cognitive deterioration. The patients usually become disinhibited in social situations and are often known for their transgressions beyond the line of propriety. In concert with this loss of social inhibition, such patients develop a pervasive lack of interest in their responsibilities and surroundings. Soon the lack of interest supersedes the inappropriate social behavior and aspontaneity and apathy pervade the clinical picture. Almost all patients with Pick's disease lack insight into their problem. This is frequently not the case in Alzheimer's disease where failing mental prowess is all too often tragically felt.

In Pick's disease, there is a relative sparing of cognitive functions during the early stage of marked behavioral change. Memory, constructional ability, geographic sense, and language are far better preserved than in the patient with Alzheimer's disease at the same stage of his illness. During the second stage, however, general cognitive changes do develop. Scant speech production is noted in a high percentage of patients with Pick's disease, while excessive rambling speech (logorrhea) by contrast is quite uncommon.[105] The patients develop an anomic aphasia (difficulty in naming objects) but do not produce paraphasias (word or letter substitutions) as do patients with Alzheimer's disease. The typical patient with Alzheimer's disease seems to suffer a much more complete disruption of language than the patient with Pick's disease, the latter producing little yet better organized speech. With progression in Pick's disease, the patients gradually lose their comprehension for language, but many retain the ability to repeat accurately. Approximately a third of the patients actually develop an echolalia where they tend to repeat, almost reflexly, all that they hear.[105] Perseveration is common in their speech and stereotyped language is also frequent.

Patients with Pick's disease demonstrate much less apraxia than do patients with Alzheimer's disease and, in general, there is a sparing of parietal lobe functions. Patients in this second stage often demonstrate a marked lack of facial expression (amimia). Some also develop an astoundingly ravenous appetite. As the disease progresses to its third stage, clear distinctions from Alzheimer's disease blur and terminal mutism, profound dementia, and paraplegia in flexion are characteristically seen.[191]

The diagnosis of Pick's disease should usually not be difficult to make, with chance strongly favoring Alzheimer's disease because of its comparative frequency. In most parts of the world, both the clinician and pathologist will see 50 to 100 cases of Alzheimer's disease to every case of Pick's disease.[132,177] Exceptions to this rule exist in Malaya, where Alzheimer's disease has not yet been reported,[192] and in Stockholm, Sweden, where there is a genetic pool of Pick's dementia.[164]

The age of onset in Pick's disease is the early to midfifties, with a life expectancy of approximately 6 to 7 years after diagnosis. Twenty percent of the patients will, however, live longer than 10 years.[164] Male and female cases have approximately equal incidence, unlike the 2:1 female predominance seen in Alzheimer's disease. There is a somewhat stronger genetic tendency in Pick's disease, with a suggested autosomal dominant pattern.

Pathologically, the disease has a very distinctive appearance. In the gross specimen, marked frontal and temporal atrophy are seen (Figs. 6-5 and 6-6). This pattern of atrophy correlates well with the clinical features of personality change (frontal atrophy) and speech abnormality (temporal atrophy). It allows the clinical diagnosis to be reinforced by CT scan or pneumoencephalography. This classic pattern of atrophy gave the disease its original name, lobar sclerosis. The pattern of atrophy is frequently not uniform, however. Pure temporal atrophy is seen

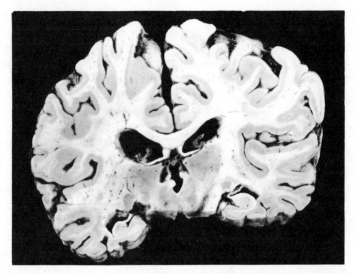

FIGURE 6–5. Brain of patient with Pick's lobar sclerosis. Note marked temporal atrophy.

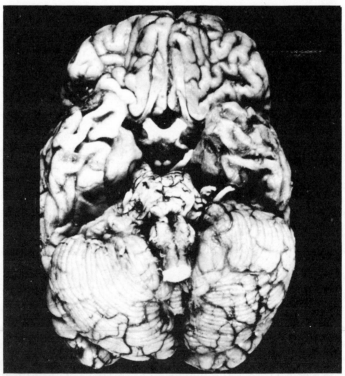

FIGURE 6–6. Brain of a patient with Pick's disease showing focal atrophy of both temporal lobes, more pronounced on the left.

in 17 percent of the cases, pure frontal atrophy in 25 percent, mixed frontotemporal atrophy in 54 percent, and atypical atrophy including occipital or parietal lobes in the remaining 4 percent.[34,192] Only one-third of the cases have symmetrical atrophy in both hemispheres, while atrophy on the left is greater in over 40 percent and on the right in less than 20 percent.[192] In all cases, there is a consistent sparing of the primary projection areas (post central gyrus, superior temporal gyrus, and the visual cortex in the occipital lobe) with the atrophy involving primarily the association areas.

Microscopically, the cortex shows cell loss, astrocytic gliosis, and many enlarged balloon-shaped cells (Pick's cells) that contain argentophilic (silver staining) intranuclear inclusions (Fig. 6-7). The outer layers of the cortex seem to be more severely involved.[189] As with Alzheimer's disease, no etiology is known, but it seems probable that the disease may start in the axons and cell processes rather than in the cell bodies themselves.[34]

DEMENTIAS WITH A STRONG SUBCORTICAL COMPONENT

There are several degenerative diseases with associated dementia in which the most prominant pathologic features are in the subcortical structures. To be precise, the substantia nigra in parkinsonism, the caudate nucleus in Huntington's chorea, the subcortical white matter in progressive subcortical gliosis,[124] the thalamus in thalamic degener-

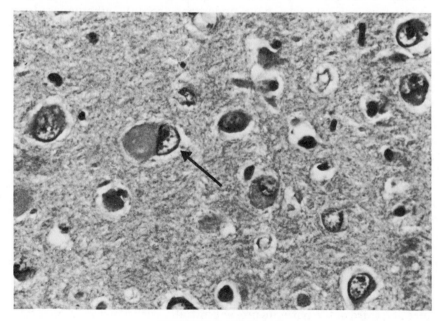

FIGURE 6–7. Pick's cell.

193

ation and subacute diencephalic angioencephalopathy[37,159,171] (not a degenerative disease, but mentioned here because of the association between subcortical lesions and dementia), and subcortical and cerebellar structures in progressive supranuclear palsy. In Huntington's disease and parkinsonism, there are also cortical lesions, but the degree of dementia seen in these patients appears more extensive than can be accounted for by the degree of cortical pathology alone.[9] Therefore, it seems evident that the degeneration of the subcortical structures is, at least in part, producing or accentuating the symptoms of intellectual and adaptive deterioration. Neurosurgeons have also noted psychologic changes in their patients after stereotactic thalamotomy, providing additional data to support the contention that subcortical structures are intimately involved in the workings of the mind.[85,127,160]

The primary clinical features of these subcortical lesions are mental sluggishness, forgetfulness, difficulty performing complex verbal abstractions, failure of high level concept formation and mental flexibility (being able to quickly switch from one way of doing something to another), and a personality change reminiscent of patients with frontal lobe damage (e.g., apathy, indifference, irritability, and euphoria).[5,6] In many of these conditions, it is quite easy to see why a certain behavioral change would be associated with a given lesion; for instance, extensive lesions in the thalamus interrupt many important input pathways to the frontal lobes and may produce many of the behaviors exhibited by patients who have undergone frontal leukotomies. Involvement of the ascending activating system above the level of the brain stem can cause impaired arousal and inefficiency in maintaining attention and concentration. It may also be true, though as yet unproven, that reticular and other subcortical inputs may in fact play a role in directing and coordinating cortical activity. Less speculative is the role of such subcortical structures as the dorsal medial thalamus and the mamillary bodies in the memory process. Any damage to these structures, particularly when associated with an interruption of frontal projections, can result in apathy which can easily explain the forgetfulness seen in these patients.

Each of the diseases in this group of subcortical dementias has its own specific clinical features. The most common types will be discussed below, while others are referenced.

Huntington's Chorea

Huntington's chorea is a familial disease with an autosomal dominant inheritance pattern. The disease has two major clinical features by which it can be readily recognized: mental deterioration and chorea. Since one third of the patients present initially with a history of mental change without chorea, Huntington's chorea is an important condition to consider in the differential diagnosis of dementia appearing in the presenile period.[130] The disease is usually manifest between ages 45 and 55; cases with an onset after 60 are distinctly uncommon and after 70 are very rare.[130]

Clinically, the early mental picture has many of the features seen in Pick's disease. Changes in emotional status and social behavior are characteristic. Apathy is very common, however, emotional instability, impulsiveness, irritability, and explosive behavior are frequently seen. Patients with Huntington's disease are usually moody, quick tempered, aggressive, even physically abusive. On occasion they can develop the psychiatric picture of manic-depressive illness or a delusional hallucinatory state resembling an acute schizophrenic episode.[115] Patients suffer a general loss of interest in work and are unmotivated to complete an assigned job.[22] They often become sloppy in their physical appearance and their living quarters. Insight is often retained early in the disease; the resultant despair coupled with poor impulse control leads to a high rate of suicide in these patients.

Despite this rather significant deterioration of emotional and social behavior, their cognitive processes typically show less dramatic alteration. The IQ, though lower than that of matched controls, may remain within the normal range.[16,25] On extensive neuropsychologic testing, performance on problem solving tasks, the trail-making test, block designs, and puzzle assembly are all significantly depressed. Controlled studies have shown that these impairments represent a degradation of performance which is greater than could be explained solely by any motor problem.[15]

As the disease progresses, chorea develops in all cases and mental deterioration continues. However, the aphasia, agnosia, apraxia, and severe amnesia that are so characteristic of Alzheimer's and Pick's diseases do not appear. Muscle stretch reflexes increase in more than two-thirds of the patients and frank pathologic reflexes or clonus are present in one-third.[130] Speech becomes dysarthric, abnormal movements more constant, and eventually the patients become bedridden, cachexic, and grossly demented. Death usually occurs within 15 years after the onset of the disease.[66]

Laboratory evaluation is not specific for making the diagnosis of Huntington's chorea. The EEG is frequently abnormal and the pneumoencephalogram often shows a rounding of the medial wall of the lateral ventricle secondary to the atrophy of the caudate nucleus. The diagnosis of Huntington's chorea is basically a clinical diagnosis based on family history and neurologic findings.

Pathologically, the gross brain usually shows mild to moderate cerebral atrophy, with frontal atrophy being most prominent. This frontal atrophy correlates well with the clinical picture of a predominantly emotional change. The caudate nucleus is markedly atrophic and the putamen and globus pallidus also show atrophy.[34] Microscopically, cell loss is prominent in the areas of atrophy, with some reactive astrocytic proliferation, but there are no specific cellular changes such as those seen in Alzheimer's or Pick's disease.

Huntington's disease, like parkinsonism and now Alzheimer's disease, has been shown neurochemically to involve rather specific transmitter systems. Glutamic acid decarboxylase (GAD), which is critical to the synthesis of the neurotransmitter gamma aminobutyric acid (GABA), and choline are reduced 85 and 50 percent respectively in the caudate nuclei of patients with Huntington's chorea. There is also a 50 percent reduction in receptor binding sites for serotonin and muscarinic acetylcholine in the Huntington patient's caudate nucleus. Binding sites in the frontal cortex are normal, however.[44] These findings suggest that a specific metabolic defect in the production and maintenance of certain neurotransmitters or transmitter systems is responsible for the eventual death of specific cells thus producing the clinical syndrome.

Parkinson's Disease

Parkinsonism is a relatively common neurologic disorder in which patients slowly develop rigidity, tremor, slowness of movement, and difficulty maintaining balance. Early studies of this disease paid little attention to any associated mental changes, but recently a number of studies have convincingly demonstrated a true dementia in many patients with parkinsonism.[11,18,78,107,108,136,139] The dementia occurs only in patients with well established disease and is not a presenting symptom. Because of this, parkinsonism need not be considered in the differential diagnosis of a patient with the initial presentation of a progressive dementia. There are some patients who develop a combined Alzheimer's/Parkinson's degeneration[68,193] and also patients with Alzheimer's, Pick's, or other dementing diseases that develop rigidity, tremor, and other parkinsonian features late in the progression of their disease. These disorders should be recognized as combined syndromes and not considered as parkinsonism alone.

Because the motor and other disabling features of Parkinsonism are always severe before the appearance of mental changes, it has been difficult to determine if the patient's mental changes represent a true dementia or merely result from a combination of physical and emotional symptoms which limit full performance on mental status and psychologic tests. Performance is slow and fraught with motor problems; speech is often inaudible or very difficult to understand; and the chronic physical disability often leads to a depressive reaction and reluctance to cooperate. All of these factors must be considered when

196

attempting to assess the intellectual functioning of the patient with parkinsonism. Despite these obstacles, it is becoming obvious that a large percentage of patients with parkinsonism (25 to 80 percent) develop true intellectual deterioration as the disease progresses.[107,108,175] In at least 50 percent of the cases, the dementia is mild and not a significant problem in the patient's management, but in 10 to 20 percent, the changes are severe and represent a major component of the patient's overall disability. In general, the severity of the dementia correlates well with the severity of other parkinsonian features; patients with severe neurologic signs (rigidity and bradykinesia) tend to have the greatest degree of dementia, whereas those with only tremor have less.[99,107,108] In addition, patients with idiopathic parkinsonism alone, either Lewy body type or Alzheimer tangle variety, have a lower incidence of dementia than those patients with parkinsonism who have a history of concomitant cerebral arteriosclerosis.[108,136]

The actual features of the Parkinson dementia have been quite consistent. Most investigators believe that there is a general lack of activation or arousal that pervades all behavior and impedes normal cognitive and social functioning.[5,18,143] Patients have difficulty with complex problem solving and concept formation, they often exhibit a lack of insight and poor judgement, and many have features of a frontal lobe syndrome with indifference and social impropriety.[11,18] On specific psychologic testing, the patient with parkinsonism often exhibits difficulty with constructional tasks, nonverbal reasoning tests such as Ravens Matrices, and a general decrease in Performance IQ.[5,78,100] Memory deficits, problems with verbal fluency, and speech perception problems have also been stressed by some investigators.[5,65] The patient with parkinsonism is also quite prone to episodes of confusional behavior. This is often related to medication but can occur in the unmedicated patient.

In addition to the cognitive changes discussed above, these patients have been shown to have a much higher incidence of depression than other physically disabled patients of the same age.[65,78] Recent theories concerning the pathophysiology of endogenous depression postulate a decrease in neurotransmitters, particularly dopamine. Since parkinsonism is primarily a disease of dopaminergic neurons, a similar mechanism may be operating to produce the depression in these patients. The very positive clinical response of these patients to the standard antidepressant medications strengthens the neurotransmitter hypothesis.

The prognosis of the dementia seen in parkinsonism is unfortunately little better than that of the other degenerative diseases. With the introduction of L-dopa therapy, it was hoped that mental symptoms would reverse as readily as the physical; however, this has not proved

197

to be true. At times there is temporary improvement, but within two years the dementia typically has continued its inexorable march.[17,70, 98,100,143] In some patients with a Parkinson-like syndrome including moderate dementia and mild extrapyramidal findings, a fairly dramatic improvement in mental state has been reported with L-dopa therapy.[40] Although these cases did not have classic parkinsonism, their response was so positive that we feel they deserve mention.

There was some early concern that L-dopa itself caused the dementia in patients with parkinsonism, but this position has not withstood careful scrutiny.[175] It is possible that the increased longevity and lessened disability that have resulted from the use of L-dopa have allowed dementia, when present, to become more apparent.

A behavioral side effect of L-dopa, discussed in Chapter 5, is the frequent precipitation of confusional behavior. In some studies, as many as 60 percent of the patients with parkinsonism developed this problem,[175] and in at least one case, a patient on L-dopa therapy developed a significant, irreversible encephalopathy after a severe confusional episode.[190] Permanent sequelae after confusional episodes can have various etiologies; the actual mechanisms are not well understood.

There is some indication that drug-related confusional episodes are much more likely to occur in the patient with parkinsonism who has evidence of dementia and slowing on his EEG.[175] The clinician should exercise caution in his use of L-dopa in such patients. When confusion occurs, we find that the only way to treat it is to decrease the dose of L-dopa.

The pathophysiology of the dementia in parkinsonism is not clear. Although some authors mention that frontal atrophy is seen in these patients, there has been very little pathologic study of the cortex in this disease.[9] The demented patient with parkinsonism does have greater cortical atrophy than age-matched normals, but the degree of atrophy does not seem sufficient to explain the degree of dementia, suggesting that many features of the dementia may relate to the subcortical lesions and not to cortical disease.

In some patients with a rather significant degree of dementia, the clinical picture suggests that a combined degenerative process with features of both parkinsonism and Alzheimer's disease is present.[95] Clinical pathologic studies verifying a complex degenerative process are few,[53,68,193] yet clinical experience indicates that the combined condition may be quite common. Since such patients have a defect both in the dopamine and acetylcholine systems, treatment of the parkinsonian symptoms with anticholinergic medications may cause deterioration in memory function. It is therefore important to be very careful in the selection of medication for the patient with both parkinsonism and significant dementia. Dopamine precursors seem to be both the safest and most effective.

Progressive Supranuclear Palsy

Progressive supranuclear palsy is a relatively uncommon Parkinson-like syndrome that was first fully described in 1964.[169] The disease usually begins in the 50s with vague emotional problems, imbalance, and difficulty with downward gaze. As the condition progresses, the patients develop a total external ophthalmoplegia with vertical gaze involved first and most severely; rigidity, with nuchal rigidity being a very prominent feature; retropulsion with a marked tendency to fall backwards; and a dementia characterized by slowness, memory loss, apathy, and difficulty with abstract reasoning, but with sparing of language and constructional ability.[6,119,169] The disease is most commonly reported in males (3:1 ratio), (although some of the reports are from Veterans Administration hospitals which would tend to bias the ratio) and runs a slow course with death occurring in 5 to 7 years.

Neuropathologic examination demonstrates extensive subcortical cell loss, gliosis, and neurofibrillary changes. The most heavily involved areas include the subthalamus, pallidum, substantia nigra, locus ceruleus, superior colliculi, and the dentate nuclei in the cerebellum. The cerebral cortex is normal.[169]

Rare Degenerative Diseases

Dementia is associated with a large group of rare degenerative diseases of the central nervous system. Most are hereditary and are found in population pockets where consanguinity is common and population mobility minimal. Several forms of spinocerebellar or olivopontocerebellar degeneration fall into this category and are often associated with a dementia. Of these, Friedreich's ataxia is probably the best known. The course of these classic abiotrophies is slow, with the dementia usually appearing late in the illness.

Familial myoclonic epilepsy is another rare condition in which dementia is a prominent symptom in most cases. The seizure state, however, is usually well established before the onset of the dementia and the diagnosis is not difficult to make.

CREUTZFELDT-JAKOB DISEASE

Creutzfeldt-Jakob disease is an uncommon (1 case per million) dementia, yet it is extremely important because of its scientific implications. The disease is caused by an unconventional (often transmissible) virus that has a very long incubation period (2 years). The disease has a relatively long clinical course (average 9 months, extremes 1 month and 6 years).[58,111] The onset and symptomatology of the disease vary considerably, with mental symptoms predominating in some cases, while neurologic signs are most prominent in others. The disease most frequently presents with nervousness, an increased startle response, anxiety, or other vague mental symptoms. Memory loss, confusional behavior, and frank psychosis are also seen.[66,111]

Neurologic signs of motor neuron involvement and cerebellar, basal ganglian, or pyramidal tract damage can all be seen either in combination or alone. Signs may be asymmetric and may undergo short periods of remission.[66] Myoclonic jerking is quite common as the disease progresses and is one of the primary distinguishing features. Severe dementia usually occurs within 6 months and progressive rigidity and mutism lead to death within 9 months in most cases.[148]

The clinical picture is usually quite clear, but atypical cases do occur. The electroencephalogram is frequently of great assistance in making the diagnosis, as it is abnormal and characteristic in 90 percent of the cases.[66] Initially, the EEG shows diffuse, often asymmetric slowing; however, the typical pattern of high voltage bursts of biphasic and triphasic slow waves soon appears (Fig. 6-8).

The disease is caused by a virus, yet 10 percent of cases have a strong dominant inheritance pattern. Transmission has been reported via surgical instruments, depth electrodes, corneal transplantation, and to surgeons and pathologists conducting surgery and autopsy, presumably through breaks in the skin.[58,181] The transmissibility of the virus

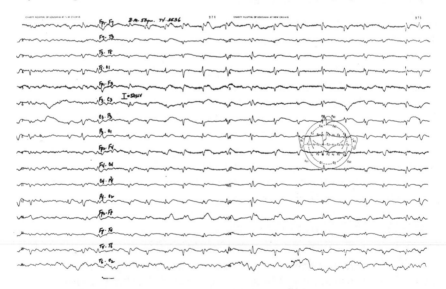

FIGURE 6–8   EEG of patient with Creutzfeldt-Jacob disease.

and the handling of infected material is more thoroughly discussed in Chapter 10.

Pathologically, the virus first causes vacuolation in the dendrite and axonal processes and the cell bodies of the neurons. Astroglia and oligodendroglia are less extensively effected. With progression, extensive gliosis occurs and finally a spongy degeneration. Unlike conventional viruses, no inflammatory response occurs, no cells are found in the spinal fluid, and the protein in the CSF is normal.[58]

DIALYSIS DEMENTIA

With the increase in the use of hemodialysis for chronic renal failure, a variety of neurologic syndromes is appearing. An unusual syndrome of mental change, speech disorder, and myoclonus has been reported in some patients who have received dialysis for several years.[7,8,24,102] The disease, at first thought rare, is the leading cause of death in the chronic, dialysis patient in some centers. Usually the condition is first noticed during the last hour or two of dialysis and is characterized primarily by a subtle personality change often associated with hesitancy in speech production and stuttering. These changes clear during the first 12 hours after dialysis. However, with successive dialysis periods, the changes progress: the speech disorder becomes more dramatic, and eventually the patients are mute by the end of the dialysis period; asterixis, facial grimacing, and myoclonus appear; confusional behavior occurs; general cognitive functioning decreases; seizures often occur; and the patients become almost immobile. This progression usually evolves over 4 to 6 months. During this time the patient is slower and slower to clear between dialysis sessions and eventually develops a chronic unremitting dementia. Focal neurologic findings are seen in 40 percent of cases, with facial and limb weakness being the most common features.

The electroencephalogram is always abnormal, with background slowing and superimposed paroxysmal high voltage, very slow waves (delta), triphasic waves, and often frank spikes.[102,122,138] In some patients, the EEG changes have been noted 6 months before the development of the dementia syndrome.[24] Treatment could logically be instituted during this early stage and development of the entire syndrome prevented.

Treatment has been hampered, in part, by the lack of agreement as to the etiology of the syndrome. The condition is not part of the disequilibrium syndrome, and the most convincing evidence points toward an accumulation of aluminum in the brain as the etiology. Some autopsy material has shown a clear increase in brain aluminum in patients dying with the syndrome,[113] and there has been clinical documentation of increased serum aluminum levels in some demented patients.[109,135] Clear reversal of the dementia has also been demonstrated in these patients when the aluminum level was reduced.[108,135] Elevated tin or calcium or decreased rubidium or phosphate have also been considered as the etiology but toxicity from aluminum seems by the far the most likely.[8,134] The source of the aluminum is varied, but in most cases it is either from exogenous aluminum gels taken by the patients[7,108,135] or from the water or purifying apparatus utilized during dialysis.[56,113]

Treatment has varied, renal transplantation showing only marginal success[24] but control of exogenous aluminum being more encouraging. Nadel[122] and Wilson were struck by the abnormal EEG findings in their patients and used diazepam (Valium) to suppress the epileptiform activity, rationalizing that the behavior change might actually be merely an epileptic state. The four patients that they reported upon did improve. Their experience is certainly encouraging when compared to the bleak prognosis experienced in most centers. An anticonvulsant regimen of diphenylhydantoin (Dilantin) and phenobarbital had been tried in earlier studies without effect.[8]

The pathology of this condition is nonspecific: the gross brain is not abnormal, but microscopically the cortex shows widespread nerve cell damage suggesting slow cell death from some adverse metabolic or toxic substance. The neurons appear shrunken and hyperpigmented with pyknotic hyperchromatic nuclei. Mild gliosis is present, and occasionally spongiform changes occur.[24]

MULTIPLE SCLEROSIS

Multiple sclerosis is a relatively common neurologic disease in which widespread distruction of myelin results in a remarkable array of neurologic signs and symptoms. Usually seen only in advanced cases, dementia may be the initial and predominant symptom in a few patients. In such cases, the disease is typically of later onset (41 to 72 years) and mimics other dementia except that the onset is quite rapid and includes memory loss, personality change, and confusional behavior as the primary symptoms.[92] Most patients show mild neurologic symptoms suggestive of myelopathy.

One of us (RLS) saw a 20-year-old male who was left with a significant recent memory defect after his initial attack. On examination, even after overheating in a hot bath, no positive neurologic signs were present. Examination during the acute phase and on subsequent follow-up[13] showed clear-cut brain stem and other findings.

Cases in which cognitive findings predominate are distinctly uncommon. In a series of 389 cases, Adams found only 7 patients in which the initial symptoms of the patient's demyelinating disease were organic mental symptoms.[1] Conversely, emotional or personality changes are often harbingers of the disease. Emotional lability, euphoria, and irritability are all rather common findings, and the multiple sclerosis patient is often diagnosed initially as being hysteric. Although clinically obvious intellectual decline is not commonly seen, a recent study utilizing a full battery of psychologic tests clearly demonstrated subtle, yet significant, cognitive impairment in a substantial number of patients with multiple sclerosis.[194] In some individuals, cognitive change accompanied minor neurologic dysfunction.

Pathologically, the major cerebral lesions are frequently in the frontal white matter closely surrounding the anterior horns of the lateral ventricles. This type of lesion disconnects many of the limbic fibers from the cingulate to the frontal lobes and has an effect similar to that of a cingulumotomy or frontal leukotomy. No pathologic studies are available on the patients with the dementia syndrome reported by Koenig[92] and a clinical pathologic correlation cannot be made on these cases.

DEMENTIA AS A REMOTE EFFECT OF CARCINOMA

The remote effect of carcinoma on the nervous system is a fascinating chapter in the study of cancer and its relation to the host. Many neurologic symptoms are seen in cancer patients—dementia being only one. In patients with nervous system symptoms, dementia is common. In one series of 42 patients, 14 (33%) were effected.[19] The dementia is described as "simple, with progressive intellectual impairment and memory failure."[19] The dementia is frequently associated with other central nervous system symptoms, particularly cerebellar findings.

Another syndrome, progressive multifocal leukoencephalopathy, produces an interesting group of neurologic symptoms but not a true dementia. This condition is caused by a viral invasion of the brain and will be discussed in Chapter 10, Infections of the Central Nervous System.

DESTRUCTIVE ENCEPHALOPATHIES

Within the symptom complex of dementia are a number of conditions more properly called encephalopathies due to specific causes. These conditions do not follow the usual gradual progression seen in dementia; but rather, their onset is quite abrupt and due to a specific widespread insult to the brain parenchyma. Serious head trauma, encephalitis, meningitis, and severe anoxia are the most common varieties. The clinical picture is usually one of mental status changes and neurologic findings that differ in each case. These conditions will be discussed in subsequent chapters as they are not involved in the differential diagnosis of dementia in the traditional sense.

Evaluation and Management

Other than specific treatment of the underlying etiology of diseases such as myxedema, the general principles of evaluation and management of dementia are the same as were outlined in the previous chapter. It is obvious that the prognosis, genetic aspects, and associated systemic and neurologic problems vary tremendously.

REFERENCES

1. Adams, D.K., Sutherland, J.M., and Fletcher, W.B.: Early clinical manifestations of disseminated sclerosis. Br. Med. J. 2:431, 1950.
2. Adams, R.D.: Acquired hepatocerebral degeneration, in Vinken, P.J., and Bruyn, G. W. (eds.): Handbook of Clinical Neurology, Vol. 6. Elsevier-North Holland Publishing Co., New York, 1968, pp. 279–297.
3. Adams, R.D., Fisher, C.M., Hakim, S., Ojemann, R.C., and Sweet, W.H.: Symptomatic occult hydrocephalus with "normal" cerebrospinal fluid pressure. N. Engl. J.Med. 273:117, 1965.
4. Adams, R.D., and Kubik, C.S.: Subacute combined degeneration of the brain in pernicious anemia. N. Engl. J. Med. 231:1, 1944.
5. Albert, M.L.: Subcortical dementia. Presented at the International Neuropsychology Society Meeting, February, 1977. Sante Fe, New Mexico.
6. Albert, M.L., Feldman, R.G., and Willis, A.L.: The subcortical dementia of progressive supranuclear palsy. J. Neurol. Neurosurg. Psychiatry 37: 121, 1974.
7. Alfrey, A.C., Le Gendre, G.R., and Kaehny, W.D.: The dialysis encephalopathy syndrome. N. Engl. J. Med. 294:184, 1976.
8. Alfrey, A.C., Mishell, J.M., Burks, J., Contiguglea, S.R., Randolph, H., Lewin, E., and Holmes, J.H.: Syndrome of dyspraxia and multifocal seizures associated with chronic dialysis. Trans. Am. Soc. Artif. Intern. Organs 18:257, 1972.
9. Alvord, E.C., Jr.: Pathology of Parkinsonism: Part II. An interpretation with special reference to other changes in the aging brain, in McDowell, F.H., and Markham, C.H. (eds.): Recent Advances in Parkinson's Disease. F.A. Davis, Philadelphia, 1971, pp. 131–161.
10. Asher, R.: Myxoedematous madness. Br. Med. J. 2:555, 1949.
11. Barbeau, A.: Long-term appraisal of levodopa therapy. Neurology 22:22 (May suppl.), 1972.
12. Bennett, R., Hughes, G.R.V., Bywaters, E.G.L., and Holt, P.J.L.: Neuropsychiatric problems in systemic lupus erthematosus. Br. Med. J. 4:342, 1972.
13. Benson, D.F.: Personal communication. August, 1978.
14. Benson, D.F., LeMay, M., Patten, D.H., and Rubens, A.B.: Diagnosis of normal-pressure hydrocephalus. N. Engl. J. Med. 283:609, 1970.
15. Bockner, S., and Cultart, N.: New cases of general paralysis of the insane. Br. Med. J. 1:18, 1961.
16. Boll, T.J., Heaton, R., and Reitan, R.M.: Neuropsychological and emotional correlates of Huntington's chorea. J. Nerv. Ment. Dis. 158:61, 1974.
17. Botez, M.I., and Barbeau, A.: Long-term mental changes in levodopa-treated patients. Lancet 2:1028, 1973.
18. Bowen, F.P., Kamienny, R.S., Burns, M.M., and Yahr, M.D.: Parkinsonism:

effects of levodopa treatment on concept formation. Neurology 25:701, 1975.

19. Brain, R., and Henson, R.A.: Neurological syndromes associated with carcinoma. Lancet 2:971, 1958.

20. Brewer, C., and Perrett, L.: Brain damage due to alcohol consumption: an air-encephalographic, psychometric, and electroencephalographic study. Br. J. Addict. 66:170, 1971.

21. Brown, D.G., and Goldensohn, E.S.: The electroencephalogram in normal pressure hydrocephalus. Arch. Neurol. 29:70, 1973.

22. Bruyn, G.W.: Huntington's chorea—history, clinical, and laboratory synopsis, in Vinken, P.J., and Bruyn, A.W. (eds.): Handbook of Clinical Neurology, Vol. 6. Elsevier-North Holland Publishing Co., New York, 1968, pp. 298–378.

23. Burger, P.C., Burch, J.G., and Kunze, U.: Subcortical arteriosclerotic encephalopathy (Binswanger's disease). Stroke 7:626, 1976.

24. Burks, J.S., Alfrey, A.C., Huddleston, J., Norenbert, M.D., and Lewin, E.: A fatal encephalopathy in chronic haemodialysis patients. Lancet 1: 764, 1976.

25. Caine, E.D., Hunt, R.D., Weingartner, H., and Ebert, M.H.: Huntington's dementia. Arch. Gen. Psychiatry 35:377, 1978.

26. Caplan, L.R., and Schoene, W.C.: Clinical features of subclinical arteriosclerotic encephalopathy (Binswanger disease). Neurology 28:1206, 1978.

27. Chawla, J.C., Hulme, A., and Cooper, R.: Intracranial pressure in patients with dementia and communicating hydrocephalus. J. Neurosurg. 40: 376, 1974.

28. Chia, B.H., and Tsoi, W.F.: A study of 136 cases of general paralysis of the insane (dementia paralytica) in a mental hospital. Singapore Med. J. 12:264, 1971.

29. Chynoweth, R., and Foley, J.: Pre-senile dementia responding to steroid therapy. Br. J. Psychiatry 115:703, 1969.

30. Clark, E.C., and Yoss, R.E.: Nervous system findings associated with systemic lupus erythematosus. Minn. Med. 39:517, 1956.

31. Coblentz, J.M., Mattis, S., Zingesser, L.H., Kasoff, S.S., Wisniewski, H.M., and Katzman, R.: Presenile dementia. Arch. Neurol. 29:299, 1973.

32. Committee of Clinical Society of London: Report on myxedema. Clinical Society's Transactions 21 (Supp.):1, 1888, Gongmans, Green and Company, London.

33. Editorial: Communicating hydrocephalus. Lancet 2:1011, 1977.

34. Corsellis, J.A.N.: Aging and the dementias, in Blackwood, W., and Corsellis, J.A.N. (eds.): Greenfield's Neuropathology. Arnold, London, 1976, pp. 796–848.

35. Courville, C.B., and Myers, R.O.: Effects of extraneous poisons on the nervous system II: the alcohols. Bull. Los Angeles Neurol. Soc. 19:66, 1957.

36. Crockard, H.A., Hanlan, K., Duda, E.E., and Mullan, J.F.: Hydrocephalus as a cause of dementia; evaluation by computerized tomography and intracranial pressure monitoring. J. Neurol. Neurosurg. Psychiatry 40: 736, 1977.

37. DeGirolami, U., Haas, M.L., and Richardson, E.P., Jr.: Subacute diencephalic angioencephalopathy. J. Neurol. Sci. 22:197, 1974.

38. Deland, F.H., James, A.E., Ladd, D.J., and Konigsmark, B.W.: Normal

pressure hydrocephalus: a histologic study. Am. J. Clin. Pathol. 58:58, 1972.

39. Denny-Brown, D.D.: Nature of apraxia. J. Nerv. Ment. Dis. 126:9, 1958.
40. Drachman, D.A., and Stahl, S.: Extrapyramidal dementia and levodopa. Lancet 1:809, 1975.
41. Drake, E.W., Jr., Baker, M., Blumenkrantz, J., and Dahlgren, H.: The quality and duration of survival in bilateral carotid occlusive disease. A preliminary survey of the effect of thromboendarterectomy, in Toole, J.F., Siekert, R.G., and Whisnant, J.P. (eds.): Cerebral Vascular Disease: Sixth Conference. Grune and Stratton, New York, 1968, pp. 242–259.
42. Dreyfus, P.M.: Amblyopia and other neurological disorders associated with chronic alcoholism., in Vinkin, P.J., and Bruyn, G.W. (eds.): Handbook of Clinical Neurology, Vol. 28. Elsevier-North Holland Publishing Co., New York, 1976, pp. 331–347.
43. Earnest, M.P., Fahn, S., Karp, J.H., and Rowland, L.P.: Normal pressure hydrocephalus and hypertensive cerebrovascular disease. Arch. Neurol. 31:262, 1974.
44. Enna, S.J., Bird, E.D., Bennett, J.P., Bylund, D.B., Yamamura, H.I., Iversen, L.L., and Synder, S.H.: Huntington's Chorea. New Engl. J. Med. 294:1305, 1976.
45. Eraut, D.: Idiopathic hypoparathyroidism presenting as dementia. Br. Med. J. 1:429, 1974.
46. Ferguson, G.G., and Peerless, S.J.: Extracranial-intracranial arterial bypass in the treatment of dementia and multiple extracranial arterial occlusion. Presented at the Congress of Neurological Surgeons, New Orleans, October 25–29, 1976.
47. Fessel, W.J., and Solomon, G.F.: Psychosis and systemic lupus erythematosus: a review of the literature and case reports. Calif. Med. 92:266, 1960.
48. Fisher, C.M.: Senile dementia—A new explanation of its causation. Can. Med. Assoc. J. 65:1, 1951.
49. Fisher, C.M.: Dementia in cerebrovascular disease, in Toole, J.F., Siekert, R.G., and Whisnant, J.P. (eds.): Cerebral Vascular Disease: Sixth Conference. Grune and Stratton, New York, 1968, pp. 232–236.
50. Fisher, C.M.: Case records of the Massachusetts General Hospital. New Engl. Med. J. 291:966, 1974.
51. Fisher, C.M.: The clinical picture in occult hydrocephalus. Clin. Neurosurg. 24:270, 1977.
52. Fisher, C.M.: Communicating hydrocephalus, Lancet 1:37, 1978.
53. Forno, L.S., Barbour, P.J., and Norville, R.L.: Presenile dementia with Lewy bodies and neurofibrillary tangles. Arch. Neurol. 35:818, 1978.
54. Fox, J.H., Ramsey, R.G., Huckman, M.S., and Praske, A.E.: Cerebral ventricular enlargement. JAMA 236:365, 1976.
55. Freeman, F.R.: Evaluation of patients with progressive intellectual deterioration. Arch. Neurol. 33:658, 1976.
56. Flendrig, J.A., Kruis, H., and Das, H.A.: Aluminium and dialysis dementia. Lancet 1:764, 1976.
57. Gado, M.H., Coleman, R.E., Lee, K.S., Mikhael, M.A., Alderson, P.O., and Archer, C.R.: Correlation between computerized transaxial tomography and radionuclide cisternography in dementia. Neurology 26:555, 1976.
58. Gajdusek, D.C.: Unconventional viruses and the origin and disappearance of kuru. Science 197:943, 1977.

59. Geagea, K., and Ananth, J.: Response of a psychiatric patient to vitamin B_{12} therapy. Dis. Nerv. Syst. 36:343, 1975.
60. Geschwind, N.: The mechanism of normal pressure hydrocephalus. J. Neurol. Sci. 7:481, 1968.
61. Godt, P., and Kochen, M.: Vitamin B_{12} deficiency due to psychotic-induced malnutrition. Lancet 2:1087, 1976.
62. Gold, A.P., and Yahr, M.D.: Childhood lupus erythematosus. Trans. Am. Neurol. Assoc. 85:96, 1960.
63. Goldstein, N.P., Ewert, J.C., Randall, R.V., and Gross, J.B.: Psychiatric aspects of Wilson's disease: results of psychometric tests during long-term therapy. Birth Defects 4:77, 1968.
64. Greitz, T., and Grepe, A.: Encephalography in the diagnosis of convexity block hydrocephalus. Acta Radiol. [Diagn.] (Stockh.) 11:232, 1971.
65. Haaland, K.V., and Matthews, G.: Cognitive and Motor Performance in Parkinsonism of Increasing Duration. Presented at the International Neuropsychology Society meeting, Sante Fe, New Mexico, February, 1977.
66. Haase, G.R.: Diseases presenting as dementia. In Wells, C.E. (ed.): Dementia. F.A. Davis, Philadelphia, 1977, pp. 27–67.
67. Hachinski, V.C., Lassen, N.A., and Marshall, J.: Multi-infarct dementia. Lancet 2:207, 1974.
68. Hakim, A.M., and Mathieson, G.: Dementia in Parkinson disease: A neuropathologic study. Neurology 29:1209, 1979.
69. Hakim, S., and Adams, R.D.: The special clinical problem of symptomatic hydrocephalus with normal cerebrospinal fluid pressure. Observations in cerebrospinal fluid dynamics. J. Neurol. Sci. 2:307, 1965.
70. Halgin, R., Riklan, M., and Misiak, H.: Levodopa, parkinsonism, and recent memory. J. Nerv. Ment. Dis. 164:268, 1977.
71. Harrison, M.J.G., and Marsden, C.D.: Progressive intellectual deterioration. Arch. Neurol. 34:199, 1977.
72. Harrison, M.J.G., Thomas, D.J., DuBoulay, G.H., and Marshall, J.: Multi-infarct dementia. J. Neurol. Sci. 40:97, 1979.
73. Hartmann, A., and Alberti, E.: Differentiation of communicating hydrocephalus and presenile dementia by continuous recording of cerebrospinal fluid pressure. J. Neurol. Neurosurg. Psychiatry 40:630, 1977.
74. Hécaen, H., and DeAjuriaguerra, J.: Les encephalopathies alcooliques subaigues et chroniques. Rev. Neurol. (Paris) 94:528, 1956.
75. Heine, B.E.: Psychiatric aspects of systemic lupus erythematous. Acta Psychiatr. Scand. 45:307, 1969.
76. Holmes, G.: Discussion on the mental symptoms associated with cerebral tumors. Proc. R. Soc. Med. 24:65, 1931.
77. Holmes, J.M.: Cerebral manifestations of vitamin B_{12} deficiency. Br. Med. J. 2:1394, 1956.
78. Horn, S.: Some psychological factors in parkinsonism. J. Neurol. Neurosurg. Psychiatry 37:27, 1974.
79. Horvath, T.B.: Clinical spectrum and epidemiological features of alcoholic dementia, in Rankin, J.G., and Lambert, S.L. (eds.): International Symposium on Effects of Chronic Use of Alcohol and Other Psychoactive Drugs on Cerebral Function, Toronto, October, 1973. Alcoholism and Drug Addiction Research Foundation of Ontario, 1975, pp. 1–16.
80. Inose, T.: Neuropsychiatric manifestations in Wilson's disease: Attacks of disturbance of consciousness. Birth Defects 4:74, 1968.

81. Jacobs, L., Conti, D., Kinkel, W.R., and Manning, E.: Normal pressure hydrocephalus. JAMA 235:510, 1976.
82. Jacobs, L., and Kinkel, W.R.: Computerized axial transverse tomography in normal pressure hydrocephalus. Neurology 26:501, 1976.
83. Jellinek, E.H.: Fits, faints, coma, and dementia in myxoedema. Lancet 2:1010, 1962.
84. Johnson, R.T., and Richardson, E.P.: The neurologic manifestations of systemic lupus erythematosus. Medicine 47:337, 1968.
85. Jurko, M.F., and Andy, O.J.: Psychological changes associated with thalamotomy site. J. Neurol. Neurosurg. Psychiatry 36:846, 1973.
86. Kahn, E., and Thompson, J.J.: Concerning Pick's disease. Am. J. Psychiatry 90:935, 1934.
87. Kass, L.: Pernicious anemia, in Smith, L.H. (ed.): Major problems in internal medicine, Vol. 7. W.B. Saunders, Philadelphia, 1976, pp. 116–122.
88. Katzman, R.: Normal pressure hydrocephalus, in Wells, C.E. (ed.): Dementia. F.A. Davis, Philadelphia, 1977, pp. 69–92.
89. Katzman, R., and Karasu, T.B.: Differential diagnosis of dementia, in Fields, W.S. (ed.): Neurological and Sensory Disorders in the Elderly. Stratton Intercontinental Medical Book, New York, 1974.
90. Keschner, M., Bender, M.B., and Strauss, T.: Mental symptoms in cases of tumor of the temporal lobe. Arch. Neurol. Psychiatry 35:572, 1936.
91. Kleinknecht, R.A., and Goldstein, S.C.: Neuropsychological deficits associated with alcoholism: a review and discussion. Q. J. Stud. Alcohol. 33:999, 1972.
92. Koenig, H.: Dementia associated with the benign form of multiple sclerosis. Trans. Am. Neurol. Assoc. 93:227, 1968.
93. Koto, A., Rosenberg, A., Zingesser, L.H., Horoupian, D., and Katzman, R.: Syndrome of normal pressure hydrocephalus: possible relation to hypertensive and arteriosclerotic vasculopathy. J. Neurol. Neurosurg. Psychiatry 40:73, 1977.
94. Levin, S.: Brain tumors in mental hospital patients. Am. J. Psychiatry 195:897, 1949.
95. Lieberman, A., Dziatolowski, M., Kupersmith, M., Serby, M., Goodgold, A., Korein, J. and Goldstein, M.: Dementia in Parkinson disease. Ann. Neurol. 6:355, 1979.
96. Littman, M.L., and Zimmerman, L.E.: Cryptococcus. Grune and Stratton, New York, 1956.
97. Logothetis, J.: Psychotic behavior as the initial indicator of adult myxedema. J. Nerv. Ment. Dis. 136:561, 1963.
98. Loranger, A.W., Goodell, H., Lee, J.E., and McDowell, F.H.: Levodopa treatment of parkinsonism syndrome. Arch. Gen. Psychiatry 26:163, 1972.
99. Loranger, A.W., Goodell, H., McDowell, F.H., Lee, J.E., and Sweet, R.D.: Intellectual impairment in Parkinson's syndrome. Brain 95:405, 1972.
100. Loranger, A.W., Goodell, H., McDowell, F.H., Lee, J.E., and Sweet, R.D.: Parkinsonism, L-dopa, and intelligence. Am. J. Psychiatry 130:1386, 1973.
101. MacNeill, A., Grennan, D.M., Ward, D., and Dick, W.C.: Psychiatric problems in systemic lupus erythematosus. Br. J. Psychiatry 128:442, 1976.
102. Mahurkar, S.D., Dhar, S.K., Salta, R., Meyers, L., Smith, E.C., and Dunea, G.: Dialysis dementia. Lancet 1:1412, 1973.

103. Malamud, N.: Neuropathology of organic brain syndromes associated with aging, in Gaitz, C.M. (ed.): Aging and the Brain, Vol. 3 in Advances in Behavioral Biology. Plenum, New York, 1972, pp. 63–87.
104. Malmquist, C.P., and Kincannon, J.C.: Psychiatric and psychological aspects of myxedema. Dis. Nerv. Syst. 21:529, 1960.
105. Mansvelt, J. V.: Pick's Disease. N.V.Voorheen Firma J.J.V.D. Loeff Enschede, Netherlands, 1954.
106. Marsden, D.D., and Harrison, M.J.G.: Outcome of investigation of patients with presenile dementia. Br. Med. J. 2:249, 1972.
107. Martin, W.E., Loewenson, R.B., Resch, J.A., and Baker, A.B.: Parkinson's disease. Clinical analysis of 100 patients. Neurology 23:783, 1973.
108. Marttila, R.J., and Rinne, V.K.: Dementia in Parkinson's disease. Acta Neurol. Scand. 54:431, 1976.
109. Masselot, J.P., Adhemar, J.P., Jaudon, M.C., Kleinknecht, D., and Galli, A.: Reversible dialysis encephalopathy: role for aluminium-containing gels. Lancet 2:1386, 1978.
110. Mathew, N.T., Meyer, J.S., Hartmann, A., and Ott, E.O.: Abnormal cerebrospinal fluid-blood flow dynamics. Arch. Neurol. 32:657, 1975.
111. May, W.: Creutzfeldt-Jakob disease. Acta Neurol. Scand. 44:1, 1968.
112. McCullough, N.B., Louria, D.B., Hilbish, T.F., Thomas, I.B., and Emmons, C.: Cryptococcus. Clinical staff conference at the National Institutes of Health. Ann. Intern. Med. 49:642, 1958.
113. McDermott, J.R., Smith, A.E., Ward, M.K., Parkinson, I.S., and Kerr, D.N.S.: Brain-aluminium concentration in dialysis encephalopathy. Lancet 1:901, 1978.
114. McHugh, P.R.: Occult hydrocephalus. Q.J.Med. 33:297, 1964.
115. McHugh, P.R., and Folstein, M.F. Psychiatric syndromes of Huntington's chorea: a clinical and phenomenologic study, in Benson, D.F., and Blumer, D. (eds.): Psychiatric Aspects of Neurological Disease. Grune and Stratton, New York, 1975, p. 267–286.
116. Meacham, W.F., and Young, A.B.: Radiological procedures in the diagnosis of dementia, in Wells, C.E. (ed.). Dementia. F.A. Davis, Philadelphia, 1971, pp. 100–110.
117. Meadows, J.C.: Normal pressure hydrocephalus. Lancet 1:618, 1973.
118. Merritt, H.H., Adams, R.D., and Solomon, H.C.: Neurosyphilis. Oxford University Press, New York, 1946.
119. Messert, B., and Van Nuis, C.: A syndrome of paralysis of downward gaze, dysarthria, pseudobulbar palsy, axial rigidity of neck and trunk and dementia. J. Nerv. Ment. Dis. 143:47, 1966.
120. Morel, F.: Une Forme anatomo-clinique particuliere de l'alcoolisme chronique: sclerose cortical laminaire alcoolique. Rev. Neurol. (Paris) 71: 280, 1939.
121. Mosberg, W.H., and Arnold, J.G.: Torulosis of the central system: review of literature and report of five cases. Ann. Intern. Med. 32:1153, 1950.
122. Nadel, A.M., and Wilson, W.P.: Dialysis encephalopathy: a possible seizure disorder. Neurology 26:1130, 1976.
123. Neubuerger, K.T.: The changing neuropathologic picture of chronic alcoholism. Arch. Path. 63:1, 1957.
124. Neumann, M.A., and Cohen, R.: Progressive subcortical gliosis: a rare form of presenile dementia. Brain 90:405, 1967.
125. Nickel, S.N., and Frame, B.: Neurological manifestations of myxedema. Neurology 8:511, 1958.

126. O'Conner, J.F., and Musher, D.M.: Central nervous system involvement in systemic lupus erythematosus. Arch. Neurol. 14:157, 1966.
127. Ojemana, G.D. (ed.): The thalamus and language. Special issue. Brain Lang. 2:1, 1975.
128. Ojemann, R.G., Fisher, C.M., Adams, R.D., Sweet, W.H., and New, P.F.J.: Further experience with the syndrome of "normal" pressure hydrocephalus. J. Neurosurg. 31:279, 1969.
129. Olszewski, J.: Subcortical arteriosclerotic encephalopathy. Review of the literature on the so-called Binswanger's disease and presentation of two cases. World Neurology 3:359, 1962.
130. Oltman, J.E., and Friedman, S.: Comments on Huntington's chorea. Dis. Nerv. System 22:313, 1961.
131. Paulson, G.W., Kapp, J., and Cook, W.: Dementia associated with bilateral carotid artery disease. Geriatrics 21:159, 1966.
132. Pearce, J., and Miller, E.: Clinical Aspects of Dementia. Bailliere-Tindall, London, 1973.
133. Petersen, P.: Psychiatric disorders in primary hyperparathyroidism. J. Clin. Endocrin. 28:1491, 1968.
134. Pieridas, A.M., Ward, M.K., and Kerr, D.N.S.: Haemodialysis encephalopathy: possible role of phosphate depletion. Lancet 1:1234, 1976.
135. Poisson, M., Mashaly, R., and Lebkiri, B.: Dialysis encephalopathy: recovery after interruption of aluminium intake. Br. Med. J. 2:1610, 1978.
136. Pollock, M., and Hornabrook, R.W.: The prevalance, natural history and dementia of Parkinson's disease. Brain 89:429, 1966.
137. Price, T.R.P., and Tucker, G.J.: Psychiatric and behavioral manifestations of normal pressure hydrocephalus. J. Nerv. Ment. Dis. 164:51, 1977.
138. Raskin, N.H., and Fishman, R.A.: Neurologic disorders in renal failure. New Engl. J. Med. 294:204, 1976.
139. Reitan, R.M., and Boll, T.J.: Intellectual and cognitive functions in Parkinson's disease. J. Consult. Clin. Psychol. 37:364, 1971.
140. Reynolds, R.H.: The neurology of vitamin B_{12} deficiency. Lancet 2:832, 1976.
141. Rice, E., and Gendelman, S.: Psychiatric aspects of normal pressure hydrocephalus. JAMA 223:409, 1973.
142. Riggs, C.E.: Some nervous system symptoms of pernicious anemia. JAMA 61:481, 1913.
143. Riklan, M., Whelihan, W., and Cullinan, T.: Levodopa and psychometric tests performance in parkinsonism—5 years later. Neurology 26:173, 1976.
144. Robertson, E.E., le Roux, A., and Brown, J.H.: The clinical presentation of Pick's disease. J. Ment. Sci. 104:1000, 1958.
145. Robinson, K.C., Kallberg, M.H., and Crowley, W.F.: Idiopathic hypoparathyroidism presenting as dementia. Br. Med.J. 2:1203, 1954.
146. Romanul, F.C., and Abramowicz, A.: Changes in the brain and pial vessels in the arterial border zones. Arch. Neurol. 11:40, 1964.
147. Roos, D., and Willanger, R.: Various degrees of dementia in a selected group of gastrectomized patients with low serum B_{12}. Acta Neurol. Scand. 55:363, 1977.
148. Roos, R. P., and Johnson, R.T.: Viruses and dementia, in Wells, C.E. (ed.): Dementia. F.A. Davis, Philadelphia, 1977, pp. 93–112.
149. Rose, F.C., Grant, H.C., and Jeanes, A.L.: Torulosis of the central nervous system in Britain. Brain 8:542, 1958.

150. Rose, M.: Why assess vitamin B_{12} deficiency due to psychotic-induced malnutrition? Lancet 2:1087, 1976.
151. Sanders, V.: Neurologic manifestations of myxedema. New Engl. J. Med. 266:547, 1962.
152. Sapira, J.D., Tullis, S., and Mullaly, R.: Reversible dementia due to folate deficiency. South. Med. J. 68:776, 1975.
153. Sargent, J.S., Lockshin, M.D., Klempner, M.S., and Lipsky, B.A.: Central nervous system disease in systemic lupus erythematosus. Am. J. Med. 58:644, 1975.
154. Sarosi, G.A., Parker, J.D., Doto, I.L., and Tosh, F.E.: Amphotericin B in cryptococcal meningitis. Ann. Intern. Med. 71:1079, 1969.
155. Scheinberg, I.H., Sternlieb, I., and Richman, J.: Psychiatric manifestations in patients with Wilson's disease. Birth Defects 4:85, 1968.
156. Schmidt, R.P., and Gonyea, E.F.: Neurosyphilis, in Baker, A.B. and Baker, L.H. (eds.): Clinical Neurology. Harper and Row, New York, 1976.
157. Schulman, R.: Vitamin B_{12} deficiency and psychiatric illness. Br. J. Psychiatry 113:252, 1967.
158. Schulman, R.: The present status of vitamin B_{12} and folic acid deficiency in psychiatric disease. Can. Psychiatr. Assoc. J. 17:205–216, 1972.
159. Schulman, S.: Bilateral symmetrical degeneration of the thalamus. J. Neuropathol. Exp. Neurol. 16:446, 1957.
160. Schulman, S.: Impaired tool-using behavior in monkeys from bilateral destruction of the dorsomedial nuclei of the thalamus. Trans. Am. Neurol. Assoc. 97:138, 1973.
161. Seltzer, B., and Sherwin, I.: Organic brain syndromes: an empirical study and critical review. Am. J. Psychiatry 13:21, 1978.
162. Shenkin, H.A., Greenberg, J., Bouzarth, W.F., Gutterman, P., and Morales, J.O.: Ventricular shunting for relief of senile symptoms. JAMA 225:1486, 1973.
163. Simpson, J.A.: The neurological manifestations of idiopathic hypoparathyroidism. Brain 75:76, 1952.
164. Sjögren, T., Sjögren, H., and Lindgren, A.G.H.: Morbus Alzheimer and Morbus Pick: genetic, clinical and pathoanatomic study. Acta Psychiatr. Neurol. Scand. Suppl. 82, 1952.
165. Slaby, A.E., and Wyatt, R.J.: Dementia in the Presenium. Charles C Thomas, Springfield, Illinois, 1974.
166. Sohn, R.S., Siegel, B.A., Gade, M., and Torack, R.M.: Alzheimer's disease with abnormal cerebrospinal fluid flow. Neurology 23:1058, 1973.
167. Sourander, P., and Sjögren, H.: The concept of Alzheimer's disease and its clinical implications, in Walstenholme, G.E.W., and O'Connor, M. (eds.): Alzheimer's Disease and Related Conditions. Churchill, London, 1970, pp. 11–32.
168. Spillane, J.D.: Nervous and mental disorders in Cushing's syndrome. Brain 74:72, 1951.
169. Steele, J.C., Richardson, J.C., and Olszewski, J.: Progressive supranuclear palsy. Arch. Neurol. 10:333, 1964.
170. Stengle, E.: A study on the symptomatology and differential diagnosis of Alzheimer's disease and Pick's disease. J. Ment. Sci. 89:1, 1943.
171. Stern, K.: Severe dementia associated with bilateral symmetrical degeneration of the thalamus. Brain 62:157, 1939.
172. Strauss, I., and Keschner, M.: Mental symptoms in cases of tumor of frontal lobe. Arch. Neurol. Psychiatry 33:986, 1935.

211

173. Stuteville, P., and Welch, K.: Subdural hematoma in the elderly person. JAMA 168:1445, 1958.
174. Sugar, O.: Central neurological complications of hypoparathyroidism. Arch. Neurol Psychiatry 70:86, 1953.
175. Sweet, R.R., McDowell, F.H., Feigenson, J.S., Loranger, A.W., and Goodell, H.: Mental symptoms in Parkinson's disease during chronic treatment with levodopa. Neurology 26:305, 1976.
176. Tarter, R.E.: An analysis of cognitive deficits in chronic alcoholics. J. Nerv. Ment. Dis. 157:138, 1973.
177. Terry, R.D.: Dementia. Arch. Neurol. 33:1, 1976.
178. Todorov, A.B., Constantinidis, J., Go, R.C.P., and Elston, R.C.: Specificity of the clinical diagnosis of dementia. J. Neurol. Sci. 26:81, 1975.
179. Tomilson, B.E., Blessed, G., and Roth, M.: Observations on the brains of demented old people. J.Neurol. Sci. 11:205, 1970.
180. Torvik, A.: Aspects of the pathology of presenile dementia. Acta Neurol. Scand. [Suppl.] 43, 46:19, 1970.
181. Traub, R., Gajdusek, D.C., and Gibbs, C.J., Jr.: Transmissible virus dementia: the relation of transmissible spongiform encephalopathy to Cruetzfeldt-Jakob disease, in Smith, W.L., and Kinsbourne, M. (eds.): Aging and Dementia. Spectrum Publications, New York, 1977, pp. 91–168.
182. Trethowan, W.H., and Cobb, S.: Neuropsychiatric aspects of Cushing's syndrome. Arch. Neurol. Psychiatry 67:283, 1952.
183. Walker, S.: The psychiatric presentation of Wilson's disease (hepatolenticular degeneration) with an etiologic explanation. Behav. Neuropsychiatry 1:38, 1969.
184. Walshe, J.M.: Wilson's disease, in Vinken, P.V., and Bruyn, G.W. (eds.): Handbook of Clinical Neurology, Vol. 27. Elsevier-North Holland Publishing Co., New York, 1976, pp. 379–414.
185. Warner, F.J.: The brain changes in chronic alcoholism and Korsakov's psychosis. J. Nerv. Ment. Dis. 80:629, 1934.
186. Wells, C.E.: Dementia. F.A. Davis, Philadelphia, 1977.
187. Wilson, S.A.K.: Neurology. Williams & Wilkins, Baltimore, 1940.
188. Wilson, S.A.K.: Progressive lenticular degeneration: a familial nervous disease associated with cirrhosis of the liver. Brain 34:296, 1912.
189. Wisniewski, N. M., Coblentz, J. M, and Terry, R. D.: Pick's disease. Arch. Neurol. 26:97, 1972.
190. Wolf, S. M., and Davis, R. L.: Permanent dementia in idiopathic parkinsonism treated with levodopa. Arch. Neurol. 29:276, 1973.
191. Yakovlev, P. I.: Paraplegias of hydrocephalics. A clinical note and interpretation. J. Ment. Defic. 51:561, 1947.
192. Yakovlev, P. I.: Pick's disease. Special Lecture given at the Boston Veterans Administration Hospital, February, 1973.
193. Boller, F., Mizutani, T., Roessmann, U., and Gambetti, P.: Parkinson's disease, dementia, and Alzheimer's disease: Clinicopathological correlations. Ann. Neurol. 7:329,1980.
194. Peyser, J.M., Edwards, K.R., Poser, C., and Filskov, S.B.: Cognitive function in patients with multiple sclerosis. Arch. Neurol. 37:577, 1980.

7

NEUROBEHAVIORAL SYNDROMES ASSOCIATED WITH FOCAL BRAIN LESIONS

A 29-year-old male was brought to the Charity Hospital in New Orleans with a two day history of abnormal behavior. The young man had been out with a group of friends the night previous to the onset of his strange behavior. The friends did not admit to the use of any drugs and said only that the patient had gone home early complaining of being tired. The following morning, he was very slow to awaken. His family reported that he was talking very strangly and did not seem to answer their questions appropriately. This abnormal behavior persisted throughout the day and the family brought him to the hospital that evening.

The patient appeared to be a normal well developed male who demonstrated no abnormalities on routine physical and neurologic examination. On mental status testing, he was awake, alert, and attentive but seemed somewhat withdrawn and uneasy. The psychiatric consultant stated that the patient was "grossly psychotic; he answers all questions totally inappropriately." Because of his inappropriate responses, withdrawal, and rather flat affect, he was admitted to the psychiatric ward with an initial diagnosis of an acute schizophrenic reaction, possibly drug related.

During the subsequent several days, the patient's condition did not improve, and a neurologic consultation was sought to rule out any organic cause for the bizarre behavior. Standard neurologic examination was again normal, but the mental status examination demonstrated striking abnormalities. The patient was alert and appeared attentive but could not repeat digits or comprehend the nature of the "A" test. Spontaneous speech was fluent, yet laconic, always off the point of the question, and contained occasional paraphasic substitutions. Comprehension was nil; he could not point to any objects on command and performed at only chance level when asked to point to one of three common objects placed in front of him. He could not answer questions requiring yes-no answers and could not follow simple verbal commands.

He could not repeat words or sentences. He was able to name only a few simple objects and even then showed considerable word searching and paraphasia.

With the demonstration of a significant aphasic disturbance, the neurologist quickly realized that the patient most likely had a left temporal lobe lesion. An extensive neurodiagnostic evaluation was then undertaken. Arteriography demonstrated a large posterior temporal lobe mass and the patient was taken to surgery. At surgery a large intracerebral hematoma with evidence of contusion and subdural blood was found in the left posterior temporal area. Postoperatively the patient's language and behavior gradually returned to normal.

This case demonstrates how a knowledge of cerebral localization and an appreciation of the clinical syndromes associated with focal brain damage, in this case aphasia, are of clinical importance in the management of many patients with acute behavioral change. Since many of the behavioral syndromes seen with focal brain damage show little, if any, evidence of abnormality on the standard neurologic testing of motor, sensory, and reflex function, it is imperative that a complete mental status examination be performed in all patients exhibiting recent behavioral change.

Focal syndromes are the manifestation of an entirely different type of lesion than those seen in the confusional states or the dementias. The focal syndrome is usually caused by a localized pathologic process such as a vascular lesion (stroke), brain tumor, abscess, or traumatic hematoma. Since many of these lesions can be removed by surgery, most cases require an extensive neurodiagnostic evaluation. Focal lesions within the brain, particularly those affecting the cortex, can often be localized accurately by careful mental status testing. This is possible because of the relatively high degree of localization of certain individual mental functions, for example: memory in the limbic structures, language in the perisylvian area of the left hemisphere, and constructional abilities in the parietal lobes. Rather characteristic clusters of neurobehavioral abnormalities have been described, and it is the recognition of these specific syndromes that allows the clinician to recognize the presence and localization of focal brain disease.

HANDEDNESS, HEMISPHERIC SPECIALIZATION, AND DOMINANCE

One of the very helpful factors in functional localization is the high degree of hemispheric specialization for language. Almost all right-handed individuals are left hemisphere dominant for language, thus an aphasic disturbance in a right-handed patient almost always indicates damage in the left side of the brain. Language function in the left-handed individual is less strongly lateralized, and we will discuss this problem more fully throughout this chapter.

Although dominance for language is the most strongly lateralized of the cognitive functions, it is not the only one. Constructional abilities, visual spatial orientation, and geographic orientation all tend to be lateralized to the right parietal lobe; the degree of dominance for these abilities is far less than for language however. Musical abilities, particularly the appreciation and production of tones and tone patterns, are dominant in the right hemisphere, principally in the temporal lobe, and the learning of skilled hand movements seems to be the province of the sensory-motor cortex opposite the preferred hand.

The degree of hemispheric specialization is similar for all right-handed individuals who are from a right-handed family. However, the situation is quite different for the individual who is not right handed or the right-handed individual with non-right-handed individuals in his immediate family. Handedness, hemispheric specialization, and dominance are all related and must be appreciated if functional localization is to be fully understood.

The situation is made much less complicated by the fact that approximately 90 to 95 percent of the population is rather firmly right handed.[74,101,118,132] However, there is a spectrum of handedness from exclusive right handedness to strong left handedness. In general, the left-handed individual is not as firmly left handed as the right handed individual is right handed; in fact, there seem to be very few individuals who are purely or exclusively left handed.[132] The average left-handed person carries out some skilled movements with the right hand or at least can demonstrate significant agility with both hands. Testing of left-handed people with a series of motor tests reveals that about 15 percent will actually show superior performance with their right hand, despite their claim of left handedness.[17,19,74] Why this should be true is unclear; it is doubtful if these individuals chose to write and throw a baseball with their left hand because it was more difficult. The point is that left handedness is less well established than right handedness and that many left-handed individuals have a strong tendency toward ambidexterity.

Several factors determine handedness and have direct bearing on the hemispheric specialization of individuals. Genetic influence is a major factor. A right-handed couple, for example, has only a 2 percent chance of having a left-handed child, whereas a left-handed couple (both parents being left handed) has a 46 percent chance of producing left-handed offspring and a mixed couple (one left handed, one right handed) has a slightly greater than 17 percent chance of having a left-handed child.[33] The family history is interesting also in that individuals who are left handed and have a family history of left handedness (parents or siblings) tend to have less strongly established left handedness than the sporadic left-handed individual. Having left-handed family members also weakens the strength of handedness in the right hander, a factor that may be important in explaining some of the mild aphasias seen in right handers with right hemispheric lesions.[101]

A second important influence on handedness is early brain damage to the dominant hemisphere. If the left hemisphere is damaged in a child who was genetically destined to be right handed, he will often, but not always, switch dominance and become left handed. This is called pathologic or symptomatic left handedness. Statistically there are probably also pathologic right-handed individuals though their number is small.[126,127] A third factor involved in determination of handedness is social pressure or identification with parents and peers. This factor has been used to help explain the high percentage of left-handed children in families in which both parents are left handed.

The specific etiology for each individual's handedness is often elusive and may be a combination of familial, pathologic, and social influences. It should be mentioned that there is a strong correlation between hand dominance and foot dominance and a positive, yet less impressive, correlation with eye preference.[132] The significance of eye dominance is somewhat suspect both because of the high incidence of refraction errors and the fact that vision from each eye is projected to both cerebral hemispheres.

The major clinical importance of handedness is its close relationship with cerebral dominance for language. In all but a few rare instances, right-handed individuals from right-handed families are completely left hemisphere dominant for language. This strong dominance is somewhat weaker if the right handed individual has a left-handed family history (usually two left-handed close family members), in such cases (approximately 16% of the population), there is a slight tendency toward bilateral language representation.[101] The left-handed individual presents a somewhat less consistent pattern: 60 to 70 percent are primarily left hemisphere dominant for language, but the incidence of some degree of bilateral language representation is 80 percent.[68] Strongly left-handed individuals with no family history of left handedness tend to have the strongest left hemisphere dominance for language of all left handers. With a family history of left handedness or a tendency toward ambidexterity, unilateral language dominance weakens and bilateral speech representation is expected.[74,101] Conversely, patients with maximum right hemisphere language dominance are usually the left handers who have had early brain damage, although 20 percent of left-handed individuals without brain damage have right hemisphere dominance.[30]

216

Although somewhat complicated and a problem in only the 5 to 10 percent of the population that is left handed, it is very important to understand these issues of cerebral dominance when evaluating and managing a left-handed patient who has a focal cerebral lesion. A generous surgical resection to expose an aneurysm which leaves the left-handed patient unexpectedly globally aphasic is tragic. In like fashion, the failure to adequately resect a tumor in the left hemisphere of a left handed individual with a family history of left handedness (such a patient has strong bilateral speech and will recover well) is equally unfortunate. With a knowledge of the intricacies of cerebral dominance in the left handed individual and the use of intracarotid sodium amytal testing to determine dominance before surgery, neurosurgical procedures will be much more satisfactorily carried out in the left-handed population.

DESCRIPTION OF THE FOCAL BRAIN SYNDROMES

The Aphasias

Aphasia is a language disturbance caused by damage to the language areas of the brain. The term aphasia does not refer to errors in pronunciation or articulation but rather to true linguistic errors in word choice, comprehension, or syntax. The brain damage resulting in aphasia is usually in the left hemisphere, but, in left-handed individuals, lesions in the right hemisphere can also produce a language disorder. Although language disturbances can be seen in demented or confusional patients, the syndromes discussed below are restricted to those seen with focal lesions.

The degree and characterization of an aphasic disturbance are largely determined by the size and location of the lesion; but also, in part, by the nature of the underlying pathologic process and how long after the onset of the aphasia the patient is examined. Patients with brain tumors and acute lesions such as trauma and stroke often have associated confusional behavior in which the aphasia may be overshadowed by the general incoherence of mental processes. In the case of a large cerebral infarction, language function is often markedly reduced for the first few hours or days but improves rapidly thereafter. Occasionally the acute aphasia is sufficiently distinct to permit determination of the exact location of the lesion within the hemisphere, but frequently definitive localization must wait. Usually within three weeks of onset, the aphasia has stabilized and detailed language testing can be carried out. Language recovery is often a slow and somewhat erratic process that can continue for months and even years. It is best to be cautious about prognosis in aphasia and not to give a final determination of linguistic competence until a clear-cut plateau of function is reached (often months after onset).

In assessing a patient's language, the clinician should conduct a full language evaluation as outlined in Chapter 3. If the patient produces language with errors of grammar or abnormal word usage (paraphasias), or fails on tests of comprehension, repetition, or naming; he should be considered aphasic and a left hemisphere lesion should be assiduously sought. The following case clearly demonstrates this point.

A 53-year-old woman was referred because of recent "confusion." Her physician felt she probably had developed a confusional state from overuse of analgesics for back pain. On examination, the patient was fully alert but had occasional word-finding pauses in spontaneous speech. Her comprehension of long or complex sentences was faulty, and she had great difficulty in correctly naming objects. Other neurologic testing was unremarkable. Because her behavioral change strongly suggested an isolated aphasia and not a confusional state, a brain scan was obtained immediately. The scan showed a questionable crescentic uptake overlying the left hemisphere which was suggestive of a subdural hematoma. Arteriography verified the presence of a subdural clot and surgery was performed. Subsequent to surgery, her language improved but unfortunately never returned to its premorbid level of adequacy.

Language testing is designed both to establish the presence of aphasia, as in the case above, and also to localize the pathology as outlined below.

GLOBAL APHASIA

Global aphasia, the most severe of the aphasic disorders, is characterized by a severe comprehension deficit and a virtual absence of speech production. Patients with global aphasia cannot read, write, repeat words, or name objects. They often produce stereotyped sounds but little else. The lesion causing a global aphasia is most commonly large, involves the entire perisylvian area of the frontal, temporal, and parietal lobes[88,138] (Fig. 7-1) and is most frequently caused by an occlusion of the internal carotid artery or the middle cerebral artery at its origin. Unfortunately, the prognosis for recovery of speech in the global aphasic is not good. Despite long term speech therapy these patients rarely recover usable language function.[98,125]

BROCA'S APHASIA

In Broca's aphasia comprehension of both spoken and written language is excellent and there are only mild problems understanding complex syntax involving sequences or relational grammar. Verbal expression,

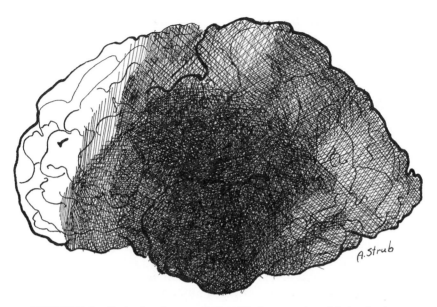

FIGURE 7-1. Brain showing composite of lesions causing global aphasia.

on the other hand, is severely impaired. The term "expressive aphasia" is often used to denote Broca's aphasia, but the term can be confusing since most aphasics, regardless of type, have some abnormalities in expressing themselves. Because of this, the inexperienced examiner tends to classify all aphasics as being "expressive aphasics."

The verbal output of a patient with Broca's aphasia is nonfluent, effortful, dysarthric, and contains mostly nouns and verbs with a paucity of other grammatical forms.[7] Repetition and reading aloud demonstrate similar deficits. Since the speaking style often has the sound of a sentientious telegram, the speech is often called telegraphic or agrammatic. A patient with Broca's aphasia describing several men loading a moving van might produce the following: "Ah. . . . chair. . . . table. . . . truck. . . . going away. . . . ah,ah, men walking, wolking, welking, oh I don't know." The patients often produce phonemic paraphasias which they have no difficulty recognizing but have great difficulty correcting. The Broca's aphasic is also impaired in object naming to confrontation and paraphasic responses are common. Writing ability is severely involved and shows similar but even more severe errors than does spontaneous speech.

The lesion causing Broca's aphasia is usually a fairly large deep lesion with maximal damage in the inferior frontal lobe; a lesion which includes the classic Broca's area 44[7,75,88,101,138] (area 2 in Fig. 7-2). Small lesions restricted to area 44 alone produce only transient mild aphasia with dysarthria and dysprosody being the principal features.[111,150] Be-

219

cause the motor cortex is involved in almost all of these patients, a right hemiplegia is usually present.

In general, prognosis for such patients is quite good because of their retained comprehension. Specific language recovery is, however, slow. These patients initially recover the ability to name objects, but fluency and grammatical complexity often remain impaired.[70] Emotionally, the Broca's aphasic frequently experiences depression, frustration and irritability[8]—important factors that must be dealt with in rehabilitation. The precise etiology of these emotional changes has not been identified but a combination of psychologic (awareness of the deficit) and organic (frontal lobe damage) factors is probably involved.

WERNICKE'S APHASIA

Wernicke's aphasia is clinically one of the most important aphasic syndromes as it often presents without evidence of either hemiparesis or a visual field defect. The patient's initial symptoms are typically those of abnormal speech production and abnormal behavior. The case presented at the beginning of this chapter is one example. The Wernicke's aphasic produces fluent, effortless, well articulated speech which is frequently out of context and smattered with paraphasias.[7, 61,70] On occasion, the spontaneous speech consists of a string of paraphasias which is completely meaningless (jargon aphasia). The Wernicke's aphasic describing a scene of moving men loading their truck might produce the following: "Well yes, there they are all doing the thing with chegles and laps or those who put it here up and there. Well yes I say how, well, you know over there and well yes I tlable flet omnit well yes."

The most outstanding feature of these patients' aphasia is the severe deficit in auditory comprehension. They are unable to comprehend their own speech or that of others, and for this reason this syndrome has often been called a receptive aphasia. Repetition, reading, and writing are all severely effected and object naming is usually grossly paraphasic. The patients often develop unusual behavioral reactions including euphoria, indifference, paranoia, and agitation.[8] At times, this behavior can be severe enough to simulate psychosis. When this occurs, the patients require sedation and occasionally must be transferred to a psychiatric ward.

Wernicke's aphasia is caused by a lesion in the posterior language zone (area 1 in Fig. 7-2). The lesion usually destroys the superior temporal gyrus (area 22 in Fig. 7-2) which is the primary auditory association cortex; this area is important in auditory comprehension as well as repetition since all basic auditory processing is accomplished there. The size and exact location of the lesion is quite variable, but it primar-

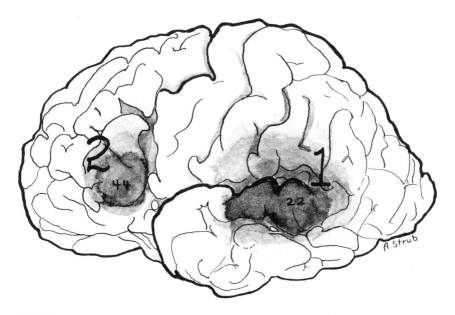

FIGURE 7–2. The lesion causing Broca's apasia occurs in area 2 and incorporates the inferior gyrus, 44. The lesion causing Wernicke's aphasia occurs in area 1, the posterior language zone, and usually destroys the superior temporal gyrus, 22.

ily destroys rather large areas of postrolandic temporal and parietal cortex.[7,75,88,101,138]

Because of the abnormal behavior often demonstrated by the Wernicke's aphasic and his bizarre speech, lack of comprehension, and paucity of expected neurologic signs; it is easy to see why these patients are at times confused with those with functional psychotic illness. The correct diagnosis is usually quite readily made, however, by carrying out a careful language examination. Schizophrenics will almost always demonstrate adequate comprehension, repetition, reading, writing, and naming whereas the aphasic will not. The evaluation of a very disorganized schizophrenic is not always easy, but persistent attempts at testing will generally yield a correct diagnosis. We recently saw a 17-year-old man who was referred because of strange language and inappropriate responses to questioning. On examination his running speech was bizarre indeed. He had extremely loose associations, mumbled considerably, and would often stop in the middle of a sentence and not continue. His language production alone sounded like a fluent aphasia. Comprehension testing, however, proved to be normal, though very difficult to assess. When asked a question such as "Is it raining today?", the patient would look puzzled, wait for a long time, and then answer, "What do you want to know that for? You can see it's not, look,

221

no rain, no rainwater, water. . . ." When asked to point to his nose, ear, and the floor; he performed accurately, but again with much suspiciousness, blocking, mumbling, and tangential thoughts. A complete language and mental status evaluation was carried out and the patient performed very well on all items except proverbs to which he gave concrete interpretations, (a typical finding in schizophrenic patients). No aphasia was demonstrated. EEG and brain scan were normal and the patient was referred to a psychiatrist for further evaluation and care.

The reason for stressing this case is that language production alone can be misleading. Therefore, the examiner is obligated to persue his initial impressions concerning a patient's language production by taking a complete history and performing a complete neurologic and mental status examination. The severely disorganized language production of schizophrenia (often called word salad) was traditionally described in patients with a long history of the disease and usually after a long period of relative isolation in a mental hospital.[13] However, as demonstrated by the case above, the language of an undiagnosed schizophrenic can initially be quite remarkably deteriorated and simulate an aphasia.

The Wernicke's aphasic and the schizophrenic have another feature in common that can be difficult to interpret at times—the use of neologistic speech. The fluent aphasic produces frequent neologistic paraphasias in running speech, however, they are quite different from those of the schizophrenic. The aphasic's neologisms tend to be random, changeable, and frequent, whereas those used by the schizophrenic are very infrequent and are consistent, systematized, and have delusional significance. The aphasic may call a comb a "clom" one time then correct it to a "come" or a "hair thing," while the schizophrenic may consider all combs to be "fleebles" that everyone carries around to monitor his thoughts.

A differential point that should be reiterated is that such neologisms are very common in aphasia, yet quite rare in schizophrenia.[58] Other types of paraphasias (i.e., letter or whole word substitutions) are strictly aphasic and not heard in the schizophrenic. Another subtle differential feature is that the schizophrenic tends to produce much longer responses to general questions than does the aphasic,[58] and the schizophrenic's discourse is also usually distinctly delusional and systematized.

Although mental status testing will almost always correctly establish the diagnosis, historical information is invaluable. A history of the age and rapidity of onset of the language disorder is important. Obviously a previous history of schizophrenia weighs heavily on the side of that diagnosis. A young patient who has gradually developed bizarre language is much more likely to be schizophrenic than aphasic (although a temporal lobe tumor can certainly produce a slowly progressive aphasia). Conversely, the acute onset of rambling, disjointed, neologistic discourse in an elderly person with no history of previous mental problems is not likely to be due to a functional psychosis but is more likely to be the result of a vascular accident in the posterior temporal area. This simple observation is not always made, however, as we have seen several elderly patients with Wernicke's aphasia who had been initially admitted to psychiatric units because of the acute onset of bizarre language and behavior.

Another disease in which abnormal language production can be confused with a Wernicke's aphasia is advanced dementia. In such patients the history and mental status examination should be sufficient to make the correct diagnosis, but a full neurodiagnostic evaluation may be necessary. Usually the demented patient's comprehension and repetition are far better than that of the Wernicke's aphasic and his general mental functioning far worse. There are cases in which a demented patient is stricken with a superimposed temporal parietal lobe infarct. In these cases, the problem of sorting out the array of linguistic problems into those due to the dementia and those secondary to the recent infarct becomes virtually impossible.

The prognosis in Wernicke's aphasia is variable and is almost completely dependent upon the degree to which auditory comprehension recovers. In patients with severe comprehension deficits, speech therapy is not useful, so therapeutic intervention must also await improvement in comprehension. If comprehension improves sufficiently, the patient's aphasia typically progresses to a level resembling conduction aphasia or frequently a simple anomic aphasia.[70]

CONDUCTION APHASIA

Conduction aphasia is a less common type of fluent aphasia in which the outstanding linguistic deficit is in the repetition of spoken language. These patients produce fairly adequate spontaneous speech which has only occasional word-finding pauses and paraphasias. Comprehension is very good, as is reading, although there may be errors in object naming and writing.

The importance of the syndrome is less practical than it is theoretical. The lesion causing this type of aphasia is usually in the cortex bordering the superior lip of the sylvian fissure yet extending deep enough to affect the arcuate fasciculus (AF)[16,60,75,88] (Fig. 7-3) which forms a direct connection from the auditory receiving area (22) to the motor speech area (44). Of considerable theoretical interest is that damage to this fasciculus and its neighboring cortex can disrupt a specific linguistic process (repetition) yet relatively spare other higher

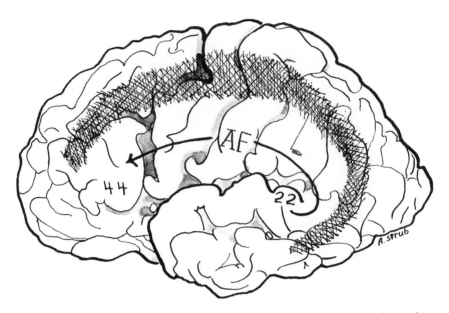

FIGURE 7–3. Lesions causing conduction aphasia are usually in the parietal area close to the Sylvian fissure. The lesion extends deep enough to effect the arcuate fasciculus (AF) which forms a direct connection from the auditory receiving area (22) to the motor speech area (44).

level language processes (i.e., conversational or propositional speech and comprehension). From observation of children during the period of speech acquisition, it is obvious that word repetition frequently precedes association of the sounds with the meaning of the words. With the study of conduction aphasia and the transcortical aphasias to be discussed next, it is now appreciated that there is a rather distinct anatomic separation between the high level language process of conversational speech which is utilized to express thought and describe the environment and the more rudimentary and mechanical process of repetition.

TRANSCORTICAL APHASIA

The transcortical aphasias are the linguistic opposite of conduction aphasia. In cases of transcortical aphasia, patients are able to repeat perfectly, yet have difficulty with comprehension, speech production, or both. These conditions, although known clinically for years, were dramatized by a recent case report of a patient with perfect repetition yet absolutely no comprehension of what was said to her and no ability to express her own wants and desires.[67] This remarkable syndrome was caused by a large crescentic infarction which spared the perisylvian tissue while destroying much of the association cortex (Fig. 7-3). Because of the destruction of the association cortex, the patient could not comprehend what was said to her and she also had inadequate association cortex for verbal reasoning or thought processes. However, the uninvolved perisylvian temporal, frontal, and parietal cortex with their interconnections, including the arcuate fasciculus, were sufficient to insure completely normal repetition.

The several varieties of transcortical aphasia depend upon the extent and location of the lesion. If the infarct involves only the anterior portion of the crescent, the patients demonstrate what is called transcortical motor aphasia: they repeat perfectly, comprehend well, yet are unable to adequately initiate spontaneous speech. Patients with posterior lesions are much the opposite: they repeat well, produce fluent, albeit paraphasic speech, yet comprehend little. These transcortical sensory aphasics are, of course, much more severely disabled because of their comprehension deficit. Those patients with the complete syndrome (isolation of the speech area) have intact repetition ability with no other language capabilities. The more severe the syndrome, the more the patients tend to echo everything they hear (echolalia). It is not difficult to demonstrate their prowess at repetition even in the face of severe comprehension deficits because of this echoing tendency. Their repetition is so mindless and slavish they are able to repeat foreign languages that they have never heard before, although their facial expressions often indicate that the language is strange and unfamiliar. Interestingly, they also tend to transpose pronouns and other grammatical structures automatically. For instance, if asked, "Is *your* name Mary Smith?" they may respond, "Is *my* name Mary Smith?"

Pathologically this unusually shaped lesion represents an infarction of the borderzone tissue between the perfusion territories of the major cerebral blood vessels. The anterior area is between the anterior and middle cerebral arteries and the posterior area falls at the border of the middle, posterior, and posterior extent of the anterior cerebral arteries. What causes ischemia to occur in these areas is either: decreased blood flow from cardiac arrest, arrythmia, or significant carotid stenosis or anoxia from insufficient blood oxygenation as with carbon monoxide poisoning.

If the clinician is aware of the transcortical aphasias, he will be able to explain the pathophysiologic mechanism of many of the aphasias he sees. This can be particularly useful in those aphasic syndromes that occur after surgery or arteriography. If a patient displays a transcortical disturbance, a drop in blood pressure or an arrythmia is more likely the cause of the aphasia than an embolus in the middle cerebral territory. Often transient ischemia in the borderzone has a more favorable prognosis than does an embolus with its resultant infarction of brain tissue. Although most transcortical aphasias are caused by ischemia or infarction, tumors of the anterior frontal lobe or the supplementary motor area have been known to cause a transcortical motor aphasia. Whether this is a true aphasia or a form of mutism from frontal damage is not known.[42,120]

ANOMIC APHASIA

Anomic aphasia is another of the fluent aphasias. The primary language deficits in such patients are a difficulty in naming objects to confrontation and word-finding problems in running speech. Comprehension, repetition, reading, and writing are all typically excellent, except when the material contains many nouns with few grammatical fillers. A sentence such as, "Let's all go over there when she comes back," for instance, will be easily repeated or read, whereas "The short fat boy dropped the china vase" will not. In all language tasks (e.g., spontaneous speech, repetition, and naming), the patient may produce pharaphasic utterances with object names but not as commonly as in Wernicke's aphasia. On confrontation naming tasks, it is more typical for the anomic aphasic to produce circumlocutory responses than paraphasias. When asked to name a comb, an anomic might answer, "Oh you know, the thing that you use to do your hair, to make you look nice when you go out." The patient also typically demonstrates the object's use to emphasize his knowledge of the nature of the object.

Anomic aphasia can result from a wide variety of lesions in the language zone. Frontal as well as parietal and temporal lesions have been shown to produce the same linguistic syndrome of anomia.[75,88] Lesions of the inferior temporal region (area 37) tend to produce the most severe word-finding difficulties without a loss of comprehension of the words or the concept of the object's use.[9] In lesions affecting the parietal language area (primarily area 39), the anomia seems to be more profound in that the patients seem also to have lost both the concept of the object *and* its name when it is presented visually. These parietal anomias have been called "semantic aphasias" because of this total loss of concept of the object as well as its associated name.[101]

Anomic aphasia is frequently associated with an alexia and agraphia in cases where the inferior parietal lobule is damaged (areas 39 and 40). This syndrome will be more fully discussed in the section on alexia.

WORD DEAFNESS

Pure word deafness is an uncommon, yet fascinating language disturbance in which patients are able to hear and recognize nonspeech sounds (e.g., dog bark or boat whistle) but are unable to understand spoken words. In sharp contrast to Wernicke's aphasia, such patients produce normal conversational speech, read without difficulty, and write normally. This is not a true aphasia since basic language processes are intact, but it is a type of disconnection syndrome in which auditory input from the primary auditory area (Heschl's gyri, areas 41 and 42) is interrupted before reaching Wernicke's area (particularly area 22).[60,82]

Pure word deafness is usually produced by a subcortical lesion (often bilateral) that disconnects the auditory radiations of the primary auditory cortex (area 41) or the primary auditory association cortex (area 42) from the secondary auditory association cortex (area 22). Since the auditory system projects bilaterally, the lesion must also disconnect the callosal fibers on their course from the right auditory area (area 42) to the corresponding area in the left hemisphere. Since such a lesion, either in the left hemisphere or symmetrically in both hemispheres, is rather unlikely, this syndrome in pure form is rare. There are, however, a number of cases in which associated damage to area 22 causes a syndrome of word deafness with concomitant paraphasic speech.

APHASIA IN THE LEFT-HANDED INDIVIDUAL

Aphasia in the left-handed patient includes several clinically important and interesting features. First, since 80 percent of left-handed individuals have some element of language in both hemispheres, the left-handed individual is more prone to develop some type of language disturbance from a brain lesion than the right-handed. The right-handed individual will develop an aphasia only with a left hemisphere lesion, but the left handed individual will most likely have an aphasia resulting from a lesion in either hemisphere.[68] This is an unfortunate aspect of being left handed, but the positive benefit is that aphasia in the left-handed individual proves to be much less severe initially, to clear more rapidly, and to have good prognosis for full language recovery.[101] In a study of soldiers sustaining missile wounds to the left hemisphere, Luria reported that 95 percent of the right-handed soldiers developed a severe aphasia acutely and 75 percent showed little improvement on follow-up evaluation. In sharp contrast, the left-handed and ambidextrous patients had a 77 percent incidence of initial severe aphasia but only a 7 percent residual severe aphasia.[101] It can be conjectured from these findings that the linguistic capacity of the right hemisphere of the left-handed patients was quite adequate to compensate for the language loss produced by the left hemisphere lesion.

The aphasic syndromes seen in left-handed individuals are somewhat different from the classic syndromes of the right handed. At least 35 to 40 percent of such cases are not classifiable, whereas only 15 percent of the aphasias in right-handed individuals are unclassifiable according to standard typology.[68] The aphasia itself very rarely involves auditory comprehension, and when it does, the comprehension loss is minimal. A true sensory aphasia is seen in fewer than 10 percent of the cases.[32,78] Expressive difficulties are common (>50%), with frequent decreased verbal fluency and dysarthria, but agrammatism is not usually seen. Repetition is seldom more than mildly involved, but anomia with its attendant word-finding difficulty is common. Anomia is much more frequently seen with left hemisphere lesions and, in fact, is rarely found with right sided lesions. Reading disturbances follow the same laterality pattern as anomia.

Anatomic correlation demonstrates that the language areas in the left handed are the same as those in the right handed, but it is the degree of bilateral representation that produces the anomalous clinical picture.[32,68] Auditory comprehension, particularly, seems to be quite strongly represented in both hemispheres in the left handed individual.

CROSSED APHASIA

Aphasia is occasionally observed in a right-handed patient with a right hemisphere lesion. The aphasia is quite different from that seen in left-handed individuals, however. The patients are often agrammatic, commonly have decreased comprehension, demonstrate good naming, and rarely have reading or writing deficits. The syndrome, like that in the left-handed individual is usually quite transient.[151] Why certain right-handed individuals show this variance from the general rule is not clear. This syndrome of crossed aphasia is seen in patients with no history of early left hemisphere damage or familial left handedness.

APHASIA WITH THALAMIC AND OTHER SUBCORTICAL LESIONS

Some rather consistent language abnormalities have been described in patients with thalamic and putamenal lesions (usually hypertension hemorrhage). Initially the patients are almost mute with little, if any, spontaneous speech. As they improve slightly, they respond to testing if the examiner makes a great effort to hold their attention. Once communication is established, the patients perform quite well for a number of seconds then deteriorate rapidly into runs of paraphasic, neologistic language.[112,122,123] In many cases, there has been comprehension difficulty as well and a diagnosis of a mixed aphasia or moderate global aphasia has been made initially.[47,49,83] In the majority of the patients, repetition has been remarkably spared and an echolalic tendency noted.[34,47,83,112,123] Naming difficulty is also usually present.

The clinical features of the syndrome have been similar in many cases, but the actual mechanism of the disorder has been much debated. Since the cerebral cortex is the basic repository of language, it has been assumed that true aphasic disturbances are produced only when the cortex itself is damaged. Because of this, it has been difficult for some investigators to consider the speech difficulty experienced by patients with these subcortical lesions to be a true aphasia.[102,112] They feel that these patients have a severe defect in attention and that their thalamic lesions prevent them from focusing on what is being said to them or on what they want to say. Because of this severe inattention and distractibility, the patients produce incoherent and garbled speech when not being strictly forced to pay close attention by the examiner. For this reason, this language disturbance has been likened to a confusional state rather than an aphasia.[41] To us, an aphasia is a clinical finding reflecting a central disturbance in language regardless of the mechanism. We would agree that the thalamus is not an actual repository of language in the brain but that damage to it can influence cortical functioning of areas with which it interacts.

Dysarthria

Articulation disturbances are commonly seen in brain disease of diverse etiology and varied location. Since they are often misconstrued by the naive examiner as being an aphasia, it is important to point out again the necessity of carrying out a full language examination on any patient with problems in speech production. Several years ago one of our junior residents presented a young hypertensive woman to us who reportedly had an expressive (Broca'a) aphasia but whose writing was entirely normal. On examination it was true that the patient could not produce any intelligible speech, yet comprehension, reading, and writing were all normal. However, she also had difficulty swallowing, could not protrude her tongue on command, and had a snout reflex. This patient had a pseudobulbar palsy from bilateral corticobulbar tract damage; her speech problem was a severe dysarthria because of an interruption of innervation to the muscles of articulation and not an aphasia.

Any lesion disrupting control of the muscles of articulation will result in dysarthria: lesions of the cortical motor area (there is considerable dysarthria in patients with Broca's aphasia), basal ganglia (Parkinson's disease, dystonia, or chorea), corticobulbar tract (pseudobulbar palsy), the motor neurons of the ninth, tenth, and twelfth cranial nerves (polio or amyotrophic lateral sclerosis), and in the muscles or muscle endplates themselves (myasthenia gravis or polymyositis). Speech disorders resulting from all of these conditions must be differentiated from the aphasias. Treatment of most of these dysarthrias with conventional speech therapy is not usually efficacious and many patients resort to writing or using flash cards to make their needs known.

Alexia

Alexia is a syndrome in which reading ability has been adversely affected by an acquired brain lesion. This is in contrast to the well-known term, dyslexia, which is applied to individuals who have normal intelligence yet are unable to learn to read effectively despite adequate educational exposure.

Several lesions can produce alexia; the most common occurs in the posterior language zone and is associated with a fluent aphasia. There is also a rather specific type of alexia seen in patients with Broca's aphasia. This alexia is often quite severe, and its major characteristics are difficulty with comprehending complex grammatical constructions and problems with maintaining the logical sequence of material read.[10]

There are, however, several alexic syndromes in which reading alone or reading and writing are affected in the absence of an associated aphasia. The classic syndrome of pure alexia without aphasia or writing disturbance (agraphia) is seen with a left posterior cerebral artery occlusion.[60] The resulting lesion damages the posterior limb of the corpus callosum as well as destroying the left visual cortex (Fig. 7-4) and prevents visual written information from entering the left hemisphere because of the damage to the corpus callosum. The language areas of the left hemisphere do not receive the written words and therefore cannot decode them. Because there is no damage to the language areas of the left hemisphere itself, the patient is not aphasic nor is he agraphic. The written message originates in the left posterior language area and is then carried out within the motor cortex in that hemisphere. It is dramatic to see such a patient spontaneously write a letter to a friend and then be totally unable to read what he has just written. There are several other interesting yet curious aspects to this syndrome: these patients seem to have little difficulty in naming objects or commenting verbally about what is going on in the world as perceived visually. This means that visual information for these tasks is transferred to the language hemisphere via more anterior callosal fibers than is written language. Along with written words, color information seems to cross in the posterior aspect of the callosum, as these patients usually lose ability to accurately name colors (they are not color blind, however, because they can match colors well, they merely cannot name them).[64] Although this syndrome of alexia without agraphia is usually seen with rather large lesions which cause an associated right homonymous hemianopia, one case has been described in the literature in which a rather small lesion deep in the occipital lobe prevented all visual information from reaching areas 39 and 40. This patient was alexic but did not have a visual field defect.[73]

The second syndrome of a relatively isolated alexia is that seen with

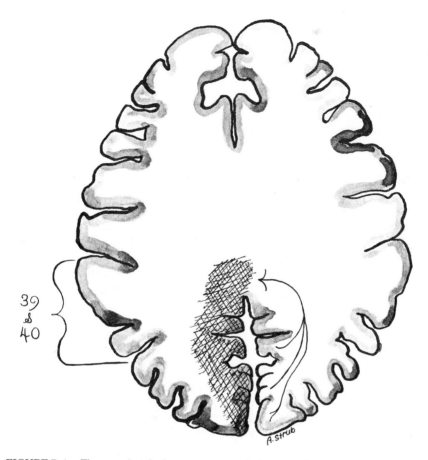

39
&
40

FIGURE 7–4. The cross-hatched area represents infarction of the left visual cortex and the posterior portion of the corpus callosum. Visual information from the right visual cortex (arrow) is unable to reach the left inferior parietal lobule (39 and 40) because of the callosal lesion. This produces the syndrome of pure alexia without aphasia or agraphia.

destruction in the inferior parietal lobule (areas 39 and 40) of the dominant hemisphere itself. In these patients, the alexia is accompanied by an equally severe agraphia and on occasion an anomia. This lesion, in essence, obliterates the patient's literacy and completely prevents the patient from using literal symbols to communicate thoughts or ideas.

Agraphia

Agraphia is a specific defect in producing written language. The term does not refer to the abnormalities in writing mechanics which are often seen in parkinsonism, limb weakness, or gross constructional

231

problems but rather to a deficit in syntax, spelling, and word choice. Agraphia is most commonly seen in conjunction with aphasia. In fact, aphasics (except those with pure word deafness) invariably demonstrate some degree of agraphia which is usually in excess of their verbal language deficit. On the other hand, agraphia is rarely, if ever, seen in isolation. Although it was once postulated that a lesion in the premotor cortex anterior to the motor area for the hand would produce an isolated writing disturbance, such a case has never been described.[46] There is one unusual situation in which a patient can develop a pure agraphia with the left hand only; this is seen in lesions of the corpus callosum and will be discussed later in this chapter.

Two syndromes have been described in which agraphia is found in nonaphasic patients, but both of these syndromes have other associated cognitive disturbances. The first is the alexia with agraphia described above and the second is Gerstmann's syndrome (a syndrome of finger agnosia, right-left disorientation, acalculia, and agraphia). Both of these syndromes are caused by lesions in the dominant inferior parietal lobe and are frequently associated with other higher cortical deficits.

Apraxia (Ideomotor)

Apraxia is a disorder in carrying out or learning complex movements that cannot be accounted for by elementary disturbances of strength, coordination, sensation, comprehension, or attention.[62] The type of movement affected is one which requires the patient to select and execute several changes in body position.[91] Examples of such praxic movements are: flipping a coin, saluting, brushing teeth, or blowing out a candle. Simple repetitious movements such as tapping the index finger on the table would not be classified as being praxic movements. Apraxia is best seen with the movement elicited by verbal command without a concrete object for the patient to use (e.g., "Show me how you would flip a coin"). It can, however, be demonstrated if the patient is asked to imitate the examiner or to use an actual object to carry out the task. An apraxic movement is one in which the various changes in position or integration of the motor pattern is distorted (e.g., the patient takes the coin in his hand and procedes to merely toss it in the air or turn the hand over and back, dropping the coin to the floor; in blowing out a candle the patient opens the mouth, cannot pucker, and coughs on the candle with variable success in actually extinguishing the flame).

The control of praxic movements, arm, leg, and mouth, is directed by the language dominant left hemisphere, and therefore ideomotor apraxia results from left brain lesions. The lesion can be localized anywhere from the inferior parietal area (B in Fig. 7-5) posteriorly to

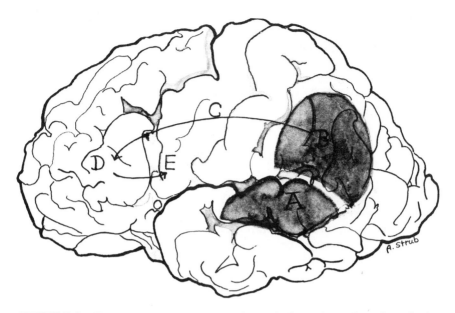

FIGURE 7–5. The lesion in ideomotor apraxia can be located anywhere from the inferior parietal area (B) to the motor association cortex (D). A = Auditory cortex. C = Intrahemispheric association fibers. E = Motor neurons.

the motor association cortex (D in Fig. 7-5) anteriorly. The movement to be executed is indicated to the patient either verbally by command via the auditory cortex (A in Fig. 7-5) or visually by imitation utilizing the visual system. The information concerning the desired movement is transferred to the inferior parietal area where kinesthetic images are evoked (B in Fig. 7-5). This kinesthetic pattern is sent to the motor association cortex (D in Fig. 7-5) via the intrahemispheric association fibers (C in Fig. 7-5). The motor association cortex effects the final motor programming before directing the motor neurons (E in Fig. 7-5) to procede with the movement.

Because of its dominant role in movement, lesions in the left hemisphere will cause a bilateral ideomotor apraxia. This is seen dramatically in Broca's aphasia where there is frequently a marked apraxia of the nonparalyzed left hand. Due to the close anatomic relationship between language and praxis, apraxia is frequently an accompanying and compounding factor in cases of aphasia. Many aphasics have difficulty with an apraxia of the buccofacial musculature and the resultant difficulty in approximating speech sounds, often called verbal apraxia, can greatly exaggerate and on occasion constitute the entirety of the patient's speech production problem. This aspect of the aphasic deficit must be appreciated by the speech pathologist and dealt with specifically during therapy.

Ideomotor apraxia of the limbs can be a complicating factor in physical rehabilitation where the patient is frequently attempting to train his left hand to take over the tasks traditionally managed by the right. With a severe apraxia of the left hand, the acquisition of skills for daily living is very difficult. Again, the therapist must appreciate this limitation in brain damaged patients and work with it as a separate problem.

Agnosia

Agnosia is a specific defect in object recognition in the absence of any disturbance in the primary sensory system. For example, a visual agnosia is diagnosed when a patient is able to see yet cannot recognize objects presented visually. Tactile agnosia and auditory agnosia are operationally defined in a similar fashion. There are also several interesting specific agnosias: prosopagnosia (face recognition), color agnosia, and finger agnosia which are all occasionally seen with focal brain lesions.

TACTILE AGNOSIA

The most common agnosia is the tactile agnosia that occurs in the hand contralateral to a hemispheric lesion. These patients appreciate primary tactile sensation in their limb, yet cannot integrate sensations sufficiently to identify an object placed in the hand (astereognosis). The lesions causing these defects in sensory integration are in the postrolandic cortex, areas 3, 1, 2, and 5 of the parietal lobes.[119]

AUDITORY AGNOSIA

Auditory agnosia is an uncommon disorder which probably never occurs alone but is associated with other auditory processing difficulties, partial cortical deafness, word deafness, and aphasia. This condition has as its primary feature the patient's inability to distinguish among various nonverbal sounds (e.g., rustling paper, bird songs, car horns, and dog barks) while being able to perceive (hear) the sounds and perform adequately on pure tone audiometry. Brain[29] claimed that all patients with auditory agnosia would, by necessity, be deaf; however, this has not proved to be true as cases of striking auditory agnosia have been reported in patients who have very good comprehension of spoken language.[4] Although it has been postulated that this condition could be seen with a single lesion in the left superior temporal lobe,[29] it seems more likely that bilateral lesions are responsible for the majority of such cases.

VISUAL AGNOSIA

In visual agnosia, the patient has adequate visual acuity yet is unable to visually recognize objects or pictures of objects. This syndrome has been better established clinically than has auditory agnosia but is an equally uncommon disorder. Two major types of visual agnosia have been described in the literature: a visual form agnosia and an associative visual agnosia. In the first type, the patient experiences a gross perceptual distortion which prevents identification of the object.[14] If the object is placed in his hand, he is able to immediately identify it kinesthetically. It has been hypothesized that this variety of visual agnosia is produced by bilateral lesions of the visual association cortex (areas 18 and 19).[14]

The second variety, associative visual agnosia, is a type of disconnection syndrome where vision and visual perception have been demonstrated to be normal in visual matching tasks, however, this intact visual information area has been disconnected from language areas. In such a case, the patient cannot name an object but clearly recognizes it and can demonstrate its use or match it with other similar objects or pictures of the object.[6,37,121] The lesion causing this type of visual agnosia is very similar to the one causing an alexia without agraphia, namely a left posterior cerebral artery occlusion and subsequent infarction of the left occipital lobe plus the posterior corpus callosum.[97] The syndrome has also been described in a patient with bilateral posterior cerebral artery lesions.[3] Because of the similarity of this lesion to that causing pure alexia, it is not surprising that many, but not all, patients with associative visual agnosia also have alexia.[2]

PROSOPAGNOSIA

Prosopagnosia is a very unusual and interesting visual agnosia in which the patient's major complaint is an inability to recognize familiar faces. These patients do not recognize family members until they speak, do not recognize famous faces in newspapers or magazines, and cannot learn to recognize new faces such as those of the doctors and nurses caring for them. The mechanism for such a discrete visual agnosia is still in question and there may be various explanations. In some of the cases, there seems to be a visual perceptual defect that is specific for this one type of visual stimulus, namely faces.[148] In other cases, the defect may not be quite that specific, however, four cases have been reported in which the patients have also lost their ability to differentiate various makes of cars or individual cows in a herd (a skill developed by some dairymen).[28] These factors suggest that the basic defect in such cases is an inability to perceive subtle discriminating features in objects that are all within the same category (e.g., faces, cars, cows). Yet another possibility is that some prosopagnosic patients have a specific type of visual memory defect which explains the agnosia.[20] As with many clinical syndromes, there seem to be various mechanisms by which a particular finding can be produced. The lesions responsible for producing prosopagnosia are usually bilateral. They are in the occipitotemporal areas with a right inferior occipitotemporal lesion being one of the necessary lesions.[106] Unilateral lesions in this right occipitotemporal junction have also been reputed, on occasion, to produce the syndrome.[148]

FINGER AGNOSIA

Finger agnosia is an unusual, yet relatively common type of agnosia. It represents a rather isolated type of failure to recognize and localize particular parts of the body. The patients demonstrate an inability to recognize, name, and/or point to individual fingers on themselves or on the examiner.[59] The agnosia is most commonly apparent when testing the middle, index, and ring fingers but can, at times, be sufficiently severe to include the thumb and little fingers.[36] The lesion most commonly causing finger agnosia is in the dominant parietal lobe, although the symptom has also been found in patients with diffuse brain disease and as a developmental finding in some people.[93,113]

Occipital Lobe Syndromes

The occipital lobes are primarily responsible for high level visual processing and the syndromes associated with their dysfunction fall within the visual sphere. Gross bilateral destruction causes cortical blindness, but partial and selected damage or stimulation produces a variety of interesting syndromes. Disconnection of visual input from the left parietal lobe results in an alexia as previously outlined. Damage to the visual association areas can produce a variety of visual agnosias including prosopagnosia. The appreciation or perception of color is also a function of the occipital lobes, and lesions damaging both occipital lobes frequently cause an acquired color blindness or color agnosia.[38,45,107] The lesions producing color agnosia are closely associated with those producing prosopagnosia, hence these two symptoms are often seen concurrently in the same patient.

There are many perceptual distortions which can occur with occipital lobe disease; such symptoms as monocular polyopia, metamorphopsia (distortion of images), persistent after-images, and loss of depth perception can all occur and are sometimes initially considered to be of hysterical rather than organic origin.[55] It is always best to investigate the visual system very carefully when a patient complains of bizarre visual symptoms rather than to grasp for a psychiatric label too quickly.

Patients with acute cortical blindness, usually secondary to bilateral posterior cerebral artery occlusion, occasionally develop a curious type of behavioral syndrome in which they actively deny *any* loss of vision.

The syndrome, often called Anton's syndrome, can be so blatant that the examiner may, at first, be completely unaware of the patient's blindness. For example, we saw a patient on rounds with a group of students. We talked to the patient, and then said that we would like to have some of the students examine him. He said, "That would be all right, but please tell me when they are coming so that I can get dressed." The students were surrounding his bed while he spoke. On the following day, one of us went back alone and the patient greeted the examiner and said "I see you have your crew here again today." Such patients are quick to confabulate, often charge about the room without regard for furniture and other obstacles in their paths, and if confronted with their problem, often evade the issue by making disclaimers about having misplaced their glasses or "having something in my eyes."

A final behavioral manifestation of occipital lobe disease that should be mentioned is the occurrence of visual hallucinations in patients with occipital epileptic foci. The type of hallucination varies depending upon the localization of the focus within the occipital lobe. Posterior lesions usually produce formless, colored, flashes of light or spots; whereas more anterior lesions will cause the hallucination of fully formed images. We have followed one patient who has an epileptogenic focus in his right occipitotemporal region. His seizures consist solely of the hallucination in his left visual field of driving down a road through a forest. Such hemihallucinations are uncommon and can be seen in the blind field of some patients with damage to the calcarine cortex. In such patients, there is preservation of the visual association areas in the anterior portions of the occipital lobe.[124]

Temporal Lobe Syndromes

The temporal lobe is a very important area of the human brain. It not only serves as the cortical area for auditory input, but it is also the auditory processor for language reception. We have discussed the aphasic disturbances in an earlier section so will only reinforce here the fact that damage to the left temporal lobe, particularly the superior-posterior portion, causes a marked defect in auditory comprehension and a general disruption in language processing.

The temporal lobes, because of their auditory function, also play a major role in the appreciation and production of music. This role is not yet as well understood nor is musical function as distinctly lateralized as is language, but many interesting observations have been made concerning this very fascinating function. After a right anterior temporal lobectomy, it is noted that patients are significantly less able to judge tone quality and remember tones over short intervals than patients with left temporal lobectomy.[109] On dichotomic listening tasks (simultaneous presentation of a different melody to each ear), it has been shown that the right hemispheric temporal lobe is much better in perceiving melodies than the left.[21,90] Removal of the entire right hemisphere or its temporary inactivation by sodium amobarbital leaves a patient unable to produce a melody, yet still capable of monotonally producing song with correct rhythm. If the same procedure is carried out in the left hemisphere, the patient can sing the melody correctly, but is unable to produce the appropriate words.[27,71] In addition to these experimental studies, there have been many examples of both musicians and individuals with no musical orientation who have lost or retained many of their musical functions subsequent to the acquisition of cerebral lesions.[1,18,39,40,53,146] From these many accounts and reviews, it appears that the right hemisphere, and particularly the temporal lobe, is very important in the appreciation and production of melody. This degree of lateralization is somewhat stronger in the naive listener who experiences melodies as entire patterns than in the trained musician who uses his left hemispheric language and analytic skills to assist him in approaching music.[21] Rhythm, conversely, seems to be adequately handled by either temporal lobe. Music is, of course, a multifaceted ability that accordingly can be affected in a myriad of ways. The interested reader is referred to Critchley and Henson's[39] recent collection of papers on the topic as an excellent review and reference source.

The right temporal lobe is also very intimately associated with high level visual processing. Removal of the lobe produces defects in visual perception and visual motor integration.[109]

The temporal lobes also contain two critical components of the limbic system: the amygdala and the hippocampus. These structures are often affected by disease and produce several remarkable behavioral syndromes. If destroyed bilaterally, amnesia results; if damaged by tumor, emotional and personality changes can occur. These clinical problems are separate topics and will be discussed later in the chapter.

The final major area of clinical interest is the behavioral changes that are seen in patients with temporal lobe epilepsy. The problem of epilepsy and especially temporal lobe epilepsy is of sufficient importance that we have devoted an entire chapter, Chapter 11, to this subject.

Parietal Lobe Syndromes

The parietal lobes contain the cross modal association areas for integrating visual, tactile, and auditory input. They also have the capacity to manipulate this high level information and are therefore a principal structure in intellectual processing within the human brain. As with the temporal lobes, there is a preferential processing in the left hemisphere for verbal material and in the right hemisphere for visual perceptual material. The left inferior parietal lobule (areas 39 and 40), as we have seen, is the specialized area for the visual/auditory integration necessary for reading, writing, and to a great extent, calculating. In addition, many of the verbally mediated activities involved in intellectual functioning are carried out in this left parietal region: verbal abstract reasoning such as proverb interpretation is but one example. Motor planning or praxis also takes place to a great extent in this left parietal lobe. Some unusual capacities of the left parietal region are more basic than the highly integrative features already mentioned. One is the appreciation of painful stimulation, and on occasion, a patient with a left parietal lesion will actually lose complete appreciation for pain, a condition which has been termed an asymbolia for pain. Also in the tactile sensory field, the left parietal lobe has a certain capacity for integrating tactile stereognosis for both sides of the body and not just for the side opposite the lesion, as is true for the right parietal area.

The left parietal lobe has many connections devoted to the integration of visual perception and the guiding of the visual-motor integrative processes needed to reproduce drawings, construct models, or to carry out any such constructional task. The left hemisphere is not, however, nearly as adept at carrying out these high level visual tasks as is the right. The right parietal area is particularly skilled at perceiving overall visual patterns, whereas the left tends to perceive things more in terms of individual specific details.[87] With damage to both parietal lobes, the disintegration of constructional abilities can be very striking.

The right parietal lobe, because of its superior ability to conceive of space and the relationships of things in space, is best able to visualize and guide us in our environment. This geographic sense also carries over to the abstract spatial orientation utilized in reading maps and blueprints. In addition, the right parietal area seems to be involved with the integration of both visual and tactile perceptions necessary for properly dressing oneself.

Both parietal lobes assist in the appreciation of right-left sense, gnosis of finger localization, and the stereognosis and localization of touch on the respective contralateral sides of the body. Both parietal lobes are also involved in helping focus attention, particularly to the side of the body or environmental field opposite it (the left is somewhat stronger in this respect).

Given this differential functioning of the two parietal lobes, the clinical syndromes associated with damage to either are easily understood.

The syndromes are rarely encountered in pure form; a combination of the various symptoms is usually seen.

I. Left parietal syndromes
   A. Alexia plus agraphia
   B. Alexia plus agraphia plus anomia
   C. Gerstmann's syndrome (agraphia, calculation difficulty, right-left disorientation, and finger agnosia)
   D. Also seen in varying combinations are:
      1. Constructional difficulty
      2. Astereognosis, right hand or sometimes bilateral
      3. Pain asymbolia
      4. Ideomotor apraxia
      5. Various fluent aphasic disorders
II. Right parietal syndromes
   A. Constructional impairment (apraxia)
   B. Dressing apraxia
   C. Geographic disorientation
   D. Astereognosis on the left side
   E. Calculation and writing problems due to grossly distorted placement or production of the actual letters and numbers.
   F. Denial and neglect of the left side, both of the body and of the environment.

This last finding deserves special attention as the syndromes of denial and neglect can be some of the most dramatic behavioral responses seen in focal brain disease. In the full-blown denial syndrome, patients steadfastly deny that they have suffered any neurologic disease. The most common situation in clinical practice is the denial of left hemiplegia. Such patients may claim that the arm or leg is perfectly well but is not moving now because it is tired. At times patients will even state that the immobile limb is not theirs at all but belongs to another person who is in bed with them.

In some cases this explicit denial is not seen, but a less dramatic implicit type of denial is expressed. We saw a 50-year-old accountant recently who had meningitis with a mild left hemiparesis. His mentation had cleared almost completely, but he told his brother-in-law that it was very nice that he was in this small hospital for people who are not too sick which was right next door to his house so he would not have too far to go when he was discharged (actually the hospital was miles from the city in which he lived). He went on to say that it was somewhat inconvenient at times because the door to his house and to the hospital were so close together that people often got into his house by mistake! This type of phenomenon was initially called reduplicative paramnesia but more recently has been referred to as a reduplication of place and called an example of implicit denial.[11,115,145] Many examples of this type of behavioral phenomenon have been described and they represent an interesting way in which patients try to minimize their illness without frankly denying it.[145]

The denial syndrome includes a spectrum of disorders ranging from marked frank denial as its most dramatic manifestation to a subtle inattention to stimuli on the contralateral side of the body during sensory testing with bilateral double simultaneous stimulation. Between these extremes is the very interesting phenomenon of unilateral neglect which can be seen both alone and in conjunction with the more dramatic forms of denial. In unilateral neglect, the patients display a variety of symptoms. They almost exclusively direct their attention toward the same side as the brain lesion, almost totally neglecting visual, tactile, and auditory stimuli to the contralateral side. If the patient is spoken to by someone standing on the neglected side, he will frequently turn toward his intact side and away from the speaker. On occasion, the neglect is so severe that the patients fail to shave or dress the neglected side. Other patients, whose lesion has not caused a hemiparesis, fail to use the contralateral arm. In drawing tasks, it is common for such patients to complete only half of the picture even when hemianopia is not present.

Many observations and experiments have been carried out over the years in an attempt to understand these curious phenomena and a number of clinical features and theoretical explanations have been reported. Firstly, these syndromes are much more common in patients with lesions in the right hemisphere than in the left.[36,60,114,144] Secondly, the full explicit denial syndrome is almost always seen primarily during the acute phase of the illness when the patient may continue to have elements of confusional behavior.[72,92,145] Thirdly, many other neurologic deficits have been noted in a high percentage of the patients with the full syndrome, including a marked reduction in cutaneous sensation at the contralateral limbs,[72,145] gross visual-constructive defects,[114] jargon aphasia in the patients in whom left hemisphere lesions have caused the syndrome,[145] and diffuse EEG slowing over the entire hemisphere containing the lesion.[140]

This syndrome is usually caused by a vascular lesion in the right parietal lobe that extends deep into the hemisphere, but the syndrome has also been seen clinically with frontal lesions and right thalamic hemorrhage[141] and experimentally produced lesions in animals in the cingulate gyrus and the reticular formation of the mesencephalon.[142]

The pathophysiology, both of the basic phenomenon and its association with right hemisphere damage, has been the object of considerable debate and speculation. Several factors seem to be important: confusional behavior in the most dramatic cases, sensory defects on the neglected side, and gross constructional defects. These elements help, in part, to explain neglect but do not explain the basic reason why right hemisphere lesions produce the syndrome more commonly and why there is active neglect of one side rather than merely a recognized sensory loss. Various explanations have been offered: (1) inability to integrate sensory stimuli from the contralateral side, giving those stimuli less importance than those from the ipsilateral side in their rivalry for attention (amorphosynthesis),[44] (2) a disconnection of visual and tactile information from the right hemisphere to the left language area, in essence rendering the left brain unable to comment on input from the right hemisphere,[60] (3) interruption of basic reticulocortical and limbocortical connections leaving the hemisphere with insufficient reticular input to concentrate attention on events entering that hemisphere,[81] and (4) a basic imbalance in the orienting response, assuming that the orienting tendency toward the right is much stronger than to the left, thus giving marked right orientation with lesions of the right side but only weak or balanced orientation with lesions on the left.[92] The reader interested in an in depth discussion of the topic is referred to a volume entitled *Hemi-inattention and Hemispheric Specialization* edited by Weinstein and Friedland.[143]

The behavioral deficits seen in parietal lobe disease are very specialized and are not readily elicited on routine neurologic testing. The parietal lobe was traditionally known as one of the "silent areas" of the brain, but during the last several decades, a tremendous amount has been learned about how to communicate with this region.

Frontal Lobe Syndrome

Bilateral damage to the premotor areas of the frontal lobes (areas 9, 10, and 11) causes a behavioral syndrome that has been recognized for well over a century. The patient, so aflicted, displays a marked change in personality and social behavior while maintaining normal or near normal intellectual and neurologic functioning. Since the syndrome is almost purely behavioral, the examiner must be thoroughly acquainted with its specific features in order to suspect the presence of frontal lobe damage. The symptom complex may vary from patient to patient, but most commonly the patients demonstrate some degree of apathy, irritability, poor judgement, uninhibited social behavior, lack of motivation and goal direction, and euphoria. The patients generally display very shallow affect and, although easily angered, do not sustain their irritation for more than a few minutes. Cognitive capabilities suffer subtle but real impairment; perseveration is present which prevents the patient from efficiently shifting his thinking or reasoning from one pattern to another when environmental changes signal the necessity for an alteration in behavior; verbal fluency is decreased (this is particularly true when the left frontal lobe has sustained the maximum insult); and there is also a tendency for the frontal lobe patient to exhibit a disturbance in the ability to efficiently sequence in temporal order.[79,100,110] Attention is also often disturbed and such patients are not only unable to sustain their attention on a specific task but are also easily distracted by irrelevant environmental stimuli.[100] Although these cognitive disruptions are not as obvious as those seen with parietal lobe damage, they nevertheless add to the overall difficulty experienced by these patients. The following case clearly demonstrates the problems encountered by some of these patients.

A 22-year-old soldier sustained a frontal lobe missile wound during his service in Vietnam. He was evacuated to the United States for recuperation and within 5 weeks had essentially recovered. The attending neurosurgeon found no gross residual neurologic abnormalities and a brief psychologic evaluation showed that his IQ, memory, and constructional abilities were within normal limits. The patient was returned to active duty at a base in the United States. Within a few weeks, complaints began to be made concerning his behavior. His wife reported that he had changed from an easy going guy to an irritable, easily angered person who would get into a fight everytime they went out socially. At work he constantly got into arguments with his supervisors and peers alike. Two months after his return to active duty, he had been jailed twice for disorderly conduct and assault. At this point he was reevaluated with a more extensive neuropsychologic battery and comprehensive neurologic examination. This evaluation brought into focus the true significance of his behavioral change, and it was finally realized that he had a rather classic frontal lobe syndrome directly attributable to his injury. He was granted a medical discharge from the army and returned to civilian life. On follow-up report this man has not been able to hold a regular job and has maintained himself only on his disability pension from the military.

The actual clinical frontal lobe syndrome varies somewhat from case to case and the symptoms appear to be somewhat related to the specific location of the lesion. Patients with lesions in the baso-orbital portion of the frontal lobe tend to display the type of behavior illustrated in the case above (uninhibited, aggressive, and pugilistic). Also seen secondary to these orbital lesions is a more pleasant form of the same disinhibition in which the patient is constantly joking, talking loudly, and acting in a generally euphoric fashion. Sexual disinhibition and irritability can be seen in both forms of the orbitofrontal syndrome.[23,100]

Patients with primary damage to the convexities of the frontal lobe tend to have more cognitive deficits and also present a more apathetic, nonmotivated, adynamic picture clinically.[23,100] Underlying the behavior of all patients with significant frontal lobe damage is an unfortunate lack of motivation, inability to plan ahead, and poor judgement. These factors, in conjunction with any personality disturbance, severely hinder these patients from leading normally productive lives.

Two critical problems in effectively diagnosing this syndrome need further elucidation. The first is the delay in recognizing the syndrome (as in the case above), and the second is the misidentification of the symptoms as being functional and not organic in origin. Failure to recognize the syndrome stems primarily from failure of the clinician to search for the specific symptoms. If the clinician has not known the patient previously, he must seek out and carefully question the patient's relatives and friends concerning any change in specific behaviors. Psychologic testing must be expanded to look for evidence of frontal disturbance on alternating sequence testing, trail making, card sorting facility, and verbal fluency. As with so many areas of medicine, one can only diagnose a disease or syndrome if one thinks of it and specifically tests for it. This is particularly true with the frontal lobe syndrome.

The second problem in diagnosis is the misconstruing of the signs of apathy, disinhibition, and short temper as being a psychiatric reaction. On first impression, apathy can mimic depression, for the depressed patient is certainly often apathetic. But apathy alone without sadness, tears, self-depreciation, and vegetative signs should strongly arouse the examiner's suspicion of organic and particularly frontal lobe disease. The frontal lobe patient who displays gross antisocial behavior and disinhibition can superficially resemble someone with psychopathic behavior unless a careful history and examination are carried out. In all cases, familiarity with the frontal lobe syndrome will make the diagnosis considerably easier.

The dramatic behavioral changes seen in frontal lobe damage led many neurosurgeons and psychiatrists to the conclusion that removal or disconnection of part or all of the frontal lobes might be useful in controlling the behavior of patients with uncontrollable psychosis or obsessional neurosis.[31,51,108,133] Over the years, these psychosurgical procedures have been refined to the use of stereotaxic lesions in the medial frontal lobe or the cingulate gyrus to disconnect limbic input to the frontal lobe. The procedures are not as widely used today because of the number of psychotropic drugs available to control abnormal behavior, but surgery can still be a useful method of controlling rare cases of severe obsessive-compulsive neurosis, severe anxiety, depression, and the affective disturbance seen in some schizophrenic patients.[31,133]

244

Limbic Syndromes

Damage or irritation to the structures within the limbic system has been shown to alter the basic instinctual, emotional, and memory functions subserved by the system. We have already discussed how certain components of the system can be affected in generalized disease such as confusional behavior or dementia, but in this section the discussion will center upon the behavioral symptoms resulting from focal lesions.

AMNESIC SYNDROME

The most common and certainly one of the most fascinating limbic syndromes is the amnesic syndrome. Clinically, the syndrome in its most extreme form is characterized by a severe deficit in recent memory in the face of normal remote and immediate memory with preservation of other intellectual functions. The amnesic patient can carry on a completely normal conversation but is totally unable to learn any new information. The patient can be told the examiner's name ten times within the space of an hour, yet 5 minutes after the last reminder the patient may say, "I don't believe I caught your name." The amnesic patient is able to initially register the information and repeat it within a few seconds but is unable to store or retrieve that information after a few minutes. Old, well established memories are spared and their retrieval is quite normal.[129] The most severe problem encountered by these patients is in new learning (anterograde amnesia), but they also usually experience an associated period of retrograde amnesia. Retrograde amnesia refers to an impaired ability to remember details that preceded the accident or illness that produced the amnesia. The memory loss causes the patients to lose orientation in time; they do not remember the date and have no way of mentally recording the passage of days and months. They also are frequently disoriented as to place. One man with Korsakoff's syndrome had settled down to the hospital routine until one day he looked out the window and reported to us that something very unusual had happened, a parking lot had been built overnight outside his window. This upset him very much and he marveled at it everytime he looked out the window. What we later found out was that he thought that the hospital was actually another hospital in which he had spent several months after the war. He felt that the hospital was familiar (they were both Veterans Administration Hospitals) but the disappearance of the garden he remembered viewing from his window upset him visibly.

As if to fill in the gap in their memory, many of the amnesic patients confabulate quite unabashedly when asked a direct question which they cannot answer. One elderly man, when asked at a conference about the location and nature of the building, said that it was a schoolroom from his old high school and that the doctors were teachers and old friends. He went so far as to single out one of the staff as having been out drinking with him the week before (a quick denial from the staff member presumably verified the confabulatory nature of the response). Spontaneous confabulation is less common, and in general these patients remain quiet rather than initiating conversation.

This curious syndrome of isolated memory difficulty is produced by restricted bilateral lesions in various limbic circuits. The case that initially demonstrated the remarkable clinical pathologic relationship between memory and the limbic system was a surgical removal of both temporal lobes in a young epileptic man.[128] This type of procedure has not been repeated because of the obvious side effects, but damage to the hippocampi with resultant amnesia is quite regularly seen in cases of severe head trauma, anoxia, and herpes simplex encephalitis. Bilateral hippocampal infarction has also been shown to cause extensive memory difficulty.[15,43] In cases of Korsakoff's syndrome, which is the amnesic syndrome seen following Wernicke's encephalopathy associated with acute thiamine deficiency (primarily in alcoholics), the limbic damage is in the mammillary bodies and the dorsomedial thalami.[137] Tumors involving the dorsomedial thalamus, midbrain, and posterior fornix have also been reported to cause amnesia, thus further strengthening the theory that limbic structures and pathways are critical in the storage and retrieval of memory traces.[80,105]

Amnesia is of sudden onset in almost all cases and of varying degrees of severity. Post-traumatic cases usually improve quite rapidly and the retrograde amnesia actually shrinks during the recovery phase.[12] Events preceding the accident return chronologically until usually it is only the few seconds before the accident that are forever lost to the patient's recall. With infectious and vascular lesions, recovery may only be partial and a mild to moderate permanent memory problem can persist. In alcoholic patients who have undergone a full Wernicke's phase with subsequent Korsakoff's amnesia, at least one-third will experience a permanent severe amnesia.[136,137] For the others, recovery ranges from full recovery (20%) to moderate disability. The possibility of progressive memory difficulty with alcoholism has not been well studied, but examination of brain specimens certainly shows atrophy in the mammillary bodies in many alcoholics. This, combined with the obvious alcoholic dementia seen in some patients, strongly supports the contention that alcohol in large quantities over time can serve as a slow poison to the neurons of the central nervous system.

In one type of amnesic syndrome, probably of vascular origin, the memory deficit is transient. This syndrome has been called transient global amnesia and is characterized by a short period, usually less than 24 hours, of confusional behavior and amnesia.[5,50,76,104] When exam-

246

ined during the acute episode, the patients repeatedly ask where they are and what they are doing. If told about their whereabouts, they soon forget and ask again. They also have a short period of retrograde amnesia as is demonstrated in the following case.

A 60-year-old housewife had been shopping the day before her amnesic episode and bought some shoes. After arriving home, she decided to return them the following day because they were the wrong color and placed them on the kitchen table so as not to forget them in the morning. The following morning she was stirring some pancake batter when she suddenly looked around and called to her husband. She asked him what she was making and whose shoes were those and what were they doing in the kitchen. The husband explained and no sooner had he finished his explanation than the patient repeated the question, seeming to obsess about the shoes. The patient was taken to the hospital where examination revealed only the confusional behavior and the memory problem. These symptoms cleared quite rapidly in the following 12 hours, and she then could remember having purchased the shoes but did not remember anything about cooking pancakes or other events of that day.

This condition is probably due to a transient ischemia of the posterior cerebral arteries. The temporal branches of these vessels supply the hippocampi, which are the postulated site of the ischemia. Many cases do not have recurrences for many years,[152] while others actually develop a progressive step-wise dementing syndrome.[104]

In transient global amnesia there is often a question as to whether the episode is of organic or psychologic etiology. The differential diagnosis between a transient organic amnesia and the dissociative type of amnesia seen in hysterical neurosis is quite easy if either the examiner or a reliable observer has seen the patient during the actual episode. In the organic cases, the patients are actively confused, continually ask where they are, and cannot store any memories during the amnesic period. Conversely, the hysterical patient acts perfectly normal during the episode, can learn things during the amnesia, and only reports a period of amnesia after the episode is over. This latter type of amnesia was illustrated in a young Peace Corps volunteer who had gone to a small town in interior Brazil to work when he soon began to "lose track of days." He returned to the capital and reported that on several occasions he had blanked out entire days. He remembered going out to buy a newspaper each morning only to awaken the following day with the paper beside his bed and no recollection of actually buying it or of the events of the previous day. Upon cautious inquiry of the townspeople he found out that he had, in fact, spent each day making appropriate contacts, talking to people, and doing all the other things expected of a volunteer during his first few months in a country. This was clearly an emotionally based amnesia and has none of the dramatic behavioral features of transient global amnesia.

OTHER LIMBIC SYNDROMES

Although memory problems are among the most common limbic disorders, some other very interesting behavioral abnormalities are seen with specific limbic lesions. When tumors arise in limbic structures, they can cause very dramatic changes in basic vegetative as well as emotional behavior. Tumors arising in and destroying the ventromedial hypothalamus produce a slowly progressive syndrome of hyperphagia, aggressiveness, and eventual confusional behavior. In one case, the patient scratched, hit, and even attempted to bite the examiner during examination.[117] In some patients, manic behavior, sloppiness, and paranoia have been reported with tumors exerting pressure on the hypothalamus from beneath.[103] Accompanying these marked behavioral abnormalities are usually a variety of other endocrine and autonomic disturbances including temperature change, menstrual abnormalities, and diabetes insipidus.

On rare occasions, tumors or demyelination have been reported in which the ventral hypothalamus has been spared and damage to the lateral nuclei has occurred.[86,147] In such instances, the patients develop an anorexia rather than hyperphagia and can easily be misdiagnosed as having anorexia nervosa. This is not to suggest that many cases of true anorexia nervosa are harboring cryptic hypothalamic tumors, as these are decidedly rare, but only to encourage the clinician to entertain this possibility, particularly if neurologic or endocrine abnormalities (other than amenorrhea) appear.

Tumors originating deep in the frontal and temporal lobes and involving the limbic structures therein have long been known to cause behavioral changes that can simulate psychiatric disease.[84,89,103,131] It is very difficult in most cases to decide if these behavioral changes represent negative phenomena (i.e., the result of loss of function from destruction of brain tissue), positive phenomena (i.e., the result of an active associated epileptic focus that stimulates the production of behavioral aberration), or the concomitant effects of increased intracranial pressure. Regardless of the specific mechanisms, it is clear that lesions in the temporal and frontal limbic tissue can lead to a variety of pseudopsychiatric states ranging from depression to schizophreniform psychosis. The specific syndromes and behavioral correlations will be discussed more fully in Chapter 11, Epilepsy, and Chapter 13, Brain Tumor.

Drs. Klüver and Bucy described a number of dramatic behavioral changes in experimental monkeys who had undergone bilateral temporal lobectomies.[94] Whether the resultant syndrome of placidity, hyperorality, amnesia, hypersexuality, and visual agnosia was secondary to removal of limbic structures or temporal neocortex is not settled, but the experiment stimulated interest in the relationship of temporal lobe structures to behavior. This syndrome (Klüver-Bucy) does appear in man in various clinical settings: bilateral temporal lobectomy,[134] head trauma,[85] and encephalitis. The full syndrome is not usually seen and, as can be seen from the nature of the etiologies, it is not always restricted to temporal lobe damage. We have seen several such cases, the most recent was an adolescent boy who had suffered herpes simplex encephalitis. During the recovery phase, he developed aggressive behavior towards his siblings, marked exploratory behavior with hyperactivity, memory difficulty, and hyperorality. When the patient entered the office he immediately began to explore every shelf and object in the room. Objects of interest such as ashtrays and staplers were immediately placed in his mouth for further investigation.

Another case was a young man who sustained a rather severe head injury during an automobile accident. Following his comatose stage, he became aggressive, amnesic, hyperoral, and sexually obsessive. He required restraint in bed because he would attack nurses sexually, fight with male staff members, and eat anything that he could get his hands on including such delicacies as his medical chart. Although the central nervous system damage was relatively diffuse in these cases, it is probable that much of the abnormal behavior stemmed from damage to limbic structures.

The syndromes discussed thus far are largely due to ablative lesions within the limbic system; there remain a number of interesting limbic syndromes associated with active epileptogenic lesions. Because much of the information on these active limbic foci comes from the study of temporal lobe epilepsy, we will discuss the entire topic of stimulating lesions in Chapter 11, Epilepsy.

Corpus Callosal Syndromes

The corpus callosum is an immense association pathway that is only infrequently involved in pathologic processes. When it is damaged, the defects produced are subtle, yet their elucidation and study has revealed a great deal concerning the functional interrelationships of the two cerebral hemispheres. We have already discussed the significant problem in reading which occurs when the left occipital lobe and posterior callosum are damaged. Visual information then reaches only the right hemisphere and is prevented from crossing to the language dominant left hemisphere. The resultant alexia clearly demonstrates the need for the callosal transmission of written language to the language area for processing.

When a lesion occurs in the anterior portion of the callosum, a far more subtle problem develops. In such cases, the right frontal and anterior parietal cortex has essentially been disconnected from the language area of the left hemisphere (Fig. 7-6). The resultant syndrome consists of the following three elements: (1) an agraphia in left-handed writing but not in right-handed writing, (2) an apraxia of the left hand, and (3) an inability to name unseen objects placed in the left hand.[65] All of these deficits are due to the fact that the right motor and sensory cortex are unable to utilize the language and praxis centers in the dominant hemisphere. Since the right hemisphere is intact, it can coordinate many activities within itself. For example, the left hand is able to copy line drawings very well, better in fact than the right hand,

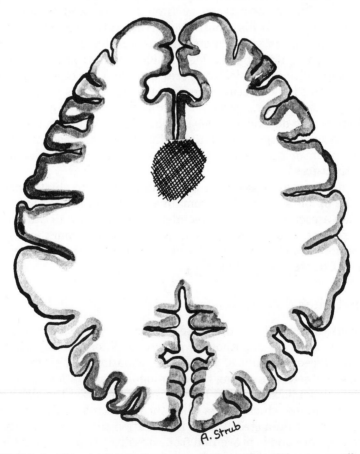

FIGURE 7-6. The cross-hatched area represents a lesion of the corpus callosum.

because of the superiority of the right hemisphere in integrating visual perceptual information.[26]

In recent years, a small number of epileptic patients have undergone complete section of the corpus callosum and anterior commissure in an attempt to control the interhemispheric spread of epileptic discharges. This has made it possible to study more precisely the role of the corpus callosum in human behavior.[24,25,56] In essence, there is no real change in bimanual motor coordination or in most general behaviors. When verbal tasks are demanded of the left hand, of course, failure is experienced. Also, the left hand under the guidance of its right hemisphere is much better at constructional tasks. An extensive series of interesting observations have been made on these surgical patients using a variety of techniques for presenting information solely to one hemisphere. These have been reported by Gazzaniga in a book entitled *The Bisected Brain*[56] and the interested reader is referred to this volume. What this work has done, more than to elucidate the function of the corpus callosum, is to help in understanding the functions of the individual hemispheres. Since in these patients the hemispheres are virtually independent, information can be presented to either hemisphere alone; tactually through the contralateral hand or visually with a tachistoscope. Thus, the functioning of each hemisphere can be assessed independently.

The studies mentioned above were all carried out on patients who had commissurotomies after the acquisition of language and many other skills. In patients born with agenesis of the corpus callosum, the interhemispheric organization is quite different. Reading capacity, for example, has been reported in both hemispheres. Some patients can name objects placed in either hand, whereas, transfer of kinesthetic learning is defective and there is some difficulty with bimanual coordination.[48] Data from these cases seem to indicate that the two hemispheres develop more independently when there are no callosal connections and lead to the contention that callosal interconnections partly account for the development of cerebral dominance. Unfortunately callosal agenesis is usually not the only cerebral anomaly in these patients and the presence of seizures and other lesions may produce many of the abnormal findings which have been demonstrated.

General Hemispheric Differences

To superficial inspection the two cerebral hemispheres appear as mirror images, but as has been demonstrated in studies of patients with lesions in one hemisphere, the initial impression of equality is functionally incorrect. By disconnecting the two hemispheres and, through ingenious testing, even greater insights have been gained as to their distinct and individual functioning. Encouraged by the obvious functional differences between right and left hemispheres, more detailed anatomic studies were begun. Basic anatomic differences which correlate well with known functional asymmetries have been discovered, the most notable being the increase in the auditory association areas in the left hemispheres of right-handed persons.[63,66,149] Despite the fact that basic anatomic asymmetries indicate that the substrate for left hemisphere language dominance is present at birth, the right hemisphere is capable of completely and efficiently taking over all language functions if the left is damaged early in life.[130] This remarkable plasticity of cortical function is one of the most interesting aspects of the developing nervous system. It is almost complete for higher cortical functions at birth and rapidly decreases as language is acquired and established. By late childhood, the degree of compensation for brain damage is much less, and in the adult, loss of the left hemisphere leaves the patient capable of producing only a few expletives under stress.

In general, the left hemisphere is most efficient in all verbal tasks including verbal memory (although it requires bilateral damage to produce a severe amnesic state, unilateral left temporal lobe damage results in a measurable decrement in verbal learning).[109] This verbal or language dominance is by far the most outstanding of all functional hemispheric asymmetries. The right hemisphere, in contrast, is nonverbal or mute, but has its prominence in the realm of visual spatial activities. This left-verbal, right-visual spatial dichotomy is consistent in most of the population, but as we have discussed, it is influenced by genetic and other factors that determine basic handedness and dominance. Although this dichotomy is the same for both male and female, the relative capacities for these functions differ according to sex. Females show a consistent superiority in verbal skills, while males show an equally strong overall strength in spatial abilities.[35] These differences are further dramatized by the much higher incidence of both delayed speech and written language problems (dyslexia) in male children (a 6 to 1 predominance).

Hemispheric differences have been examined in many ways; currently it is popular to discuss the mode of functioning of the individual hemispheres rather than the specific function being carried out. The term "cognitive style" has been adopted to indicate this functional concept. The right hemisphere, because of its superior capacity for appreciating patterns or overall spatial concepts, has a so-called synthetic or holistic style, whereas the left hemisphere has a more analytic and logical style which is attentive to detail but inadequate for rapid synthesis.[96] This style of functioning is well demonstrated in patients with right or left hemisphere lesions when they attempt to complete block designs. When the left hemisphere is working alone (right hemisphere damage) the patient is unable to approximate the overall outline of the design. In the left hemisphere damaged patient, the outline of the design will be correct, but the details of the internal structure will be faulty.[87] This type of observation has also been made in patients after commissurotomy (corpus callosal section) where each hemisphere can be tested individually.[24,25,26]

The differential role of the hemispheres has been shown to extend beyond pure cognitive capacities and into the field of emotional behavior. Again, both studies of hemisphere damage as well as the observation of commissurotomy patients have elucidated the varying roles of the two hemispheres. One of the earliest observations was made in aphasic patients who, upon being asked to perform demanding linguistic tasks such as verbal arithmetic, would suddenly show an intense anxiety reaction.[69] This catastrophic reaction, as it has been called, occurs whenever the patient begins to fail on a task that was previously within his capability. The reaction often develops so rapidly that it appears to be an actual intrinsic aspect of the inability to carry out the task rather than a secondary emotional reaction of the patient after the realization of his failure. This observation of the emotional reactions of the aphasic patient has led to many systematic studies of patients with unilateral brain lesions, the results of which have verified the initial impression and refined the concept in many ways. Left hemisphere damage has been repeatedly shown to give a much higher incidence of both the catastrophic anxiety reaction and depression. This observation has been made by clinical observation[52,78] and on psychologic testing using the Minnesota Multiphasic Personality Inventory.[22,99] Within this group of left hemisphere damaged patients, it is the aphasics and most particularly the Broca's aphasics, that show the greatest abnormality.[8,52] Wernicke's aphasics, conversely, demonstrate a very different personality reaction. These patients show indifference rather than anxiety, and paranoia rather than depression.[8,52]

Damage to the right hemisphere causes quite a different clinical picture than does similar left hemisphere damage. Such patients demonstrate a remarkable lack of emotional response and often display the type of apathy seen in patients with frontal damage.[52,77] They are indifferent to their surroundings and, in general, seem to have lost the ability to appreciate and produce appropriate emotional subtleties. Their appreciation of humorous situations is greatly affected and they tend to respond either with an exaggerated response or none at all.[54] They are largely unable to discriminate and identify the emotional quality or tone of someone's voice and also are reduced in their ability to evoke specific emotional expression.[135] From these observations, it appears that the right hemisphere develops, in addition to its cognitive synthetic abilities, a superior ability to synthesize limbic emotional responsivity to environmental experience.

As knowledge of hemispheric function has become more sophisticated, it is now possible for the neuroscientist to ask philosophical questions concerning the anatomic substrate for such concepts as the self-conscious mind. Is self-consciousness a discrete function which is lateralized to one hemisphere or is it a capacity contained by both hemispheres? In the study of commissurotomy patients, it has been observed that each hemisphere is able to analyze sensory input and guide the behavior of the opposite limb, but it is only the left hemisphere that can actually discuss and verbalize its decisions and actions.[57,95] The right hemisphere is a mute worker whose thoughts and feelings can only be inferred verbally by the left hemisphere's observation of the right's behavior.[57] As is fitting, the workers in this field are split on their interpretation of these observations. Some say that it is only the verbal left hemisphere that is truly self-conscious because of its ability to verbally reflect on its activity,[57] while others claim that the mute right hemisphere can make decisions involving judgements and goal setting and therefore is also conscious in its own right.

Popper, the philosopher, and Eccles, the Nobel lauret in neurophysiology, have recently queried this same issue in an interesting new book entitled, *The Self and Its Brain.*[116] These men are also divided, Eccles feels strongly that the verbal reflectiveness of the left hemisphere is the necessary feature of mans self-conscious mind; whereas Popper, fully realizing that the self-consciousness of the mute hemisphere is not as developed as the questioning and rhetorical left hemisphere, feels that the right hemisphere has a level of true self-consciousness that may in some ways be similar to the crude self-consciousness experienced by higher animals. The issue is fascinating and exciting in the fact that the study of the brain's activity has now reached a level when these age old questions of the philosopher can now be discussed in more than mere abstraction.

NEUROBEHAVIORAL EVALUATION

A complete mental status examination, as outlined in Chapter 3, is particularly useful in diagnosing the focal syndromes. Focal brain disease tends to cause isolated defects in behavior or typical symptom clusters while frequently completely sparing other functions. With a complete examination, the defects stand out sharply against the background of normal functioning and suggest the focal lesion.

Again, it is necessary to evaluate handedness and familial handedness when localizing focal lesions. This is of greatest importance in assessing disorders involving language but should be ascertained in all cases.

MEDICAL EVALUATION

A complete medical and neurologic history and examination are necessary. Specific attention should be paid to the following factors:

I. Onset of symptoms: Acute onset suggests a vascular accident; a slowly progressive onset indicates an expanding mass in most cases.

II. History of
   A. Hematologic disease or anticoagulant use
   B. Cardiac disease: Arrhythmia, failure, myocardial infarction of endocarditis
   C. Vascular disease including the symptoms and signs of vasculitis
   D. Cancer or symptoms suspicious of cancer
   E. Head trauma
   F. Chronic infection
   G. Alcoholism
   H. Drug abuse

III. Seizures

IV. Focal neurologic signs

DIFFERENTIAL DIAGNOSIS

Unilateral Hemispheric Lesions

The differential diagnosis of unilateral hemispheric lesions is quite straightforward and is well discussed in most standard neurologic texts. The primary lesions are:

I. Acute
   A. Cerebral vascular accidents
      1. Occlusive: Either from thrombosis or embolism from heart and great vessels
      2. Hemorrhagic: Due to aneurysm, arteriovenous malformation, hypertensive hemorrhage, spontaneous hemorrhage from blood dyscrasia, or anticoagulant use
   B. Migraine: Usually very short lived (< 12 hours)
   C. Bleeding into tumor
   D. Trauma

II. Slowly progressive deficit
   A. Tumor: Primary or metastatic
   B. Abscess
   C. Cyst
   D. Subdural lesion, such as a hematoma

Bilateral Hemispheric Lesions

The differential diagnosis of the bilateral syndromes is somewhat different. The frontal lobe syndrome can be caused by various conditions including: frontal tumors (gliomas, metastatic lesions, subfrontal and perisaggital meningiomas, and large pituitary tumors), hydrocephalus, general paresis, Huntington's chorea, Pick's disease, alcoholic and Parkinson's dementia, other frontal masses such as abscess or cyst, and head trauma. The amnesic syndrome from bilateral limbic damage is most commonly seen secondary to trauma but can occur with alcoholism, encephalitis, discrete vascular lesions, and rarely, a tumor in the region of the posterior third ventricle and upper midbrain.

LABORATORY EVALUATION

Laboratory tests will consist primarily of brain scans and cerebral contrast studies, but certain general screening tests should also be obtained.

1. Complete blood profile
2. Sedimentation rate
3. Coagulation studies
4. Sickle cell preparation or hemoglobin electrophoresis if indicated
5. Serologic test for syphilis
6. Chest and skull x-rays
7. Electrocardiogram

The specific neurodiagnostic test in evaluating focal intracranial lesions is the computerized tomography (CT) scan. If this diagnostic tool is not available, a standard brain scan should be obtained. The electroencephalogram is sometimes helpful in focal disease, but only in cases where no clear-cut lateralizing signs are found on other components of the evaluation. Spinal puncture should be used with great caution in focal lesions, particularly if a mass lesion is suspected. In general, a spinal tap is done to identify infection or subarachnoid hemorrhage. At this point in the evaluation it is best to consult a neurologist or neurosurgeon to assist in further evaluation. Cerebral arteriography under the supervision of the neurologist or neurosurgeon is required in many cases of focal cerebral lesions. When evaluating a left-handed patient or one with a strong family history of left handedness, the intracarotid sodium amytal (Wada) test should be carried out during arteriography.[139]

CONSULTATIONS

Neurologic or neurosurgical consultation should be obtained in most cases of focal brain disease if such services are readily available. Early in the course of the patient's illness and certainly before any nonemergency neurosurgical procedure is carried out, a full neuropsychologic evaluation should be completed. This evaluation serves many purposes: it can further delineate the deficit diagnosed on the mental status exam, it quantifies the extent of the deficit, and it outlines the patient's residual strengths. The psychologist can also be extremely helpful in interpreting the nature and significance of the behavioral deficit to the family.

In the aphasic patient, it is often useful to have the speech pathologist see the patient early in the evaluation, even though therapy may not be initiated at that time. The speech pathologist can assess the language problem and help the patient, his family, and the medical personnel understand the patient's language restrictions. This often relieves anxiety and a helps establish a sensible communication system.

PATIENT MANAGEMENT

The medical or neurosurgical management of strokes, brain tumors, and other such focal brain lesions is a broad subject and is described in more general medical, neurologic, and neurosurgical texts. Here we will emphasize the elements of comprehensive rehabilitation rather than the basic medical management. Since many focal lesions are isolated events in the lives of the patients (and do not represent progressive diseases) the prognosis for survival is good. The direction of longterm management then is rehabilitative rather than medical. This rehabilitation is a lengthy process that usually starts with a period of intensive inpatient evaluation and therapy.

Initially, a comprehensive evaluation should be carried out by the rehabilitation physician, the neuropsychologist, the speech pathologist, and the physical and occupational therapists. This evaluation will outline both the physical and cognitive strengths and weaknesses so that a full rehabilitation program can be instituted. This extensive evaluation and treatment program is usually begun several weeks after the initial hospitalization (physical therapists may be seeing the patient much earlier; but a comprehensive rehabilitative effort usually awaits the passing of the acute medical or surgical period).

In the rehabilitation setting, the physical therapist is involved primarily in gross motor and gait training, while the occupational therapist is concerned mostly with fine motor control of the hands and the skills involved in the routine activities of daily living. The speech pathologist can be of assistance in articulation problems, buccofacial apraxia, and certain aphasic disturbances. Global aphasia and severe Wernicke's aphasia do not respond well to standard speech therapy, therefore any speech pathologist working with these patients should concentrate on other communication systems within the family (e.g., picture cards, sign language).

A number of specific behavioral deficits that may not be obvious at first can significantly interfere with the rehabilitative effort and cause considerable frustration and wasted time if not recognized. The apathy and lack of motivation associated with frontal lobe damage is one such factor. Trauma, postoperative aneurysm, or tumor patients with frontal lobe damage often do not put an enthusiastic effort into therapy and thus gain nothing. Frequently the therapist misinterprets the organically based apathy as a depression, laziness, or lack of cooperation; such a misunderstanding often engenders an unjustifiable hostility and makes an already difficult situation impossible. Unfortunately, rehabilitation, particularly vocational rehabilitation, of patients with damaged frontal lobes is frequently unsuccessful.

Another problem is caused by the neglect or unilateral inattention seen with right hemisphere lesions. When these patients have a hemiplegia, their unilateral neglect causes them to attempt full use of the affected limb and fall. Such a patient must be continually cajoled into moving only after he has gotten himself into a secure standing position with his brace on. These patients may take many months to achieve what may take only a few weeks in a patient without unilateral neglect. Patients with right hemisphere lesions may also have some of the features of apathy and euphoria seen in the frontal lobe patient; these emotional changes add yet another obstacle to rehabilitation.

Ideomotor apraxia is a behavioral deficit that can be a problem in retraining fine motor control. Since the apraxia can be present in both hands, switching to the nonpreferred hand does not always solve the problem. Fortunately, the use of real objects is the simplest possible level of fine motor control for the apraxic, so many can carry out actual daily living activities while they cannot follow limb movement commands on verbal request or by imitation. However, in severely apraxic patients fine motor coordination as well as gross movements may be affected and cause a lasting disability in carrying out complex movements.

A significant memory deficit almost precludes any type of rehabilitation effort that requires learning. Paralyzed limbs can be worked with and basic exercises can be done, but there will be little if any carry over from session to session. In general, the amnesic patient requires custodial care regardless of the level of his motor functioning. He can never be independent because he cannot remember to pay bills, go to a job, find his way home or keep in order any of the thousands of details necessary for daily living.

A further problem which should not go unnoticed, if an adequate evaluation has been completed, is the presence of an underlying dementia or bilateral hemispheric disease. Bilateral disease greatly increases the general disability and decreases the chances for successful recovery. If the underlying disease is a progressive cerebral atrophy, rehabilitative efforts should be limited to basic self-care activities and not include vocational rehabilitation. Other bilateral disease, such as that after trauma, must be recognized as a possible impediment to recovery, but an effort should be made to maximize all existing capacities.

A final element that frequently impairs full effort and benefit from therapy is the patient's superimposed emotional responses, usually a reactive depression. Although many of the emotional changes seen in brain damage are organic, a significant proportion are undoubtly due to the patient's emotional reaction to his illness. In such cases, it is best to consult a psychiatric colleague to assist the patient in dealing with his loss. This is a very important aspect of rehabilitation which is all too often left to the therapist to try and cure with mere encouragement and friendly reinforcement.

In any rehabilitation effort, particularly those dealing with young patients, serious attention must be paid to the eventual vocational possibilities of the patient. In some patients the disability is obviously too great for the patient to return to work, but in many cases careful planning and counseling can lead to gainful employment. Vocational services should become involved with the patients from their entrance into the program and gather background information on premorbid education and training and carefully assess the psychological test scores in order to help the patient choose a suitable and realistic vocation. In many cases, it is impossible to judge in the abstract setting of the hospital how a patient will readjust vocationally. In those cases where recovery seems to be quite good, we arrange for the patients to return to work or try a new job for awhile and have their supervisors report on the adequacy of their performance.

Throughout the rehabilitation period, it is very important to carefully discuss the progress, goals, and future plans for the patient with both the patient and his family. This family counseling is very important and should be a continual dialogue after discharge. If social workers are available, they can be very helpful in working with the family and should become involved early in the patient's hospitalization. So-

cial service workers are acquainted with the facilities and other resources in the community and can coordinate care and training following the period of hospitalization.

Rehabilitation after a focal brain lesion is often slow, with improvement seen over many months to a year's time. Periodic reassessment
is necessary to determine when a plateau is reached and maximum
hospital benefits have been achieved. By this time, an outpatient plan
should have been made and the patient should be discharged before the
syndrome of chronic overhospitalization sets in and the patient begins
to lose ground from sheer boredom.

REFERENCES

1. Alajouanine, T.: Aphasia and artistic realizations. Brain 71:229, 1948.
2. Albert, M., Reches, A., and Silverberg, R.: Associative visual agnosia without alexia. Neurology 25:322, 1975.
3. Albert, M., Soffer, D., Silverberg, R. and Reches, A.: The anatomic basis of
   visual agnosia. Neurology 29:876, 1979 and 30:109, 1980.
4. Albert, M., Sparks, R., Von Stockert, T., and Sax, D.: A case study of
   auditory agnosia: Linguistic and non-linguistic processing. Cortex 8:-
   427, 1972.
5. Bender, M.: Syndrome of isolated episode of confusion with amnesia. J.
   Hillside Hospital 5:212, 1956.
6. Bender, M., and Feldman, M.: The so-called "visual agnosias." Brain 95:-
   173, 1972
7. Benson, D.F.: Fluency in aphasia: Correlation with radioactive scan localization. Cortex 3:373, 1967.
8. Benson, D.F.: Psychiatric aspects of aphasia. Br.J.Psychiatry 123:555, 1973.
9. Benson, D.F.: Varieties of anomia. Presented at the Academy of Aphasia,
   Miami, October, 1976.
10. Benson, D.F.: The third alexia. Arch. Neurol. 34:327, 1977.
11. Benson, D.F., Gardner, H., and Meadows, J.C.: Reduplicative amnesia
    Neurology 26:147, 1976.
12. Benson, D.F., and Geschwind, N.: Shrinking retrograde amnesia. J. Neuroi.
    Neurosurg. Psychiatry 30:539, 1967.
13. Benson, D.F., and Geschwind, N.: Psychiatric conditions associated with
    focal lesions of the central nervous system, in Arieti, S. (ed.): American
    Handbook of Psychiatry, Vol. 4. Basic Books, New York, 1975, pp. 208–
    243.
14. Benson, D. F., and Greenberg, J.P.: Visual form agnosia. Arch. Neurol.
    20:82, 1969.
15. Benson, D. F., Marsden, C., and Meadows, J.: The amnesic syndrome of
    posterior cerebral artery occlusion. Acta Neurol. Scand. 50:133,
    1974.
16. Benson, D.F., Sheremata, W.A., Bouchard, R., Segarra, J.M., Price, D., and
    Geschwind, N.: Conduction aphasia. Arch. Neurol. 28:339, 1973.
17. Benton, A.L.: Clinical symptomatology in right and left hemisphere le-
    sions, in Mountcastle, V.B. (ed.): Interhemispheric Relations and Cere-
    bral Dominance. The Johns Hopkins Press, Baltimore, 1962, pp. 253–
    264.

18. Benton, A.L.: The Amnesias, in Critchley, M., and Henson, R.A. (eds.): Music and the Brain. Heinemann, London, 1977, pp. 378–397.
19. Benton, A.L., Meyers, R., and Polder, G.J.: Some aspects of handedness. Psychiatr. Neurol. (Basel) 144:321, 1962.
20. Benton, A.L., and Von Allen, M.W.: Prosopagnosia and facial discrimination. J. Neurol. Sci. 15:167, 1972.
21. Bever, T.G., and Chiarello, R.J.: Cerebral dominance in musicians and nonmusicians. Science 185:537, 1974.
22. Black, F. W.: Unilateral brain lesions and MMPI performance: A preliminary study. Percep. Mot. Skil. 40:87, 1975.
23. Blumer, D., and Benson, D.F.: Personality changes with frontal and temporal lobe lesions, in Benson, D.F., and Blumer, D. (eds.): Psychiatric Aspects of Neurologic Disease. Grune and Stratton, New York, 1975, pp. 151–170.
24. Bogan, J.E.: The other side of the brain I: Dysgraphia and dyscopia following cerebral commissurotomy. Bul. Los Angeles Neurol. Soc. 34:73, 1969.
25. Bogan, J.E.: The other side of the brain II: An appositional mind. Bul. Los Angeles Neurol. Soc. 34:135, 1969.
26. Bogan, J.E., and Bogan, C.M.: The other side of the brain III: The corpus callosum and creativity. Bul. Los Angeles Neurol. Soc. 34:191, 1969.
27. Bogan, J.E., and Gordon, H.W.: Musical tests for functional lateralization with intracarotid amobarbital. Nature 230:524, 1971.
28. Bornstein, B., Sroka, H. and Munitz, H.: Prosopagnosia with animal face agnosia. Cortex 5:164, 1969.
29. Brain, W.R.: Speech Disorders. Aphasia, Apraxia, Agnosia, ed. 2. Butterworth, London, 1965.
30. Branch, C., Milner, B., and Rasmussen, T.: Intracarotid sodium amytal for the lateralization of cerebral speech dominance. J. Neurosurg. 21:399, 1964.
31. Bridges, P.K., and Bartlett, J.R.: Psychosurgery: yesterday and today. Br. J. Psychiatry 131:249, 1977.
32. Brown, J.W., and Hécaen, H.: Lateralization and language representation. Neurology 26:183, 1976.
33. Chamberlain, H.D.: The inheritance of left handedness. J. Hered., 19:557, 1928.
34. Clemins, V.A.: Localized thalamic hemorrhage: A cause of aphasia. Neurology 20:776, 1970
35. Cohen, D., Schaie, K.W., and Gribbin, K.: The organization of spatial abilities in older men and women. J. Gerontol. 35:578, 1977.
36. Critchley, M.: The Parietal Lobes. Edward Arnold & Co., London, 1953.
37. Critchley, M.: The problem of visual agnosia. J. Neurol. Sci. 1:274, 1964.
38. Critchley, M.: Acquired anomalies of colour perception of central origin. Brain 88:711, 1965.
39. Critchley, M., and Henson, R.A.: Music and the Brain. Heinemann, London, 1977.
40. Damasio, A.R., and Damasio, H.: Music faculty and cerebral dominance, in Critchley, M., and Henson, R.A. (eds.): Music and the brain. Heinemann, London, 1977, pp. 141–155.
41. Damasio, A.R., Ferro, J., and Dimasio, H.: Language processing and the thalamus. Presented at the Academy of Aphasia, Miami, October, 1976.

261

42. Damasio, A.R., and Kessel, N.F.: Transcortical motor aphasia in relation to lesions of the supplementary motor area. Presented at the American Academy of Neurology, Los Angeles, April, 1978.
43. DeJong, R., Itabashi, H., and Olson, J.: Memory loss due to hippocampal lesions. Arch. Neurol. 20:339, 1969.
44. Denny-Brown, D., Meyer, J.S., and Horenstein, S.: The significance of perceptual rivalry resulting from parietal lesions. Brain 75:433, 1952.
45. DeRenzi, E., Faglioni, P., Scotti, G., and Spinnler, H.: Impairment in associating colour to form, concomitant with aphasia. Brain 95:293, 1972.
46. Exner, S.: Untersuchungen Über die lokalizationen in der Grosshirnrinde des menschen. Wien Wilhelm Braumuller, 1881.
47. Fazio, C., Sacco, C., and Bugiani, O.: The thalamic hemorrhage. Eur. Neurol. 9:30, 1973.
48. Ferriss, G.S., and Dorsen, M.M.: Agenesis of the corpus callosum. Cortex 11:95, 1975.
49. Fisher, C.M.: The pathologic and clinical aspects of thalamic hemorrhage. Trans. Am. Neurol. Assoc. 84:56, 1959.
50. Fisher, C.M., and Adams, R.D.: Transient global amnesia. Trans. Am. Neurol. Assoc. 83:143, 1958.
51. Freeman, W., and Watts, J.W.: Psychosurgery. Charles C Thomas, Springfield, Illinois, 1950.
52. Gainotti, G.: Emotional behavior and hemispheric side of lesion. Cortex 8:41, 1972.
53. Gardner, H.: The shattered mind. Knopf, New York, 1975.
54. Gardner, H., Ling, P.K., Flamm, L., and Silverman, J.: Comprehension and appreciation of humorous material following brain damage. Brain 98: 399, 1975.
55. Gassel, M.M.: Occipital lobe syndromes (excluding hemianopia), in Vinken, P.J., and Bruyn, G.W. (eds.): Handbook of Clinical Neurology, Vol 2. 1969.
56. Gazzaniga, M.S.: The Bisected Brain. Appleton-Century-Croffts, New York, 1970.
57. Gazzaniga, M.S., LeDoux, J.E., and Wilson, D.H.: Language, praxis, and the right hemisphere: Clues to some mechanisms of consciousness. Neurology 27:1144, 1977.
58. Gerson, S.N., Benson, D.F., and Frazier, S.H.: Diagnosis: Schizophrenia versus posterior aphasia. Am. J. Psychiatry 134:966, 1977.
59. Gerstmann, J.: Some notes on the Gerstmann-syndrome. Neurology 7:866, 1957.
60. Geschwind, N.: Disconnection syndromes in animals and man, Part I. Brain 88:237, 1965; Part II. Brain 88:585, 1965.
61. Geschwind, N.: Current concepts in aphasia. N.Engl.J.Med. 284:654, 1971.
62. Geschwind, N.: The apraxias: Neural mechanisms of disorders of learned movement. Am. Sci. 63:188, 1975.
63. Geschwind, N.: Implications of the anatomical asymmetry of the brain. Presented at the Academy of Aphasia, Montreal, October, 1977.
64. Geschwind, N., and Fusillo, M.: Color-naming defects in association with alexia. Arch. Neurol. 15:137, 1966.
65. Geschwind, N., and Kaplan, E.: A human cerebral disconnection syndrome. Neurology 12:675, 1962.
66. Geschwind, N., and Levitsky, W.: Human brain: Left-right asymmetries in temporal speech region. Science 161:186, 1968.

67. Geschwind, N., Quadfasel, F., and Segarra, J.: Isolation of the speech area. Neuropsychologia 6:327, 1968.
68. Gloning, K.: Handedness and aphasia. Neuropsychologia 15:355, 1977.
69. Goldstein, K.: Aftereffects of Brain Injuries in War. Grune and Stratton, New York, 1942.
70. Goodglass, H., and Kaplan, E.: Assessment of Aphasia and Related Disorders. Lea & Febiger, Philadelphia, 1972.
71. Gordon, H.W., and Bogan, J.E.: Hemispheric lateralization of singing after intra-carotid amylobarbitone. J. Neurol. Neurosurg. Psychiatry 37:727, 1974.
72. Green, J.B., and Hamilton, W.J.: Anosognosia for hemiplegia: Somatosensory evoked potential studies. Neurology 26:1141, 1976.
73. Greenblatt, S.H.: Alexia without agraphia or hemianopsia: Anatomical analysis of an autopsied case. Brain 96:307, 1973.
74. Hardyck, C., and Petrinovich, L.F.: Left-handedness. Psychol. Bull. 84:385, 1977.
75. Hayward, R.W., Naeser, M.A., and Zatz, L.M.: Cranial computed tomography in aphasia. Radiology 123:653, 1977.
76. Heathfield, K.W.G., Croft, P.B., and Swash, M.: The syndrome of transient global amnesia. Brain 96:729, 1973.
77. Hécaen, H.: Clinical symptomatology in right and left hemispheric lesions, in Mountcastle, V.B. (ed.): Interhemispheric relations and cerebral dominance. Johns Hopkins Press, Baltimore, 1962, pp. 215–244.
78. Hécaen, H., and Ajuriaguerra, J.de: Left Handedness. Grune and Stratton, New York, 1964.
79. Hécaen, H., and Albert, M.L.: Disorders of mental functioning related to frontal lobe pathology, in Benson, D.F., and Blumer, D. (eds.): Psychiatric Aspects of Neurologic Disease. Grune and Stratton, New York, 1975, pp. 137–149.
80. Heilman, K.M., and Sypert, G.W.: Korsakoff's syndrome resulting from bilateral fornix lesions. Neurology 27:490, 1977.
81. Heilman, K.M., and Watson, R.T.: Mechanisms underlying the unilateral neglect syndrome, in Weinstein, E.A., and Friedland, R.P. (eds.): Hemi-inattention and Hemispheric Specialization. Raven Press, New York, 1977, pp. 93–106.
82. Hemphill, R.E., and Stengle, E.: A study on pure word-deafness. J. Neurol. Psychiatry 3:251, 1940.
83. Hier, D.B., Davis, K.R., Richardson, E.P., and Mohr, J.P.: Hypertensive putamenal hemorrhage. Ann. Neurol. 1:152, 1977.
84. Holmes, G.: Discussion on the mental symptoms associated with cerebral tumors. Proc. R. Soc. Med., 24:65, 1931.
85. Hooshmand, H., Sepdham, T., and Vries, J.K.: Klüver-Bucy syndrome: Successful treatment with carbamazepine. JAMA 229:1782, 1974.
86. Kamalian, N., Keesey, R.E., and ZuRhein, G.M.: Lateral hypothalamic demyelination and cachexia in a case of "malignant" multiple sclerosis. Neurology 25:25, 1975.
87. Kaplap, E.: Personal communication, 1972.
88. Kertesz, A., Lesk, D., and McCabe, P.: Isotope localization of infarcts in aphasia. Arch. Neurol. 34:590, 1977.
89. Keschner, M., Bender, M.B., and Strauss, I.: Mental symptoms in cases of tumor of the temporal lobe. Arch. Neurol. Psychiatry 35:572, 1936.

90. Kimura, D.: Left-right differences in the perception of melodies. Quart. J. Exp.Psychol. 16:355, 1964.
91. Kimura, D.: Studies in apraxia. Presented at the Academy of Aphasia, Montreal, October, 1977.
92. Kinsbourne, M.: Hemi-neglect and hemisphere rivalry, in Weinstein, E.A., and Friedland, R.P. (eds.): Hemi-Inattention and Hemispheric Specialization. Raven Press, New York, 1977, pp. 41–50.
93. Kinsbourne, M., and Warrington, E.: A study of finger agnosia. Brain 85:47, 1962.
94. Klüver, H., and Bucy, P.C.: "Psychic blindness" and other symptoms following bilateral temporal lobectomy in rhesus monkeys. Am. J. Physiol. 119:352, 1937.
95. LeDoux, J.E., Wilson, D.H., Gazzaniga, M.S.: A divided mind: Observations on the conscious properties of the separated hemispheres. Ann. Neurol. 2:417, 1977.
96. Levy-Agresti, J., and Sperry, R.W.: Differential perceptual capacities in major and minor hemispheres. Proc. Natl. Acad. Sci. 61:1151, 1968.
97. Lhermitte, F., and Beauvois, M.F.: A visual-speech disconnection syndrome. Brain 96:695, 1973.
98. Lomas, J., and Kertesz, A.: Patterns of spontaneous recovery in aphasic groups: A study of adult stroke patients. Brain Lang. 5:388, 1978.
99. Louks, J., Calsyn, D., and Lindsay, F.: Personality dysfunction and lateralized deficits in cerebral functions as measured by the MMPI and Reston-Halstead battery. Percept. Mot. Skills 43:655, 1976.
100. Luria, A.R.: Frontal lobe syndromes, in Vinken, P.J., and Bruyn, G.W. (eds.): Handbook of Clinical Neurology, Vol. 2. Elsevier-North Holland Publishing Co., New York, 1969. pp. 725–757.
101. Luria, A.R.: Traumatic Aphasia. Mouton, The Hague, Netherlands, 1970.
102. Luria, A.R.: On quasi-aphasic disturbances in lesions of the deep structures of the brain. Brain Lang. 4:432, 1977.
103. Malamud, N.: Psychiatric disorders with intracranial tumors of the limbic system. Arch. Neurol. 17:113, 1967.
104. Mathew, N.T., and Meyer, J.S.: Pathogenesis and natural history of transient global amnesia. Stroke 5:303, 1974.
105. McEntee, W.J., Biber, M.P., Perl, D.P., and Benson, D.F.: Diencephalic amnesia: A reappraisal. J. Neurol. Neurosurg. Psychiatry 39:436, 1976.
106. Meadows, J.C.: The anatomical basis of prosopagnosia. J. Neurol. Neurosurg. Psychiatry 37:489, 1974.
107. Meadows, J.C.: Disturbed perception of colours associated with localized cerebral lesions. Brain 97:615, 1974.
108. Mettler, F.A. (ed.): Selective Partial Ablation of Frontal Cortex. Hoeber, New York, 1949.
109. Milner, B.: Laterality effects in audition, in Mountcastle, V.B. (ed.): Interhemispheric relations and cerebral dominance. Johns Hopkins Press, Baltimore, 1962, pp. 177–195.
110. Milner, B.: Interhemispheric differences and psychological processes. Br. Med. Bull. 27:272, 1971.
111. Mohr, J.P.: Broca's area and Broca's aphasia, in Whitaker, H., and Whitaker, H.A. (eds.): Studies in Neurolinguistics, Vol. 1 in Perspectives in Neurolinguistics and Psycholinguistics. Academic Press, New York, 1976.

112. Mohr, J.P., Watters, W.C., and Duncan, G.W.: Thalamic hemorrhage and aphasia. Brain Lang. 2:3, 1975.
113. Nielsen, J.: Gerstmann syndrome: Finger agnosia, agraphia, confusion of right and left, and acalculia. Arch. Neurol. Psychiatry 39:536, 1938.
114. Oxbury, J.M., Campbell, D.C. and Oxbury, S.M.: Unilateral spatial neglect and impairments of spatial analysis and visual perception. Brain 97:551, 1974.
115. Pick, A.: On reduplicative paramnesia. Brain 26:242, 1903.
116. Popper, K.R., and Eccles, J.C.: The Self and Its Brain. Springer-Verlag, New York, 1977.
117. Reeves, A.G., and Plum, F.: Hyperphagia, rage, and dementia accompanying a ventromedial hypothalamic neoplasm. Arch. Neurol. 20:616, 1969.
118. Roberts, L.: Aphasia, apraxia, and agnosia in abnormal states of cerebral dominance, in Vinken, P.J., and Bruyn, G.W. (eds.): Handbook of Clinical Neurology, Vol. 4. Elsevier-North Holland Publishing Co., New York, 1969, pp. 312–326.
119. Roland, P.E.: Astereognosis. Arch. Neurol. 33:543, 1976.
120. Rubens, A.B.: Aphasia with infarction in the territory of the anterior cerebral artery. Cortex 11:239, 1975.
121. Rubens, A., and Benson, D.: Associative visual agnosia. Arch. Neurol. 24:305, 1971.
122. Rubens, A., and Benson, D.: Aphasia with thalamic hemorrhage. Presented at the Academy of Aphasia, Miami, October, 1976.
123. Samarel, A., Wright T.L., Sergay, S., and Tyler, H.R.: Thalamic hemorrhage with speech disorder. Trans. Am. Neurol. Assoc. 101:283, 1976.
124. Sanders, M.D., Warrington, E.K., Marshall, J., and Wieskrantz, L.: "Blindsight:" Vision in a field defect. Lancet 2:707, 1974.
125. Sarno, M.T., Silverman, M., and Sands, E.: Speech therapy and language recovery in severe aphasia. J. Speech Hear. Res. 13:607, 1970.
126. Satz, P.: Pathological left-handedness: An explanatory model. Cortex 8: 121, 1972.
127. Satz, P.: Left handedness and early brain insult: An explanation. Neuropsychologia 11:115, 1973.
128. Scoville, W., and Milner, B.: Loss of recent memory after bilateral hippocampal lesions. J. Neurol. Neurosurg. Psychiatry 20:11, 1957.
129. Selzer, B., and Benson, D.F.: The temporal pattern of retrograde amnesia in Korsakoff's disease. Neurology 24:527, 1974.
130. Smith, A.: Dominant and nondominant hemispherectomy, in Kinsbourne, M. and Smith, W.L. (eds.): Hemispheric disconnection and cerebral function. Charles C Thomas, Springfield, Illinois, 1974, pp 5–33.
131. Strauss, I., and Keschner, M.: Mental symptoms in cases of tumor of the frontal lobe. Arch. Neurol. Psychiatry 33:986, 1935.
132. Subirana, A.: Handedness and cerebral dominance, in Vinken, P.J., and Bruyn, G.W. (eds.): Handbook of Clinical Neurology, Vol 4. Elsevier-North Holland Publishing Co., New York, 1969, pp. 248–272.
133. Sweet, W.H.: Treatment of medically intractable mental disease by limited frontal leucotomy—justifiable? New Engl.J. Med. 289:1117, 1973.
134. Terzian, H., and Ore, G.D.: Syndrome of Klüver and Bucy: Reproduced in man by bilateral removal of the temporal lobes. Neurology 5:373, 1955.
135. Tucker, D.M., Watson, R.T., and Heilman, K.M.: Discrimination and evocation of affectively intoned speech in patients with right parietal disease. Neurology 27:947, 1977.

136. Victor, M.: The Wernicke-Korsakoff syndrome, in Vinken, P.J., and Bruyn, G.W. (eds.): Handbook of Clinical Neurology, Vol. 28. Elsevier-North Holland Publishing Co., New York, 1976, pp. 243–270.
137. Victor, M., Adams, R., and Collins, G.: The Wernicke-Korsakoff Syndrome. F.A. Davis, Philadelphia, 1971.
138. Vignolo, L.: The localization of aphasia-producing lesions: clinical-anatomical correlations with computerized axial tomography (EMI scanning). Presented at the Academy of Aphasia, Montreal, October, 1977.
139. Wada, J., and Rasmussen, T.: Intracarotid injection of sodium amytal for the lateralization of cerebral speech dominance. Experimental and clinical observation. J. Neurosurg. 17:266, 1960.
140. Watson, R.T., Andriola, M., and Heilman, K.M.: The electroencephalogram in neglect. J. Neurol. Sci. 34:343, 1977.
141. Watson, R.T., and Heilman, K.M.: Thalamic neglect. Neurology 29:690, 1979.
142. Watson, R.T., Heilman, K.M., Miller, B.O., and King, F.A.: Neglect after mesencephalic reticular formation lesions. Neurology 24:194, 1974.
143. Weinstein, E.A., and Friedland, R. P. (eds.): Hemi-inattention and Hemispheric Specialization, Vol. 18 in Advances in Neurology. Raven Press, New York, 1977.
144. Weinstein, E.A., and Friedland, R.P.: Behavioral disorders associated with hemi-inattention, in Weinstein, E.A., and Friedland, R.P. (eds.): Hemi-inattention and Hemispheric Specialization Vol. 18 in Advances in Neurology. Raven Press, New York, 1977. pp. 51–62.
145. Weinstein, E.A., and Kahn, R.L.: Denial of Illness. Charles C Thomas, Springfield, Illinois, 1955.
146. Wertheim, N.: The amusias, in Vinken, P.J., and Bruyn, G.W. (eds.): Handbook of Clinical Neurology, Vol. 4. Elsevier-North Holland Publishing Co., New York, 1969, pp. 195–206.
147. White, L.E., and Hain, R.F.: Anorexia in association with a destructive lesion of the hypothalamus. Arch. Path. 68:275, 1959.
148. Whiteley, A.M., and Warrington, E.K.: Prosopagnosia: A clinical, psychological, and anatomical study of three patients. J. Neurol. Neurosurg. Psychiatry 40:395, 1977.
149. Witelson, S.F., and Pallie, W.: Left hemisphere specialization for language in the newborn: Neuroanatomical evidence of asymmetry. Brain 96:641, 1973.
150. Zangwill, O.L.: Personal communication, 1977.
151. Zangwill, O.L.: Aphasia associated with lesions of the right hemisphere. Presented at the Academy of Aphasia, Montreal, October, 1977.
152. Shuping, J.R., Rollinson, R.D., and Toole, J.F.: Transient global amnesia. Ann. Neurol. 7:281, 1980.

SECTION III

NEUROBEHAVIORAL SYNDROMES OF SPECIFIC ETIOLOGIES

8

CLOSED HEAD TRAUMA

A 48-year-old woman was involved in an automobile accident approximately 7 months prior to our seeing her. The accident had been relatively mild; she had struck her head on the windshield of the car and was unconscious for only a few minutes. She had virtually no retrograde amnesia and a post-traumatic amnesia of less than 15 minutes. Her major complaint after the accident was a rather persistent headache of several months duration. As the headache lessened, however, she claimed, "I just don't feel right." She complained of not having the energy that she previously did, and she described herself as being generally quite apathetic about everything since the injury. Formerly, she was very active in many social activities, but she has given up much of this since the accident. Even though she is generally less concerned about major events, she finds herself irritated by minor problems. She says that she "just cannot cope" with certain situations. In addition to this personality change, she complains of mild memory problems and a definite problem with calculating. She says that she always kept the household accounts because she was good at such matters and enjoyed doing it. Now she is not as quick to do the work and has been "messing up the check book" regularly. She previously was able to go shopping, write a series of checks, and then return home and record them accurately but is now unable to do this.

Standard neurologic testing revealed no abnormalities, and she had no complaints other than the previously stated behavioral ones. On mental status testing she was attentive, nonaphasic, and learned new material relatively well but when asked about recent events in the local, national, and world news, her response was very sketchy. Although not aphasic, her discourse was somewhat vague. Not having known the woman before the accident, we were not certain that this was a departure from her normal style of conversation. Calculation was accurate but very slow, as was her drawing. Proverb interpretation and similarities were also within normal limits.

The changes in this patient are typical of the cognitive and behavioral changes that can be seen after mild head trauma. Such subtle behavioral changes frequently are not recognized by physicians, especially when the standard neurologic examination is normal. In cases in which the patient or his family have specific behavioral complaints, it is not uncommon for the physician to ascribe these to an emotional reaction from the accident. The patient with a mild concussion, for instance, may experience difficulty concentrating for several weeks. If such a patient returns to work prematurely, the difficulty he experiences in carrying out his work can easily be very frustrating to him and will often be misinterpreted by his employer as being a deliberate attempt to receive additional compensation or time off from work.

This failure to recognize behavioral sequelae may at times be a problem in major head trauma as well. We were called quite frantically one day by an exasperated physical therapist who told us that she was working with a young woman who absolutely would not cooperate and follow instructions. On examination, the patient had evidence of imbalance and spasticity but in addition had a moderately severe ideomotor apraxia and a substantial problem with auditory comprehension. Not only did the patient fail to understand much of what was requested of her, but what she could understand verbally, she could not execute motorically. In both of these examples, a great deal of frustration and misunderstanding could have been avoided if the behavioral problems had been recognized early in the post-traumatic period.

Before embarking upon a detailed description of the specific clinical post-traumatic syndromes, it is important to define some of the basic terms used in discussing head trauma. The first, and in many ways the most complicated, is *concussion.* No definition can satisfactorily encompass all variations of concussion, but two central features are constant: (1) concussion results from a mechanical impact to the head and (2) there is an immediate impairment of neural function.[1,13] However, the nature of the impairment of neural function has been difficult to define. Loss of consciousness has often been given as the essential feature and, when present, certainly does indicate concussion. But, many significant blows to the head merely daze or stun the patient and do not render him unconscious (football games and boxing matches often produce such instances). Immediately after the trauma, these patients experience varying periods of confused thinking or lethargy but maintain consciousness. Certainly blows disrupted normal neural functioning, and we maintain that these patients sustained a concussion.

Another aspect of concussion, which has been considered the requisite feature by some, is a period of absolute amnesia.[19,55,57,66] The amnesic period is measured from the last memory before the trauma (retrograde amnesia) to the point of complete return to continuous memory (anterograde or post-traumatic amnesia). Recovery must be to the point of full orientation not merely a return to consciousness. In almost all patients with concussions, there is a period of amnesia that extends beyond the period of unconsciousness. Although a period of permanent memory loss, with or without loss of consciousness, is found in most cases of concussion, there are some unusual cases in which neither amnesia nor loss of consciousness is present. The following case illustrates this point.

A 27-year-old woman was driving on the highway at 55 miles per hour when her car hit the middle divider and she lost control. The car rolled over several times, and her left occiput was struck with sufficient force to give her a traumatic neuropathy of the occipital nerve but not to render her unconscious. She was dazed and very lethargic for at least twelve hours. During this period, she could not remember the accident or what was done at the hospital. She was also somewhat disoriented as to time. The following day, however, the patient was fully alert, oriented, and could clearly remember all details of the accident and the events subsequent to it. She had no period of permanent amnesia, either retrograde or anterograde. In our opinion, this patient suffered a mild concussion, although there was neither a loss of consciousness or a permanent period of amnesia.

Another feature of concussion that has been debated is the question of its reversibility. Many standard definitions of concussion require that the patient's neurologic impairment return completely to pre-morbid levels and that there be no residual brain damage. We, however, agree with Symonds[61] that this is too rigid a definition and feel that persons sustaining simple concussive injuries may have mild resultant neurologic and cognitive impairment.[1] Being cognizant of the limitations discussed above, we define a concussion as an acute impairment of cerebral function secondary to an impact injury to the head in which the following are usually, but not invariably, present: amnesia, loss of consciousness, and complete recovery.

Once concussion is defined, another problem is the establishment of parameters by which to determine the degree of severity. This is so very important since prognosis is closely allied to the severity of the injury. Again, considerable dispute is reflected in the literature. In general, there is a direct relationship between both the length of coma (unconsciousness) and post-traumatic amnesia and the subsequent prognosis. The relationship between post-traumatic amnesia (PTA) and prognosis has received the most attention in the literature.[33,45,55] The correlation between amnesia and prognosis has been found to be much greater in patients over the age of thirty[7] but can still be a useful clinical indicator with younger patients. We use the following classification system:

Degree of Severity	Duration of PTA
Slight concussion	0 to 15 minutes
Mild concussion	15 minutes to 1 hour
Moderate concussion	1 to 24 hours
Severe concussion	1 to 7 days
Very severe concussion	> 7 days

Another term commonly used in describing patients with head trauma is *cerebral contusion.* This diagnostic label is often applied to any patient who has a residual neurologic deficit after closed head trauma. We feel that this is a misapplication of the term for two reasons: (1) contusion is not a clinical term but refers to a pathologic condition in which superficial damage has been done to the crests of the cortical convolutions secondary to trauma, literally a "brain bruise,"[60] and (2) all patients with contusions do not have residual neurologic signs nor do all patients with residual neurologic signs have cortical contusions. As will be discussed later, most of the brain damage resulting from severe closed head trauma is in subcortical structures.

The final term to be considered is *traumatic encephalopathy.* This is used in cases with residual clinical evidence of brain damage from trauma. The term is not restricted to closed, uncomplicated head trauma but may be applied to the sequelae of hematomas (extradural, subdural, and intracerebral), brain lacerations, or open head wounds.

It is unfortunate that standard definitions are not consistently applied by each investigator, for the resultant looseness in terminology makes comparing results from one study to the next virtually impossible. Although admittedly all cases cannot neatly fit within any one group of definitions or classification scheme, an effort toward standardization will yield significant clinical and scientific rewards.

DESCRIPTION OF THE CLINICAL SYNDROMES

Minor Head Injury (without Gross Neurologic Findings)

In less serious concussive injuries, patients experience a fairly standard series of events during the initial and early post-traumatic period. With the initial impact, there is usually a general paralysis of nervous function which is characterized by loss of muscle tone causing the patient to drop to the ground motionless. Consciousness, reflexes, and respiration are lost concomitantly.[15,55]

In most cases of minor injury, the unconscious patient lies motionless for only a few seconds to a few minutes. Respiration quickly returns, and the patient soon thereafter becomes restless and begins to regain consciousness. During the initial period of consciousness, the patient is usually irritable, apathetic, confusional, and occasionally uncontrollable and abusive. Autonomic dysfunction is common with nausea, vomiting, hypothermia, and alterations of pulse and blood pressure being the principal vegetative phenomena. This unstable confusional period usually lasts less than 24 hours. During this time, the patients act somewhat purposefully but will frequently question what has happened and will not recall anything concerning the injury. Behavior is often similar to that displayed by a patient during an episode of transient global amnesia. The patients are unable to learn during this time and most have a retrograde amnesia covering hours, days, or even years prior to the accident.

In cases where the blow does not render the recipient unconscious, he appears dazed and may go through the motions of purposeful activity but is actually both confused and disoriented. This latter situation is best exemplified in sports injuries where a player may continue the game or boxing match even though he may have no memory of it the following day. Dazed boxers have been known to complete a fight without anyone realizing that they were concussed (probably because boxing is an overlearned almost automatic activity). With the football player (North American football) who must remember plays and signals called at the beginning of each play, the extent of the head injury is soon realized when he commits an obvious error.

The confusional period fades to the point of normal functioning in most cases, but at times the patients seem to suddenly "snap out of it" and say, "Hey, what am I doing here, and what's going on?" The concussive period is considered over when the patient becomes fully oriented and full consciousness has been achieved. Full consciousness refers to the ability to remember all ongoing events and to maintain orientation.[61] At this point, the patient can be questioned concerning his memory of the preceding events and both retrograde and post-traumatic amnesia can be established. The retrograde amnesia is usually short, almost always less than 30 minutes, and usually only a few seconds in duration.[55] The post-traumatic amnesia is usually much longer but in the majority of cases of minor injury lasts less than 24 hours.

Several interesting features of these amnesic periods are of both practical and theoretical importance. The first is the period of retrograde amnesia. In most cases, this period of amnesia shortens as the patient recovers.[4] Events prior to the injury are at first unknown or indistinct, but with the passage of time, the patient is able to retrieve details which are closer and closer in time to the point of impact. In the typical case, it is only the few seconds immediately before the accident that are lost forever. Some cases have been reported, however, in which the retrograde amnesia actually lengthens. This has been described in both severe injuries[58] and in the minor concussions without loss of consciousness seen in football players.[67] In several football players, the memory of the play that resulted in injury was present on initial examination immediately following their head injury but was lost on subsequent examination after conclusion of the game.[67] In these latter cases, it is most probable that the memories of the play were retained in short term or immediate memory but, due to trauma to the limbic system, could not be consolidated and stored in long term or permanent memory. In cases with more severe injuries, this explanation would not hold, since the time for recovery of consciousness is longer than the period for which information can be held in short term memory. It must be remembered that the patient's account of an automobile accident or blow to the head by an assailant is often of critical legal importance. If initial questioning does not reveal the pertinent information, in some cases where the amnesia shrinks, the facts may be retrievable.

The period of post-traumatic amnesia is not always absolute. The patient's memory for events occurring during the confusional period is usually permanently lost, but the confusional behavior characteristically fluctuates so dramatically, that lucid periods may leave islands of memory in the sea of amnesia.[55] Even after the confusion has cleared and the patient appears to be remembering normally during examination, memories may still not be fully consolidated and events of one day may be forgotten on the next. In such cases, the post-traumatic amnesia can actually lengthen after consciousness has been regained.

After return to full consciousness and assurance by the physician that the neurologic examination is normal, the patient with a concussion of mild or moderate degree is usually discharged from the emergency room or hospital. He is encouraged to remain at home for several days and then to slowly return to a normal working routine. During this post-traumatic period, subtle organic behavioral defects may be unappreciated for what they are and blamed on the patient's emotional reaction or his desire for compensation. Most patients with head injuries will have some post-traumatic symptoms, and it is extremely important for the physician to discuss these with the patient before discharge. By being understanding and sympathetically supportive, many of the problems can be easily handled without undue anxiety.

One of the more common problems that we encounter clinically is the patient with complaints of continuing memory and concentration difficulties. The patient feels well enough to return to work but finds that he cannot keep his mind on the job and forgets details that were easily retained previously. Because the medical release mentions no neurologic abnormalities, employers often interpret the patient's complaints as a deliberate attempt to avoid work or get a greater amount of compensation. The patient is caught between his very real problems and the normal neurologic examination. Gronwall and his associates[21,22] have studied this problem extensively and have convincingly demonstrated the difficulty that the post-concussive patient has in processing incoming information. The deficit, which they demonstrated in a paced serial addition test, correlated positively with the length of post-traumatic amnesia. Performance gradually returned to normal levels 35 days after injury in all patients with amnesia of less than 1 hour and 54 days after injury in those with amnesia of 1 to 24 hours. The difficulty experienced by the patients during the recovery period was attributed to fatigue, inattention, and defects in rapid information processing. As with many sequelae of head trauma, older patients fared poorly in contrast to those who were younger.

Persistent memory difficulty is also a major complaint and shows a relationship to post-traumatic amnesia and age. In patients with no amnesia, no symptoms of memory difficulty are found. With amnesia of less than 5 minutes duration, approximately 1 patient in 20 will complain; with 5 to 15 minutes of amnesia, 1 in 10 will complain; and with 1 to 4 hours of amnesia, 40 percent will have both memory and concentration problems.[27] Again, these complaints in the patient with mild or moderate concussion are usually transient with full recovery over time.

In conjunction with memory and concentration problems, many patients experience one or more other psychologic symptoms. Anxiety, fear, insomnia, restlessness, fatigue, and nervousness have been described in as many as 80 percent of patients with recent head injury.[13] These symptoms tend to be more prominent during the second week after the injury[40] and usually subside, as do the other symptoms, during the first month to six weeks after the injury.

Other than memory difficulty, disturbances of higher cognitive function are rare with minor head trauma unless a subsequent subdural hematoma develops. Aphasia, for example, was seen in only 13 of 750 patients with closed head injury admitted to a large neurosurgical service.[25] The aphasia was usually not severe and was primarily anomic. Such cognitive deficits are much more frequent in cases of penetrating brain wounds or severe closed head injury with or without concomitant hematoma formation or brain laceration.

Two other nonbehavioral symptoms that very commonly occur after closed head injury should be mentioned to complete the description of the post-traumatic syndrome. These are headache and dizziness. These symptoms usually appear during the first 24 hours after injury but may be delayed in their onset for days or even weeks. Headache is a very prominent symptom and is reported in 60 to 95 percent of all such patients.[11,13,27] Dizziness, though relatively less common, is seen in over half of the patients during the initial post-traumatic period.

Concentration difficulties, memory problems, emotional changes, insomnia, headache, and dizziness in the weeks following closed head trauma are sufficiently common that these symptoms, in various combinations, have been labeled the "post-traumatic or post-concussive syndrome." The syndrome varies in intensity and complexity and no specific cluster of symptoms appears to be more common than any other.[11,13,27] In general, half of these patients will be symptom-free in six weeks, conversely there are patients whose complaints persist for over a year.[57] Many factors influence the prognosis and speed of recovery and must be appreciated when treating the individual patient. It is well known that physical exercise, mental aggravation, and use of alcohol can all exacerbate or cause a resurgence of problems. At least two-thirds of the patients will have additional trouble in the first few days after discharge from the hospital.[40] This may be due to physical and/or mental stress but also is partly due to the patients' perception that they are "supposed" to be well, while actually they do not feel completely normal. This unfortunate situation arises primarily because of the physician's failure to adequately advise the patients regarding the possible resurgence of their post-traumatic symptoms.

The definition of this post-traumatic syndrome and the determination of its etiology have been and remain very problematical. The neurologic examination and skull x-rays are usually normal, as are the EEG and other neurodiagnostic tests. For this reason, some physicians consider any patient who has symptoms lasting longer than a few weeks or a month after injury to have emotional or other reasons (e.g., a desire for compensation) for the perpetuation of symptoms.[45,51] Conversely, other investigators have found no correlation between the preinjury personality and the development of a post-traumatic syndrome and have concluded that the syndrome is not a neurosis but is, in fact, organic.[62]

We tend to agree with Symonds[61] and Peterson[50] who concur that a combination of organic, emotional, and social factors are responsible for the subacute and chronic symptoms after head trauma. Supporting this position is the finding of transient and permanent pathologic changes in both experimental animals and human patients dying of other causes after mild head injury.[48] This will be discussed later in this chapter.

Age also appears to be significant. There is definitely an increase in symptoms in older patients, a finding which may be of multifactorial etiology but certainly suggests that the older, less plastic brain, cannot adjust to trauma as well as the younger one. These observations, combined with the fact that the syndrome occurs in many patients without preexisting neurosis and no hope of compensation or other pending legal matters, give us a strong suspicion that an organic brain disturbance is at the seat of many of these symptoms.

Although pretraumatic neurosis does not generally seem to be a significant factor in development of the post-traumatic syndrome, it is definitely the case in some.[24] However, other personality factors may exist which may be more important than a neurotic process, (e.g., a history of parental rejection or overprotection, chronic maladjustment, alcohol abuse, and proneness to accidents[49,54]).

The context in which the injury occurs also seems to influence the prognosis of the post-traumatic symptoms. Work-related injuries and automobile accidents where compensation and legal awards are predicated upon such abstract considerations as "pain and suffering" often lead patients either consciously or unconsciously to prolong symptoms in order to receive the maximum financial settlement. All physicians know patients who regularly visit the office with bitter complaints after an accident which disappear or miraculously improve after their legal case is settled. Some physicians are convinced that most cases of extended post-traumatic symptoms are frank malingering to increase financial reward. Miller reported that 90 percent of his cases completely improved after settlement had been rendered.[45] Other evidence in support of Miller's view is provided by the comparison of the incidence of post-traumatic symptoms in individuals concussed on the job or in their cars with those receiving equally severe injuries during sports contests. While the initial post-traumatic symptoms are similar in both groups, sports injuries have been found to produce far fewer prolonged complaints;[11] the theory being that in sports injuries, the participant expects an occasional bump on the head and cannot seek any compensation for it (unless he is a professional athlete, of course). We find the reported figures to be significantly higher than we have experienced in our own practice. The curious finding that the post-traumatic syndrome is more common in patients after minor head injuries than in those sustaining severe injuries has been used by some as additional support for the importance of psychogenic factors.[18,45]

Other factors that have been noted to have a high incidence in patients with lengthy post-traumatic symptoms are those related to the social problems that existed in these individuals' lives before the accident. A combination of job difficulty, difficulty in marriage, and declining economic status was found to be present in more than 90 percent of the symptomatic patients in one study and in only 35 percent of the patients with no prolongation of symptoms after minor head trauma.[49]

In essence, the post-traumatic syndrome must be viewed as the sequela of a complex combination of organic, emotional, and social factors. The initial symptoms of concentration and memory difficulty, headache, and dizziness are very likely organic. The insomnia, fatigue, nervousness, and other psychologic symptoms may very well be organic but emotional and social overtones are certainly present. The worsening or perpetuation of these symptoms after several months seems less likely to be purely organic than to be a combination of the patient's personality, specific fears about the accident, compensation and legal claims, other intangible social factors, and some persistent organic dysfunction.

Regardless of the exact etiology or blend of etiologies in each patient, post-traumatic symptoms are a major medical, economic, and legal problem in our society. The accurate prediction of prognosis is complicated and must be based on all of the factors discussed above. Generally, the patient with a mild head injury (post-traumatic amnesia of less than 24 hours) is back to full work in 2 months. Russell's study[55] showed that 93 percent of patients under the age of 40 and 78 percent of those over 40 were working two months following injury. Lidvall[40] found that less than 25 percent of his patients had any symptoms after 3 months. However, one must never forget that minor head trauma does occasionally lead to serious complications such as subdural hematoma. In one series of 275 cases of "trivial" head injury, 1 percent died and 1.7 percent had hematomas.[51] In the same series, 93 percent had no residual signs and symptoms. Accordingly, in most cases, the minor head injury is an aggravating yet relatively benign event.

Repeated Minor Head Trauma

If a person is sufficiently unlucky as to sustain several or even many blows to the head over time, the effect of each injury becomes more significant, recovery is slower, and eventually permanent brain damage can result. Gronwall and Wrightson[23] studied a group of individuals who had sustained 2 concussions, an average of 4½ years apart. Although both injuries were mild, the concentration and information processing deficit experienced by the patients after the second concussion was as great as that seen in patients after a severe first concussion. Even though all of Gronwall and Wrightson's patients did ultimately recover to normal levels on the tests used, their recovery was significantly slower than that of patients who had sustained only one concussion.

Professional sportsmen have provided the best opportunity to study the cumulative effects of multiple closed head trauma. Boxing subjects

278

its participants to by far the most gruesome display of continuing head trauma; but football players, steeplechase riders, wrestlers, and others have also been reported to have suffered the lasting ill effects of repeated head trauma.[16] The plight of these athletes is typified by the following case.

A 41-year-old boxer was first seen some 12 years after retirement from his professional boxing career. He complained that he was having difficulty walking and had noticed that his memory was not as sharp as it previously was. He worked as a dealer in a Las Vegas casino and was having trouble keeping track of the players' cards. His boxing career had started at a young age. In fact, he had stretched the truth a bit and began fighting professionally at the age of 16. He was very successful and won the world title in his weight class at the height of his career. He fought steadily for 13 years. He did not remember exactly how many fights he had had, but he claimed never to have been knocked out (he was knocked down 10 times and lost 3 fights on technical knockouts).

He retired at age 29 and functioned adequately until age 36 when he was hospitalized for "paranoid behavior." When we first saw him at age 41, he was employed and doing quite well except for problems with his gait and minor memory problems. On examination he had rather pronounced slurring and scanning of speech which he reported was normal for him and "not like those punch-drunk guys that hang around the gym." In fact, throughout the examination, though admitting that he had some trouble that he attributed to his boxing, he vehemently denied that he was like "those other punchy guys."

His gait was slightly ataxic and on finger to nose testing he displayed mild clumsiness and dysmetria (left worse than right). Rapid alternating movements were carried out poorly, tone was slightly increased in the legs, the right biceps reflex was increased, and there was a questionable extensor toe sign on the left. Sensation and cranial nerve examinations were within normal limits. Memory was poor: he did not remember the name of the doctor who had sent him to our office one hour before, he knew the name of the present president but not the previous one, and he had great difficulty learning any new material. He was not aphasic and calculations, drawings, and proverb interpretation were good.

This clinical syndrome, often called dementia pugilistica or the punch drunk syndrome, consists of both motor and behavioral signs. Motorically, patients develop a scanning dysarthric speech, striatal tremor, mixed pyramidal and extrapyramidal signs, cerebellar trunkal and limb signs, seizures, and sometimes a parkinsonism syndrome.[53] The behavioral change is often equally dramatic with slowness of thought processes, fatuousness, euphoria, emotional lability, dementia, paranoia, swings of mood that can often lead to violence, temper outbursts, and a generally disinterested attitude towards the environment and those in it.[14,65] We saw one 51-year-old retired veteran of 163 fights who told us with glee how he "punched out" the bellman in his building because our patient did not think that the man was being sufficiently helpful to a lady guest at the hotel. In conjunction with their erratic behavior, patients with dementia pugilistica usually have memory and concentration problems and are very sensitive to the effects of alcohol.[12]

This syndrome is unfortunately quite common in professional fighters who have fought for at least 3 years. Roberts[53] found 28 percent of over 200 British pugilists examined to be suffering from central nervous system damage. The condition is regrettably nonreversible and in a surprising number is actually slowly progressive after the fighter retires. For example, Roberts found evidence of encephalopathy in 47 percent of all retired fighters over the age of 50 who had fought for at least 10 years during their lifetime, but in only 25 percent of younger fighters with the same number of fights.

The chance of becoming demented from an athletic career correlates highly with the severity and frequency of head trauma. Again the best statistics are obtained from the study of boxers who show a marked increase in encephalopathy in instances of long careers that encompassed many fights. A 10 year career with 150 fights results in a 50 percent chance of developing dementia, while a shorter fighting career with less than 50 fights only results in a 5 to 10 percent risk.[53] The severity of the head injuries sustained, as judged by the length of post-traumatic amnesia, also correlates strongly with outcome. In general, a fighter with a period of amnesia greater than 24 hours has a 72 percent chance of becoming demented, while amnesic periods of up to one hour carry only a 21 percent risk.[53]

Although the boxer may be the extreme example of repeated minor head trauma, one wonders how truly benign any trivial head trauma is over time.

Severe Closed Head Trauma

The definition of a *severe closed head injury* varies somewhat from investigator to investigator, but the patient must have a post-traumatic amnesic period of at least 24 hours. In most studies of patients with severe head injuries, the average period of amnesia has been greater than 7 days[7,8,30] and in some centers a minimum of 7 days is used as the criterion for severe concussion.[30] Length of coma is another factor often included in the definition, yet again there is a discrepancy as to the duration of coma required to define an injury as severe. A coma of

1 hour is used by some[17] and of 6 hours by others.[30] Because of the difference in opinion concerning this parameter, it is quite difficult to compare the results of various investigators and to arrive at any firm consensus regarding prognosis (both for the degree of expected disability and the projected length of the recovery period). However, we will attempt to summarize the available data, so that when faced with a specific case, the clinician will be able to provide the patient and his family with some sensible expectations regarding recovery and rehabilitation.

Many aspects of the severe injury are similar to those of the minor head injury but are extended over time. The initial coma is longer and the period of post-traumatic amnesia is much longer as is the period of confusional behavior during the return to full consciousness. Unfortunately, with the lengthy recovery process come significant neurologic and behavioral deficits which are often irreversible. Some of these are quite obvious, such as hemiparesis or aphasia, while others of equal significance are more difficult to recognize and may go unnoticed by the inexperienced physician. It is these unsuspected factors that can interfere with full rehabilitation, particularly with vocational and social readjustment. The following case exemplifies some of the problems that are frequently encountered.

A 32-year-old female, who had sustained a severe closed head injury in a motorcycle accident (coma of 5 weeks), was referred for neurologic examination because of a residual left sided weakness and "unwillingness to cooperate in therapy." More specifically, the therapists found the patient immature, demanding, disinterested, irritable, inattentive to instructions, hyperactive, and generally unable to remember what was expected of her in therapy. When we talked to the therapists about the patient, it was apparent that they had become very hostile toward her because her behavior had been interpreted as being a deliberate attempt to resist help.

On examination, a very different impression was gained. She did demonstrate some resistance to the examination, but her inattention, apathy, irritability, and total lack of insight were obviously organic in nature and not intentional. An interview with the patient's friend verified that these personality traits were totally unlike the patient's premorbid personality. She previously had been an outgoing, cheerful individual who had many friends. She was described as being a dependable employee who took an active interest in her work. On neuropsychologic testing, she showed significant cognitive deficit: WAIS Full Scale IQ of 73 (Verbal, 80; Performance, 67), the Memory Quotient was only 63, and Trail-making Test performance showed marked impairment. Language and constructional ability were normal.

This young woman experienced many of the behavioral changes commonly seen in severe head injury; memory difficulty[9] and a personality change characteristic of frontal lobe damage being the most prominent. Because these changes are not as readily apparent as is weakness or aphasia, they must be specifically sought in examination. The personality change can be particularly difficult to recognize because the main features of apathy, euphoria, irritability, and inappropriate behavior often appear to be or are misinterpreted as being intentional. The identification of the behavioral change as organic makes it much easier for the staff to work with the patient but, unfortunately, means the prognosis is less favorable.

Levin and Grossman,[39] in a well studied sample of patients with closed head injury, found a rather distinct profile of behavioral disturbance in their moderately to severely injured patients (coma of less than 24 hours with or without concomitant neurologic deficit). The outstanding features were: cognitive disorganization manifested by disconnected thought processess, disorientation and conceptual disorganization, emotional withdrawal, various affective disturbances including excitement and blunting of affect, and motor retardation. The degree of behavioral disturbance was directly related to the severity of neurologic disturbance and the length of coma.

Other cognitive disturbances are also seen as sequelae of severe head injury, although these are less common unless an associated hematoma or brain laceration is present. Aphasic disturbances are reported in a third of the patients with very severe closed head injury (mean posttraumatic amnesia period of 43 days),[8] and a decline in overall intellectual functioning is also expected in this group.[6] Early in the recovery period, the performance (nonverbal) IQ suffers the greatest drop. The Performance IQ improves during recovery, and by 6 months after the injury, both verbal and performance scores have generally stabilized at approximately equal levels.[43] This pattern is true only for uncomplicated closed head trauma; if the patient sustains a depressed skull fracture or a localized hematoma, the cognitive disturbance has the additional features secondary to the focal lesion.

During the period of recovery from a severe closed head injury, some patients go through a very bizarre stage in which their behavior is very much akin to that described by Drs. Klüver and Bucy in monkeys after bilateral temporal lobectomy.[36,37] We saw one young man 5 months following injury who had to be tied to his bed or chair because of violent behavioral outbursts and sexual advances to the nursing staff. He also displayed marked hyperorality. Although this clinical picture is uncommon, elements of the syndrome are seen in some patients as they recover from significant head trauma. On occasion, these behaviors have been reported to persist and appear to be related to bilateral temporal lobe seizure activity.[26]

In severe head trauma, considerable torsional and shearing forces are directed at the deep white matter of the cerebral hemisphere and the structures in the upper brain stem, principally the midbrain.[10,38,59] The resultant injuries can produce several syndromes that have direct behavioral manifestations. Bilateral damage to the corticobulbar tracts, particularly in the region of the striatum, frequently results in a pseudobulbar syndrome with a marked lability of emotional expression. The patients cry or laugh with the least provocation, frequently in neutral or inappropriate situations. These outward expressions of emotion are involuntary and usually do not represent an expression of true emotion. It is important for the personnel working with the patients with pseudobulbar syndrome to recognize the involuntary nature of these emotional outbursts and also to help the family realize that they do not reflect depression. Family members often feel very guilty if their every remark makes the patient cry; accordingly it is important to discuss these pseudobulbar features frankly with them.

Damage to the midbrain secondary to significant head injury is quite common. During the actual injury, as the head is moved violently, the brain twists and turns within the cranial vault, causing tremendous distortion to the midbrain structures. It is damage to the brain stem reticular substance that results in the prolonged coma in these cases, but many other structures in this area are concomitantly damaged. The resultant syndrome is fairly stereotyped; the patients have marked dysarthria, imbalance, ataxia, limb tremor with dysmetria, occasionally signs of occulomotor nerve damage, and pyramidal tract signs, particularly early in the recovery period.[5,38] In those patients with severe dysarthria as well as other neurologic abnormalities, it is very easy to conclude that the patients are also demented. This is frequently not the case, however. Often the brain stem has borne the brunt of the damage and the higher cortical functions are relatively spared. The dysarthria makes the patient appear demented, but with patient questioning and use of a nonverbal response modality such as nodding the head, it is frequently possible to help them demonstrate their cognitive capacities. Since these patients have sustained significant trauma, they often have some memory deficits and also some frontal lobe behavioral changes, but their basic intellectual processes are often remarkably intact.

Emotional disturbance of a functional nature can also be present in the patient with severe head injury. This seems to be somewhat related to the patient's insight as to the extent and implications of his disability. Genuine depression (as opposed to mere apathy) with anxiety is less likely to be organic and generally is a reactive emotional response to the injury.[41] Such patients require psychiatric care as a component of their general rehabilitation. In many cases, depression is seen in patients with a premorbid predisposition toward depression or personality imbalance, but this is not universally true.[41] Although depression is the most common emotional reaction to head injury, psychotic reactions are known to occur, however, they are distinctly uncommon.[2,41]

A curious feature in patients with severe injuries is the paucity of headache, dizziness, and the other features of the post-traumatic syndrome.[18,46] This may be merely a selection artifact, but it has been reported frequently enough that we feel there may well be a decreased incidence of these findings in such patients. The mechanism resulting in the post-traumatic syndrome in cases of mild head injury is so unclear that to venture an explanation for its absence in severe injury would be sheer speculation.

The question of prognosis, both of survival per se and of the quality of survival of those who do survive a severe head injury, is an important one. Various investigators have used different methods of reporting their case material; accordingly, we will be unable to fully summarize all the available information in a single table. We can provide a number of statistics, however, that will give an overall impression of prognosis in terms of time lost from work, percentage of patients able to work, and some of the factors determining quality of survival and eventual social and vocational readjustment. A severity scale established by Jennet and Bond[31] is useful in categorizing patients after injury. The most severe level on the scale is, of course, death. Next is *the persistent vegetative state*[34] in which the patients recover from coma to the point that their eyes open and appear to search the room, but they remain in a state which has been described as "unresponsive, speechless wakefullness with only primitive postural motor activity".[29] The next level is *severe disability;* the patients are conscious but are totally dependent upon others. With a *moderate disability,* the patients are sufficiently independent to ride public transportation and to work in a sheltered work situation but have prominent neurologic abnormalities. In the category of *recovery* (good outcome), the patients are completely independent and able to return to their regular employment although there may be some minor neurologic signs.

Favorable outcome has a consistent inverse relationship to age, duration of coma, and length of post-traumatic amnesia.[6,29] This is true for quality of survival as well as basic survival. In general, the cognitive and behavioral handicap is the limiting factor both in vocational readjustment and in the successful reestablishment of social and family relationships. Mental problems including personality change, intellectual deficit, and memory problems improve rapidly in the initial six months after the injury but tend to improve less dramatically or to stabilize after that point.[6,9] The physical handicap has a much more gradual recovery course and can show continued improvement over a number of years.[46] Estimates of overall functional recovery can be given quite accurately at 6 months, whereas a prognosis after 3 months or less is often unnecessarily pessimistic. In one study, it was reported that one third of the patients rated severely or moderately disabled at 3 months following injury had improved to the moderate and good categories respectively when tested after one year.[31] However, none of the severe patients had changed to the good category.

Although the prognosis can be accurately given in many cases 6 months after injury, some individuals will continue to improve over a number of years.[42,46] The exact mechanism of this long term recovery is not known but much of it must represent compensatory mechanisms and strategies employed by the patient rather than actual neurologic recovery.

In general, the overall outcome from severe head injury is as follows: death occurs in 50 to 52 percent of cases before leaving the hospital, another 19 percent die during the initial 5 years after the accident, 3 percent remain in a persistent vegetative state and usually die within 1 year, 10 percent are severely disabled, 20 percent are moderately disabled, and 17 percent have a good recovery.[35,46] Age plays an important part in mortality as can be seen in the statistics reported by Russell[55] from a series of patients with less severe injuries: death rate under 40 years of age was 3 to 4 percent; between 40 and 50 years of age, 12 percent; and over 50 years of age, 27 percent. A similar age-related trend is seen for all levels of severity in those patients who survive the initial injury.

Studies relating prognosis to coma and amnesia demonstrate that for patients with coma of over 2 months duration, the full recovery rate is only 6 percent; whereas it is 57 percent in cases of coma of less than 2 months.[35] Patients with an amnesia of over 3 to 4 weeks generally have been reported to have significant mental problems and persistent memory deficits.[6,31]

A final group of statistics important in the assessment of prognosis in head injured patients is the time lost from work and the ultimate job level after severe injury. Guttman[24] reports means of 4.5 weeks lost time with injuries with 24 hours of amnesia, 8.8 weeks lost with 1 to 7 days amnesia, and 13.7 weeks work lost in patients with over a one week period of post-traumatic amnesia. Miller and Stern[46] found that their patients averaged 13 months away from work. In Brook's[8] series of patients with an average amnesia of 43 days, 65 percent had returned to work after one year. Russell[55] reported that two-thirds of his patients with an amnesia of greater than 3 days did not return to work for 6 months and that only 14 percent were back at work within 2 months. Approximately half of the patients suffered no earning loss when returning to work, but 25 to 35 percent were required to take a less responsible job because of their disability.[18,46]

It is obvious from these statistics that severe head injuries are not always hopeless when a full rehabilitative effort is put forth.

Some secondary complications of closed head and general trauma must be mentioned because they frequently are heralded by behavioral changes in a patient who has apparently recovered from the initial concussive incident. One is the development of a post-traumatic communicating hydrocephalus. The primary features are gait difficulty, frontal lobe behavior changes, incontinence, and in the acutely developing case, a progressive decrease in the level of consciousness. The symptoms of this condition have been discussed at length in Chapter 6, Other Dementias. Hydrocephalus is always an important differential consideration in any victim of head injury who begins to regress during the recovery period. A second complication that should always be considered is subdural hematoma. We have seen several patients in whom a fluctuating mild aphasia was the only clue that their recovery was atypical. Whenever a patient is recovering normally and then takes a downward turn, an epidural and subdural clot must be assiduously sought.[20] A third post-traumatic problem, one which is associated with bone fracture with or without head trauma, is fat embolism. The patient with fat embolism typically experiences an uneventful recovery for the first 24 to 72 hours and than rapidly develops a classic acute confusional state. Fat droplets are dispersed throughout the body and are seen on microscopic examination of the urine. Fortunately a rapid recovery is experienced by most patients with this complication.

NEUROBEHAVIORAL EVALUATION

If a patient is seen shortly after awakening from a head injury, he will generally show signs of confusional behavior. During this confusional period, the patient will be unable to establish new memories and will be able to give only sketchy details about the events leading up to his trauma. With the passage of time, his mind will clear and, at some point, he will be fully conscious and remember all ongoing events. At this point, the post-traumatic amnesia has ended and the length of time elapsed since the trauma can be used as a gauge of the severity of the injury. It is not always easy to determine the exact time of return to full consciousness as confusional behavior fluctuates and what would appear to be a total clearing of mentation at 8:00 A.M. might not remain constant throughout the day and night. Multiple determinations must be made and the true length of the amnesia may be quite difficult to establish. As we pointed out in the clinical section of this chapter, there will often be subtle memory and concentration problems for a month, even in patients with minor head injury. These problems, however, should not be taken into account in calculating the amnesic period. The post-traumatic amnesia must represent a period of rather significant memory loss.

During the initial confusional period, it is important to watch for any significant, sustained decrease in level of alertness as this may be the only clinical sign of a developing hematoma or hydrocephalus. Periodic mental status screening is useful. Although it is expected that patients will have many mild cognitive deficits, the appearance of a significant specific defect or a sudden worsening of one function (e.g., language or drawing) may suggest the development of a focal lesion.

When the patient with a minor head injury has recovered from the initial traumatic period and is ready for discharge, it is advisable for the clinician to be prepared and to prepare the patient for the appearance of post-traumatic symptoms and problems. We take a brief history to assess most of the factors that influence the appearance and prolongation of a post-traumatic syndrome: (1) is a lawsuit likely to ensue? (2) does the patient hold someone else responsible for the accident? (3) was the patient experiencing financial or personal problems before the accident? and (4) is there any indication of a pretraumatic neurosis or character problem? It is also important to inquire about previous trauma, since multiple trauma often significantly extends the period of recovery.

Prior to discharge, a complete mental status examination should be carried out and specific attention must be given to eliciting any behavioral change, anxiety, and concentration or memory problems. Frequently the entire management plan for a given patient will be predicated on the results of this examination.

With patients who have survived a severe head injury, a more complete neurobehavioral evaluation is required. To gain an initial estimate of prognosis, the examiner must know the patient's age, the length of coma, length of amnesia, and whether any surgery was performed or an associated focal lesion identified. The mental status examination that follows should be comprehensive since the examiner is attempting to document areas of cognitive and emotional deficit as well as residual strengths. Again, the specific search for frontal lobe personality change is very important. It is essential that the clinician contact someone who knew the patient well prior to the accident to verify any personality change. We recently saw a teenage boy who had been in a motorcycle accident. We felt that he was acting unusually silly, disinhibited, and immature subsequent to his injury. We were very interested to hear his mother rather disgustedly report, "He was always like that!" Had we not checked with the mother, we could easily have reported that the boy had suffered significant frontal lobe damage with a subsequent behavioral change.

A careful evaluation of memory, language, praxis, and abstract reasoning is also an important aid in planning the comprehensive rehabilitation program. Signs of depression should be carefully sought as the success or failure of a patient's rehabilitation and readjustment is often directly related to the presence of significant emotional/behavioral factors.

MEDICAL AND LABORATORY EVALUATION

The question of when to obtain a skull x-ray of a patient with a head injury is a difficult one; certainly any patient who is unconscious for more than a few seconds should have a skull series, but there is no universally accepted rule. With the increasing amount of litigation in cases of head injury, it is more and more important to obtain appropriate diagnostic tests to ensure that no possibility is overlooked. The skull x-ray is a good screening test for subdural hematomas. In one recent series, only 5 percent of the patients with hematomas secondary to head injury did not have either positive neurologic signs or a skull fracture.[20]

The use of the electroencephalogram (EEG) is more equivocal, particularly in cases of minor head injury. Many studies have demonstrated that the incidence of abnormal EEGs in patients with minor concussion is similar to that of the normal population.[40] Repeating the EEG in those patients with abnormalities frequently shows no improvement, since the abnormality was actually related to a premorbid variation and not to the head trauma. These "false positive" cases can lead to the erroneous conclusion that such patients had really sustained lasting brain damage. In cases of more severe trauma, the EEG will be abnormal in proportion to the severity of the injury. In such cases, the EEG can be used to follow the patient's improvement and can at times detect subdural hematomas. Again, the legal aspects of head trauma have caused physicians to order far more EEGs than are realistically necessary. This situation has resulted in the label of "post-traumatic brain damage" being applied to many patients who actually do not have it.

The computerized tomography scan (CT) has been extremely useful in cases of head trauma. The CT scan can differentiate hematoma, edema, and contusion, as well as demonstrate communicating hydrocephalus or post-traumatic atrophy.[3,47] The CT scan, because of its expense, should probably not be routinely used in cases of minor head

288

trauma unless the patient is unduly slow to recover or if neurologic signs are present or develop in the post-traumatic period. The development of this remarkable neurodiagnostic tool has dramatically decreased the need for arteriography in cases of trauma, and it has gained an excellent reputation in identifying subdural hematomas. In one recent series, the CT scan clearly identified 57 of 60 hematomas and inferred their presence in the remaining 3, which were isodense, by virtue of ventricular distortion.[33] In this series, there were no false positive or false negative scans. The CT scan has replaced the pneumoencephalogram for follow-up studies of cases of severe head injury, as the CT scan can demonstrate either atrophy or hydrocephalus with no patient risk. Cerebral arteriography is still used in evaluating some cases of acute head trauma, but this procedure should always be either completed by or supervised by a neurosurgeon.

Recently, some investigators have measured serum-myelin-basic-protein levels in patients with severe head injuries and have reported some encouraging initial results.[63] In patients with a poor prognosis, the levels of the myelin protein were higher during the first week and stayed higher for a longer period (over two weeks) than in the patients who had a good outcome. While experimental at present, this type of test could become a very useful parameter for the early evaluation of the degree of brain damage.

CONSULTATIONS

There are many occasions in the evaluation and management of head trauma cases when consultation with specific colleagues is strongly indicated. After the acute injury, particularly if it is severe, a neurosurgeon should be asked to see the patient and should share the responsibility for early patient care. The neurosurgeon is the best person to decide when and what neurodiagnostic laboratory tests are indicated and whether immediate hospitalization is necessary. The neurosurgeon, of course, is the only one qualified to provide surgical management when necessary.

During the management of the patient with a post-traumatic syndrome from minor head trauma, it is sometimes comforting to the patient to see a neurologist or to revisit the neurosurgeon. Usually, however, any competent physician can help the patient cope with the headache, dizziness, insomnia, and nervousness which are parts of the syndrome. If the patient complains of concentration and memory problems, it is frequently advisable to refer the patient to a psychologist for evaluation and assistance in management. Serious or persistent minor cognitive problems must be documented and honestly discussed with the patient in regards to their social and vocational implications.

In case of severe head trauma, full rehabilitation resources are necessary. Physical therapy is generally the mainstay, but a number of other services are often required. Every patient with severe head injury requires a full neuropsychologic evaluation. Information gained from that evaluation can be essential in helping the patient during the therapeutic process as well as during the period of adjustment following hospitalization. A neurologist does not have to see all patients with severe brain injury but can often make useful suggestions, particularly by assessing the extent of the injury and localizing its greatest areas of damage. We find that the bilateral brain damage present in many patients is not always fully appreciated by the therapists working with them and a good neurologic examination can usually highlight these deficits and thereby provide crucial information.

MANAGEMENT

The management of the patient with a head injury depends to a major degree upon the severity of the trauma. Therefore, we will discuss the management of the patient with minor trauma and then that of the patient with severe injury, realizing that there is a continuum between them. We will concentrate our discussion on the elements in the management plan that directly relate to the behavioral aspects of the trauma and not concentrate on the specific medical or surgical management of such conditions as subdural hematomas or depressed skull fractures as this material is adequately handled in other basic texts.

With cases of minor head trauma, the basic plan is: bed rest, symptomatic medication, and supportive sympathy with gentle encouragement to resume regular activities. The general principals are quite straightforward, but the specifics as to when to admit the patient to the hospital, how long he should remain in bed, and when he should be encouraged to resume work are impossible to standardize. In most cases, we let the patients set their own pace with some encouragement and let them return to work when they feel sufficiently well.

As a rule, the first question is when to hospitalize a patient for observation. Although some physicians advocate admitting all patients for one week,[51] we consider this unnecessary. Patients who have been dazed for only a few seconds to minutes and who are neurologically and cognitively clear upon arrival at the hospital can usually go home safely after the initial examination. Those patients who have a documented period of unconsciousness or who are still lethargic or confusional upon arrival at the hospital are best admitted for at least one night. Patients who live alone or at a great distance from the hospital are best admitted. The adult who is vomiting or has a skull fracture should also be admitted in almost all cases.

290

In general, there is a tendency to overadmit. Several recent reports bear this out and firmly state that precautionary admission in minor head injury is unnecessary.[32,64] When the patient is fully conscious and has a negative neurologic examination and skull x-ray, he may safely go home. Admitting such patients does not seem to have increased the early detection of hematoma formation.[32]

During the first few days after an injury, other than checking the patient for any developing signs of intracranial hematoma, bed rest is the most efficacious treatment. Two to four days of rest is generally necessary for most patients, but depending upon the age of the patient (older patients require additional rest) and the severity of the trauma, some patients require several weeks of supervised rest. If a patient is kept in bed overly long, he will begin to develop additional post-traumatic symptoms, so in most cases it is best to err on the side of less treatment rather than to be overly cautious.[66] We usually spend some time during the first few days reassuring the patient and also preparing him for the possible post-traumatic symptoms that he may experience. They are told that headache, dizziness, insomnia, fatigue, nervousness, and concentration difficulties are common and that they will be understood and treated if they do occur. The patients are encouraged to sit up when they feel able and also to ambulate at will. Since exercise and any effort, either mental or physical, can exacerbate symptoms; the patient is warned about this possibility, told to take it easy for a bit longer if symptoms become troublesome, and to report such symptoms to the physician.

When the patient leaves the hospital or is preparing to return to work, it is important to warn both the patient and his employer that he should start with part-time or light work for an initial period. In the young patient with an uncomplicated course, two weeks should be sufficient to have him back to a full work schedule, but again this prognosis is related to many factors. Patients should also be warned that alcohol will have the same tendency to reactivate post-traumatic symptoms as heavy work.

The most common mistake that we see in the management of cases of minor head trauma is that which Courville[13] warned against a quarter of a century ago—the quick "brush off." In such cases, the x-ray is negative and the neurologic examination is negative and so the patient is declared to have no sequelae from the head injury and told to go back to work. The patient tries to do so, does not function adequately, and is sent back to the doctor who then reaffirms his earlier opinion. Neither the doctor nor the employer believe that the patient is still symptomatic, and the patient is frequently told to either work or to take off from work at his own expense. Understandably this situation breeds tremendous anger and such patients develop many additional tension-related symptoms. They then become hostile and aggressively seek medical or financial compensation. At this point, what could have been a minor accident resulting in a two week loss of work becomes a complicated situation that drags on for many months. It is much easier and more efficacious to warn the patient and employer of possible sequelae, put the patient on a graduated work schedule, and treat them with analgesics, mild tranquilizers if necessary, and sympathy for their plight. Thus, the emotional agony and time lost from work can be minimized. Unfortunately this simple plan does not always work because of the long drawn out legal proceedings involved in many such cases. In these cases, one can only do the best one can and hope that an early settlement is made.

The management of the severely brain damaged patient requires more intensive and comprehensive efforts. After survival has been assured and the patient is conscious and able to begin a comprehensive rehabilitation program, it is important to undertake a complete neurologic and neuropsychologic evaluation. With an accurate conception of the patient's disabilities and residual strengths, it is then possible to outline a realistic program. Evidence of frontal lobe damage, memory problems, and specific cognitive disturbances are all very important to note, as these defects are so often the limiting factors in the patient's rehabilitation. As previously mentioned, the mental symptoms improve rapidly during the first 6 months following trauma. Accordingly, it is best not to attempt to predict the patient's eventual level of recovery too early in the post-traumatic period. Unfortunately, there is currently no effective therapy for most of these mental deficits and one must await spontaneous recovery while working diligently on the physical impairments. During this initial recovery period, emotional reactions such as depression or anxiety should be treated as they would in any setting. Psychiatric consultation can frequently be of major importance and should be requested at the first signs of a significant mood disturbance.

When the patient's mental status begins to stabilize, the next major step in the comprehensive rehabilitation program is to devise a logical vocational plan. This is often the most difficult and least satisfying part of the entire rehabilitation process. These patients have both physical and mental disabilities and career plans are very difficult to formulate and then even more difficult to realize. The final blow is often the presence of frontal lobe damage. Thus afflicted, the patient loses his basic drive and the resultant apathy makes a productive career impossible even when the cognitive and physical problems have been overcome.

Because of his multiple handicaps, the patient with a severe head trauma must rely very heavily on family resources, both personal and financial, and family counseling is a critical part of the patient's total rehabilitation program. The family must understand the patient's deficits and capabilities if they are to work effectively with the patient after discharge. Without the family's support, the patient will flounder. Social workers are of inestimable value in preparing the family for the patient's return home, in arranging community resourses and financial aid, and in providing continuing support.

NEUROPATHOLOGY

There are several mechanisms by which the brain is damaged both directly and indirectly in trauma. There is cortical contusion both at the point of impact and, in contrecoup fashion, on the opposite side of the head. There is also extensive subcortical white matter injury from the rotational and torsional forces in effect while the head is recoiling from the blow.

These torsional forces which are generated by a freely movable head lead to the actual concussion.[15] The midbrain is one of the points of maxium rotation and accordingly this structure suffers an initial and often prolonged injury. The ascending activating system at this level is thereby paralyzed and loss of consciousness ensues. If significant damage is done at this level, a prolonged coma is seen. In mild injuries, where consciousness is quickly regained, it is very possible that dysfunction of these ascending fibers is responsible for the attention and concentration problems experienced by some patients.

Secondary damage can occur when the injury is complicated by hematoma formation, vasospasm, massive cerebral edema, and penetrating fragments. Here we will consider these factors in a very general fashion and not attempt an exhaustive discussion of the pathophysiology or experimental models.

With mild head injury, it has been the consensus in the literature that the condition is relatively benign pathologically. Recent studies, however, have shown that there is considerable pathologic change even in patients with post-traumatic amnesia of 10 to 15 minutes or less.[48,56] Tiny capillary hemorrhages, severed nerve fibers, surface shearing, and contusion are all seen in these minor injuries. Some axons are torn and there is considerable distortion of synaptic connections. Although clinical recovery usually occurs, Russell[56] seriously questions whether complete recovery is ever achieved in such patients.

In individuals with repeated minor trauma, the pathologic effects are clearly documented. The demented pugilist, for example, has evidence of multiple cortical contusions, petechial hemorrhages that have scarred, a marked decrease in white matter resulting in enlargement of the lateral ventricles, and rupture of the septem pellucidum.[12,44]

Alzheimer's tangles are seen diffusely throughout the brain stem and substantia nigra as well as cortex. Nerve fiber degeneration is also significant.[60] The prominent changes in the substantia nigra, which are responsible for the parkinson-like syndrome, are due to cell loss and neurofibrillary degeneration. The neurofibrillary changes seen in the brain are concentrated in the medial temporal grey matter, though they are seen throughout the brain. Unlike Alzheimer's disease, the trauma patient does not develop the characteristic senile plaques of Marinesco.[12] Once initiated, the dementia often progresses even without further trauma, therefore, the trauma itself must trigger some aberrant physiologic process that can then become self perpetuating.

In cases of severe head injury, patients have multifocal lesions. Contusions are seen in almost all patients, many (40 to 60%) have evidence of intracranial hemorrhage, and white matter degeneration is extensive.[28] In patients with prolonged coma, the deeper structures are more prominently involved. In patients with persistent vegetative states, the white matter destruction is the primary feature, with lesions in the posterior walls of the third ventricle also present in some cases.[28,59] In those patients with better levels of recovery, the deep lesions are less frequent. It is in these more serious injuries that secondary pathologic processes occur and greatly add to the morbidity and mortality.

The recovery process in these severe cases is slow. The pathophysiologic nature of the recovery process is uncertain, but recent work gives some hope that actual regeneration within the central nervous system does occur.[52] If such regeneration can be stimulated and guided, it is possible that the outlook for the patient with severe head injury will be more encouraging in the future than it is today.

REFERENCES

1. Ad Hoc Committee of the Congress of Neurological Surgeons: Head injury nomenclature: a glossary of head injury. Clin. Neurosurg. 12:386, 1966.
2. Aita, J.A., and Reitan, R.M.: Psychotic reactions in the late recovery period following brain injury. Am. J. Psychiatry 105:161, 1948.
3. Ambrose, J., Gooding, M.R., and Uttley, D.: E.M.I. scan in the management of head injuries. Lancet 1:847, 1976.
4. Benson, D.F., and Geschwind, N.: Shrinking retrograde amnesia. J. Neurol. Neurosurg. Psychiatry 30:539, 1967.
5. Boller, F.C., Albert, M.L., LeMay, M., and Kertesz, A.: Enlargement of the sylvian aqueduct, a sequel of head injury. J. Neurol. Neurosurg. Psychiatry 35:463, 1972.
6. Bond, M.R.: Assessment of the psychosocial outcome after severe head injury, in Outcome of Damage to the Central Nervous System. Ciba Foundation Symposium 34 (new series), Elsevier-North Holland Publishing Co., New York, 1975, pp. 141–155.
7. Brooks, D.N.: Memory and head injury. J. Nerv. Ment. Dis. 155:350, 1972.

8. Brooks, D.N.: Recognition memory and head injury. J. Neurol. Neurosurg. Psychiatry 37:794, 1974.

9. Brooks, D.N.: Weschler Memory Scale performance and its relationship to brain damage after severe closed head injury. J. Neurol. Neurosurg. Psychiatry 39:593, 1976.

10. Compton, M.R.: Brainstem lesions due to closed head injury. Lancet 1:669, 1971.

11. Cook, J.B.: The effects of minor head injuries sustained in sport and the postconcussion syndrome, in Walker, A.E., Caveness, W.F., and Critchley, M. (eds.): The Late Effects of Head Injury. Charles C Thomas, Springfield, Illinois, 1967, pp. 408–413.

12. Corsellis, J.A.N., Bruton, C.J., and Freeman-Browne, D.: The aftermath of boxing. Psychol. Med. 3:370, 1973.

13. Courville, C.B.: Commotio Cerebri. San Lucas Press, Los Angeles, 1953.

14. Critchley, M.: Medical aspects of boxing, particularly from a neurological standpoint. Br. Med. J. 1:357, 1957.

15. Denny-Brown, D., and Russell, W.R.: Experimental cerebral concussion. Brain 64:93, 1941.

16. Editorial: Brain damage in sport. Lancet 1:401, 1976.

17. Evans, C.D.: Discussion of scale, scope and philosophy of the clinical problem, in Outcome of Severe Damage to the Central Nervous System. Ciba Foundation Symposium 34 (new series), Elsevier-North Holland Publishing Co., New York, 1975, pp. 12–18.

18. Fahy, J.T., Irving, M.H., and Millac, P.: Severe head injuries: A six year follow-up. Lancet 2:475, 1967.

19. Fisher, C.M.: Concussion amnesia, Neurology 16:826, 1966.

20. Galbraith, S., and Smith, J.: Acute traumatic intracranial hematoma without skull fracture. Lancet 1:501, 1976.

21. Gronwall, D.M.A., and Sampson, H.: The Psychological Effects of Concussion. Auckland/Oxford Press, New Zealand, 1974.

22. Gronwall, D.M.A., and Wrightson, P.: Delayed recovery of intellectual function after minor head injury. Lancet 2:605, 1974.

23. Gronwall, D.M.A., and Wrightson, P.: Cumulative effect of concussion, Lancet 2:995, 1975.

24. Guttman, E.: The prognosis in civilian head injuries. Br. Med. J. 1:94, 1943.

25. Heilman, K.M., Safran, A., and Geschwind, N.: Closed head trauma and aphasia. J. Neurol. Neurosurg. Psychiatry 34:265, 1971.

26. Hooshmand, H., Sepdham, T., and Uries, J.K.: Klüver-Bucy syndrome, successful treatment with carbamazepine. JAMA 229:1782, 1974.

27. Jacobson, S.A.: Mechanisms of the sequelae of minor craniocervical trauma, in Walker, A.E., Caveness, W.F., and Critchley, M. (eds.): Late Effects of Head Injury. Charles C Thomas, Springfield, Illinois, 1969, pp. 35–45.

28. Jellinger, K., and Seitelberger, F.: Protracted posttraumatic encephalopathy: Pathology and clinical implications, in Walker, A.E., Caveness, W.F., and Critchley, M. (eds.): The Late Effects of Head Injury. Charles C Thomas, Springfield, Illinois, 1969, pp. 168–181.

29. Jennett, B.: Scale, scope and philosophy of the clinical problem, in Outcome of Severe Damage to the Central Nervous System. Ciba Foundation Symposium 34 (new series) Elsevier-North Holland Publishing Co., New York, 1975, p. 7.

30. Jennett, B.: Assessment of severity of head injury. J. Neuro. Neurosurg. Psychiatry 39:647, 1976.
31. Jennett, B., and Bond, M.: Assessment of outcome after severe brain damage. Lancet 1:480, 1975.
32. Jennett, B., and Galbraith, S.L.: Head injury and admission policy. Lancet 1:552, 1979.
33. Jennett, B., Galbraith, S.L., Teasdale, G.M., and Steven, J.L.: EMI scan and head injuries. Lancet 1:1026, 1976.
34. Jennett, B., and Plum, F.: Persistent vegetative state after brain damage. Lancet 1:734, 1972.
35. Jennett, B., Teasdale, G., Braakman, R., Minderhoud, J., and Knill-Jones, R.: Predicting outcome in individual patients after severe head injury. Lancet 1:1031, 1976.
36. Klüver, H., and Bucy, P.C.: "Psychic blindness" and other symptoms following bilateral temporal lobectomy in rhesus monkeys. Am. J. Physiol. 119:352, 1937.
37. Klüver, H., and Bucy, P.C.: Preliminary analysis of functions of the temporal lobes in monkeys, Arch. Neurol. Psychiatry 42:979, 1939.
38. Kremer, M., Russell, W.R., and Smyth, G.E.: A midbrain syndrome following head injury. J. Neurol. Neurosurg. Psychiatry 10:49, 1947.
39. Levin, H.S., and Grossman, R.G.: Behavioral sequelae of closed head injury. Arch. Neurol. 35:720, 1978.
40. Lidvall, H.F., Linderoth, B., and Norlin, B.: Causes of the post-concussional syndrome. Acta Neurol. Scand. [Supp.] 56:3, 1974.
41. Lishman, W.A.: The psychiatric sequelae of head injury: a review. Psychol. Med. 3:304, 1973.
42. Lishman, W.A.: Organic Psychiatry. Blackwell Scientific Publications, Oxford, 1978, pp. 191–261.
43. Mandleberg, L.A., and Brooks, D.N.: Cognitive recovery after severe head injury. J. Neurol. Neurosurg. Psychiatry 38:1121, 1975.
44. Mawdsley, C., and Ferguson, F.R.: Neurological disease in boxers. Lancet 2:795, 1963.
45. Miller, H.: Mental after-effects of head injury. Proc. R. Soc. Med. 59:257, 1966.
46. Miller, H., and Stern, G.: The long-term prognosis of severe head injury. Lancet 1:225, 1965.
47. New, P.F.J., and Scott, W.R.: Computed Tomography of the Brain and Orbit. Williams & Wilkins, Baltimore, 1975, pp. 426–439.
48. Oppenheimer, D.R.: Microscopic lesions in the brain following head injury. J. Neurol. Neurosurg. Psychiatry 31:299, 1968.
49. Ota, Y.: Psychiatric studies on civilian head injuries, in Walker, A.E., Caveness, W.F., and Critchley, M. (eds.): Late Effects of Head Injury. Charles C Thomas, Springfield, Illinois, 1969, pp. 110–118.
50. Peterson, G.C.: Organic brain syndromes associated with brain trauma, in Freedman, A.M., Kaplan, H.I., and Sadock, B.J. (eds.): Comprehensive Textbook of Psychiatry. Williams & Wilkins, Baltimore, 1975, pp. 1093–1108.
51. Plaut, M.R., and Gifford, R.R.M.: Trivial head trauma and its consequences in a perspective of regional health care. Milit. Med. 141:244, 1976.
52. Raisman, A.: What hope for repair of the brain? Ann. Neurol. 3:101, 1978.
53. Roberts, A.H.: Brain Damage in Boxers. Pitman, London, 1969.

54. Ruesch, J., and Bowman, K.: Prolonged post-traumatic syndromes following head injury. Am. J. Psychiatry 102:145, 1945.
55. Russell, W.R.: The Traumatic Amnesias. Oxford Press, London, 1971.
56. Russell, W.R.: Recovery after minor head injury. Lancet 2:1315, 1974.
57. Rutherford, W.H., Merret, J.D., and McDonald, J.R.: Sequelae of concussion caused by minor head injuries. Lancet 1:1, 1977.
58. Sisler, G., and Penner, H.: Amnesia following severe head injury. Can. Psychiatr. Assoc. J. 20:333, 1975.
59. Strich, S.J.: Shearing of nerve fibers as a cause of brain damage due to head injury. Lancet 2:443, 1961.
60. Strich, S.J.: Cerebral trauma, in Blackwood, W., and Corsellis, J.A.N. (eds.): Greenfields Neuropathology. Arnold, London, 1976, p. 329.
61. Symonds, C.: Concussion and its sequelae. Lancet 1:1, 1962.
62. Taylor, A.R.: Post-concussional sequelae. Br. Med. J. 3:67, 1967.
63. Thomas, D.G.T., Palfreyman, J.W., and Ratcliff, J.A.: Serum-myelin-basic-protein assay in diagnosis and prognosis of patients with head injury. Lancet 1:113, 1978.
64. Totten, J., and Buxton, R.: Were you knocked out? Lancet 1:369, 1979.
65. Unterhornscheidt, F.J.: Injuries due to boxing and other sports, in Vinken, P.J., and Bruyn, G.W. (eds.): Handbook of Clinical Neurology, Vol 23. Elsevier-North Holland Publishing Co., New York, 1975, pp. 527–593.
66. Verjaal, A., and Van T. Hooff, F.: Commotio and contusio cerebri (cerebral) concussion), in Vinken, P.J., and Bruyn, G.W. (eds.): Handbook of Clinical Neurology, Vol. 23. Elsevier-North Holland Publishing Co., New York, 1975, pp. 417–444.
67. Yarnell, P.R., and Lynch, S.: The "ding": Amnesic states in football trauma. Neurology 23:196, 1973.

9

TOXIC SUBSTANCES

N.K. is a 35-year-old artist who was cleaning brushes in her low ceilinged closed studio when she began to feel very light-headed and to see double. She sat down to rest and was found in that spot shortly thereafter by a friend. The friend reported that the patient was quite confusional and could not express herself at all clearly. He opened the windows and within several minutes, the patient felt much better, had clearing of the double vision, and was more coherent.

Although subjectively and clinically much improved, the patient continued to have difficulty in thinking clearly and felt that her memory was faulty. The next day in her job as an art teacher she attempted to write a simple report but found that her writing ability had deteriorated remarkably. Her friend described her mental function during this period as being "very fuzzy." These symptoms generally improved over the course of 5 to 6 weeks. However, she still complained of mild memory problems when we saw her 6 months later. Her friends also felt that she still did not think clearly and stated that she was quite forgetful and anxious.

On examination (6 months after exposure), the patient's routine neurologic examination was completely normal. Neuropsychologic testing, however, showed distinct abnormalities. She was anxious and quite apprehensive throughout the evaluation and had difficulty concentrating on tasks for sustained periods. Her affect was generally appropriate, although, on occasion, emotionality in the form of nervous laughter was exhibited in what appeared to be inappropriate situations. She had mild difficulty in naming objects to confrontation and also had noticeable word finding difficulty in free conversation. She often resorted to circumlocution when unable to retrieve a specific word. Articulation and comprehension were normal.

Intelligence testing revealed a WAIS Full Scale IQ of 103, with the Verbal IQ being 98 and Performance IQ being 110. There was considera-

ble scatter among the subtest scores, with the lowest scores achieved on tests of attention and concentration. Her memory, as objectively tested by the Wechsler Memory Scale Form II, showed a significantly disproportionate impairment in performance when compared to her general level of intelligence. The Memory Quotient was 69. Visual memory was excellent, with most of her memory difficulties being with verbal material. Verbal abstract reasoning as tested by the Shipley-Hartford Test was grossly impaired (Conceptional Quotient = 50), but visual reasoning was shown to be within normal limits by performance on the Raven's Coloured Progressive Matrices. An MMPI was normal. Both an EEG and brain scan were normal.

The above case represents some of the behavioral sequelae of exposure to toxic materials. In today's society, there are many similar potential risks: the accidental or inadvertent risk of a single overwhelming exposure as was true in this case, the insidious repeated exposure experienced by workers who habitually use hydrocarbon solvents or organic insect sprays, the tragic mass poisonings with heavy metals (in particular, mercury) when such metals are mistakenly introduced into the food chain, and finally the intentional repeated insults of alcohol and all manner of other noxious chemicals abused by some members of our culture to cope with the stress of day to day living.

In this chapter, we cannot and do not intend to make a general review of toxicology nor do we wish to discuss at length the many acute intoxication syndromes and their clinical management; rather we will limit this presentation to some of the lasting behavioral side effects that can occur with both a single heavy exposure and with repeated exposure whether intentional or accidental. In many such cases, the effects upon memory, intellectual performance, and emotionality can be devastating, while the effect upon basic motor and sensory systems can be nil. Diagnostic tests such as the EEG and CT scan are often normal, therefore many cases of mild to moderate encephalopathy have probably been considered to be hysterical or malingering. We feel that with careful mental status testing and neuropsychologic evaluation, this error can be avoided and adequate precautions can be provided for those individuals coming into contact with these compounds.

DESCRIPTION OF THE CLINICAL SYNDROMES

Organic Solvent Inhalation

Numerous volatile hydrocarbon substances have been produced since the beginning of the industrial revolution and all of us are exposed to them in one form or another almost every day.[46] Gasoline, cleaning fluids, and paint solvents are commonly found in the home. In industry, a vast array of similar chemicals is used to process synthetic materials, clean machines, and as solvents in many products. If properly used in adequately ventilated spaces, their toxicity to workers is minimal. With carelessness or disregard for safety precautions, however, acute intoxication or subtle insidious behavioral changes can develop. With little thought for their deleterious effects, scores of young people have embraced the toxic side effects of many substances as being enjoyable and have repeatedly exposed themselves to highly concentrated noxious fumes. Sniffing glue, in which toluene is the major solvent, and inhaling the fumes of gasoline have been the most popular. Although such abuse is a negative and dangerous practice, by studying the abuser one can gain valuable information concerning the potential toxicity of chronic exposure to these substances.

The clinical picture of acute intoxication is similar for most of these agents: general inebriation, giddiness, confusion, dizziness, nausea, and vomiting if the exposure is extreme. With overwhelming exposure, stupor, coma, and even death can occur. A description of the comprehensive management of the acute intoxication syndrome is beyond the scope of this work and the reader is referred to a standard text on toxicology for specific details. The general consensus in the literature is that, barring significant anoxia, complete recovery from an acute episode is expected. Our experience, an example of which was presented at the beginning of the chapter, suggests that such exposures are not nearly as benign as was previously believed. It is possible that patients with mild memory or behavioral changes after a single exposure have been considered in much the same way that post-traumatic patients have: as malingering, seeking compensation, or emotionally unstable. We have examined several patients with rather significant neuropsychologic deficits after inhalations and feel that the true toxicity of these substances has not been fully appreciated.

In individuals who suffer repeated subacute intoxicating levels of exposure (e.g., the spray painter who works in a poorly ventilated enclosed space), a chronic syndrome develops which is related to the cumulative total exposure. Such individuals become progressively depressed, weak, anorexic, increasingly sensitive to the effects of alcohol, and experience difficulty in concentrating.[39] They also become easily fatigued and frequently experience headache.[15] Psychomotor agility is decreased both in terms of basic dexterity and speed of performance;[41] and verbal reasoning and memory also show significant decrements in performance.[19,26] Workers who are suspected of having a problem of toxic exposure demonstrate the most significant abnormalities, but asymptomatic workers at the same facilities tested at random also show significant cognitive difficulties.[26] These changes, while being statistically significant, are not pronounced enough to be noted by the casual observer and because of their nature (i.e., cognitive and behavioral) are usually not detected in routine medical examinations. Nonetheless the risk is present, and the full effects of a working lifetime of 30 years exposure to these solvent fumes have not yet been fully documented. In one study of 50 factory workers exposed to trichloroethylene for an average of 4 years, 66 percent had overt complaints. Careful psychiatric and psychologic evaluation of the 50 patients demonstrated a slight to moderate "psycho-organic syndrome" in 34 percent.[15] Although these symptoms are often reversible when the person is withdrawn from the toxic environment, cases have been reported in which significant symptoms were still present after 14 months.[39]

The population with the most extensive toxic exposure is that of the intentional "sniffers" who utilize glue or paint to induce repeated intoxication. Permanent severe encephalopathy has been frequently reported in this population.[12,24] The results are difficult to interpret in many instances, as the patient population is typically drawn from a low socioeconomic group of young people with poor cognitive and educational backgrounds. Many of these individuals have significant personality problems, have previously experienced serious head trauma, and also use a variety of other drugs. It has been, therefore, difficult to use this population to extrapolate the possible effects of repeated industrial exposure in the normal worker. However, many investigators in this field are convinced that irreversible central nervous system damage does occur in young people who chronically misuse these solvents.[33]

Heavy Metals

Mental symptoms either preceding or accompanying other neurologic symptoms are commonly seen in many of the heavy metal intoxications. By far the most frequent and important offenders traditionally have been lead and mercury. In most cases of chronic exposure, the patients display irritability, apathy, headache, dizziness, weakness, and fine tremor. In lead toxicity, peripheral neuritis is common, particularly of the radial nerve resulting in wrist drop. In mercury poisoning, ataxia, stomatitis, dermatitis, and blue gum lines assist in making the diagnosis clinically.[13]

Two rather different syndromes result from mercury poisoning with the presentation being determined by the chemical form of mercury to which the patient has been exposed. When the toxicant is methylmercury (i.e., organic mercury) such as that which polluted Minamata Bay in Japan and was used as a fungicide on the grain consumed in Iraq in 1972, the syndrome consists primarily of motor and sensory abnormalities: cerebellar ataxia, slurred speech, paresthesias, visual field constriction, tremor, pyramidal signs, and often complete cortical destruction.[13,25,28,36] Although depression and dementia are common, these are not the outstanding features of the clinical manifestation of organic mercury poisoning.

Inorganic mercury, conversely, is well known for its ability to cause a primary psychiatric condition immortalized in the character of the "mad hatter" in Lewis Carroll's, *Alice's Adventures in Wonderland*. The main symptoms include irritability, excitability, a tendency to lose control in public which causes a withdrawal from society, memory difficulty, and often a full-blown psychosis.[28,34] Headaches, fine tremor, and weakness, while frequently present, are minor in comparison to the behavioral aspects.

Exposure to heavy metals is a constant threat in an industrial society and it is only through careful adherence to safety precautions and alertness on the part of industrial medicine personnel that such horrors as those which occured in Minamata and Iraq can be avoided.

Alcohol

Alcohol abuse and its frequent companion, malnutrition, are the cause of a wide variety of neurobehavioral syndromes. Because alcoholism is such a major problem in the world, all physicians should become familiar with its various toxic manifestations and their management.

The acute stage of alcoholic intoxication is all too familiar to most of us, whether from personal experience or from working in a hospital emergency ward. Little elaboration of its symptoms seems necessary other than to mention that it can frequently appear as an acute confusional state and must be considered in the differential diagnosis of that state.

All individuals, however, do not follow the usual course of inebriation. There are a number who undergo a rather remarkable personality and behavioral transformation after only a few drinks. This so-called alcoholic idiosyncratic intoxication[2] or pathologic intoxication[3] is a very dramatic event, one that has been viewed with a jaundiced eye by some clinicians.[22] The typical history is that of a young to middle-aged male who may or may not be a habitual drinker who, usually after only a few drinks, becomes suddenly disoriented, paranoid, anxious, and violent. The individuals frequently state that they feel extraordinarily strong and often are physically very violent. In many reported cases, the individuals have actually severely injured or killed people unfortunate enough to be in their immediate environment.[3] After the sudden explosive outburst, the individual is usually fatigued and falls easily to sleep. Upon awakening he typically has little or no memory of the

303

episode. Many of these individuals basically have rather pathologic personalities, and it is difficult to totally excuse the behavior as occurring as a completely unconscious and uncontrolled act. However, the exact pathophysiology of these reactions is not known. They may represent a type of alcohol induced dissociative episode, but this is currently only one speculation.

The habituated alcohol user runs the risk of developing one or a variety of more serious organic brain disorders. Once addicted, the individual may suffer the acute symptoms of withdrawal should he abruptly stop drinking, or more significantly, he can develop irreversible amnesia (Korsakoff's syndrome) or dementia. The most familiar syndrome secondary to alcohol withdrawal is delirium tremens. Already discussed in Chapter 4, this state is a syndrome of tremulousness and agitated confusion that develops during the first few days of abstinence and can last from a few days to a week. Visual and tactile hallucinations, paranoia, and wild agitation are present in severe cases. Generalized seizures occur in a few cases, with status epilepticus being one of the most serious problems encountered in management. As with any confusional state, the course will fluctuate during the day, with nocturnal exacerbations being characteristic. Treatment regimens vary, but vitamins, adequate nutrition, sedation (chlordiazepoxide [Librium] up to 400 mg./day), anticonvulsants (diphenylhydantoin [Dilantin], 300 mg. day), and physical restraint when absolutely necessary have been the most satisfactory for us.

A fascinating, rare withdrawal syndrome is seen in a very small number of alcoholics—chronic alcoholic hallucinosis.[47] The hallucinations are usually auditory, unlike the vivid visual and tactile hallucinations of delirium, and are present in an individual with an otherwise completely clear sensorium. The syndrome most frequently occurs after a delirium and while usually lasting only a few weeks, it can persist for years. Whether this syndrome is totally an effect of alcohol or is really a schizophrenic syndrome in an alcoholic is not yet known.

The central nervous system of the alcoholic is subjected to various insults: the toxic effects of alcohol itself; repeated head trauma; the secondary effects from liver disease; and, in many alcoholics, severe nutritional deficiency. In those individuals with inadequate nutrition, the vitamin thiamine often becomes grossly deficient. Thiamine deficiency results in one of the most devastating syndromes associated with the abuse of alcohol, the Wernicke-Korsakoff syndrome.[43] The condition appears in a small percentage of the alcoholic population and recent experimental evidence strongly suggests that those affected have an inborn predisposition.[45] They have been shown to have a genetic defect in the enzyme transketolase that prevents thiamine binding. This leaves them particularly vulnerable to thiamine deficiency. This syndrome is seen in chronically malnourished alcoholics and usually develops over a period of a few days to a few weeks.

The acute phase of the condition, the Wernicke's encephalopathy or hemorrhagic polioencephalitis, is heralded in two-thirds of the cases by a state of mental confusion, often called a global confusional state.[43] Unlike the patient in active delirium tremens, the patient with a confusional state secondary to Wernicke's encephalopathy is most often quiet or lethargic. The condition has all of the features of a confusional state described at length in Chapter 4, except that the alcoholic more frequently shows the physical appearance of dereliction and is somewhat less likely to have hallucinations. In association with the mental changes, the patients demonstrate nystagmus (85%), various occular rotation abnormalities (lateral rectus palsy [54%]), conjugate gaze difficulty (44%) and complete ophthalmoplegia [rare]), ataxia (87%), and polyneuropathy (82%).[43] The diagnosis is not difficult to make clinically if suspected, and treatment of the acute episode is relatively simple.

Once diagnosed, the specific treatment is intramuscular or intravenous thiamine, 50 to 100 mg./day for several days, then oral thiamine 50 mg./day for one month or until such time as the patient resumes a normal diet. Avoid using concentrated glucose solutions *particularly before* administering thiamine because the metabolism of the glucose further depletes the patient's thiamine stores, thus causing an acute deterioration of the patient's status. Seizures are not a usual problem nor is severe agitation; accordingly sedatives and anticonvulsants should only be used when necessary.

Recovery from the neurologic deficits and the mental confusion is usually quite rapid and the mortality rate during the acute stage is less than 20 percent.[43] Lateral gaze problems may regress in a matter of hours and are almost always clear within a week's time.[43] The gaze palsy clears more slowly, with restitution of function being complete in 95 percent of the patients within four weeks. Nystagmus and ataxia may linger in 31 and 52 percent of patients respectively[43] after one month's treatment. Confusional behavior is present in 33 percent of the patients after one month, but this has usually cleared after 2 months.

As the confusional behavior and neurologic abnormalities clear, a high percentage of patients with Wernicke's encephalopathy are found to have a significant residual memory deficit—84 percent according to Victor and associates.[43] This memory defect is a typical organic amnesia with recent memory (ability to learn new material) significantly affected, while immediate recall and remote memory are unimpaired.[49] At this stage, such patients are diagnosed as having a Korsakoff's syndrome. It is often very difficult to ascertain when the patient passes from the acute Wernicke's encephalopathy into the chronic amnesic Korsakoff stage. The amnesic patient often appears confusional because of his memory trouble; similiarly, the patient in the last throes of a confusional state often has difficulty with memory whether he eventually develops a Korsakoff's syndrome or not. There is no specific laboratory test to help with the differential diagnosis; accordingly the examiner must rely on his clinical acumen to make the distinction.

The Korsakoff syndrome when fully developed is a profound amnesic state. The patients are literally suspended in time. No new experiences can be recorded for more than a few moments, and patients are hopelessly incapable of maintaining an independent existence. During the first weeks or months of his amnesia, the patient with Korsakoff's syndrome has a strong tendency to confabulate whenever specific information is asked of him. This phase passes in time and the chronic patient is generally apathetic, somewhat withdrawn, and as a salubrious side effect, no longer addicted to alcohol. This spontaneous cure of the alcoholism may be a direct effect of hypothalamic lesions or possibly a behavioral effect relating to a general lack of concern. As was pointed out in Chapter 7, the patient's general intelligence does not suffer significantly during the course of the disease with the cognitive defect being restricted to memory processes.

The prognosis for the patient with Korsakoff's syndrome is not hopeless as at least 20 percent ultimately recover completely according to Victor and associates.[43] An additional 25 percent show significant improvement in memory function. Unfortunately the remaining 55 percent demonstrate either no or only slight improvement in memory processing. Those that do recover usually do so over a period of months, though occasionally the period of recovery can be as short as a few weeks or as long as two years.

The pathology of Korsakoff's syndrome is primarily in the midline structures in the diencephalon, most frequently the mamillary bodies and the dorsomedial nucleus of the thalamus. Lesions are also found with regularity throughout the brain stem and cerebellum as well as in the cerebral cortex and a complete discussion of the neuropathology in such cases can be obtained from the work of Victor and associates.[43]

The Wernicke-Korsakoff syndrome is a dramatic acute condition that frequently leaves the patient with an equally dramatic chronic neurobehavioral change. It has been known for over 100 years that significant brain damage can occur acutely in the alcoholic, but the question of a gradual deterioration of mental and neurologic function in the alcoholic has been less adequately documented. In Chapter 6, we discussed much of the evidence to support the hypothesis that an alcoholic dementia does exist, and we will not reiterate the arguments here. As with most dementias, deterioration is slow, and in the case of alcoholism, can be arrested at any time if permanent abstinence is achieved.

A series of recent neuropsychologic studies of alcoholics has amply demonstrated that the chronic alcoholic without overt dementia does in fact demonstrate impairment on a number of psychologic tests.[5,10,14,27,30,31] With abstinence, test performance tends to show improvement over a period of a few weeks.[4,30] After this initial period of improvement, however, the alcoholic continues to show significantly lower scores than do matched controls on tests of nonverbal functioning, memory, and abstract reasoning.[4,5,30] The degree of residual permanent mental deficit seems to be directly related to the amount of alcohol consumed and the cumulative years of alcohol abuse, though all studies do not agree.[30,50,51] Most investigations were carried out on older men (midforties and older) which favored the hypothesis that many years of heavy drinking were necessary to produce mental change. Two recent reports concerning alcoholics in their midthirties gave differing results.[50,51] One study showed significant intellectual impairment in 59 percent of those studied and cerebral atrophy (maximal frontal) on CT scanning in 49 percent;[50] while the other study, equally carefully done, failed to demonstrate any significant neuropsychologic deficit in these young alcoholics.[51] Regardless of the actual number of years of alcoholism necessary to cause mental impairment, the fact remains that heavy, chronic alcohol intake is not uniformly well tolerated by the brain. Normal social drinkers seem to be immune to these effects, at least we hope so.

Drugs

The literature covering the untoward effects of prescription and illicit drugs is voluminous and virtually impossible to summarize briefly. Therefore, in this section we will review only some of the recent opinions concerning the possible long-term behavioral side effects of chronic drug abuse. Comprehensive reviews of the acute effects, pharmacology, management, and social aspects of drug abuse are available and the interested reader is referred to the work of Brecher,[6] Hofmann,[21] Inciardi and associates,[23] and Pradham and Dutta.[32] We have discussed in Chapter 4 the fact that many drugs, licit or illicit, can produce an acute confusional state as a symptom of intoxication. This intoxication syndrome varies somewhat (e.g., the strange mute state with phencyclidine [PCP][11] and the active paranoiac hallucinatory states with LSD), but it basically can be characterized by an altered sensorium, clouded consciousness, inattention, and a fluctuating course.

Chronic misuse or overuse of any psychoactive substance can produce a state that looks very much like dementia because of its chronicity but actually is more akin to a chronic confusional state. This condition usually reverses quite promptly with cessation of use of the drug. The contention that chronic misuse of either prescribed psychotropics or illicit street drugs results in permanent brain damage has not yet been firmly substantiated. Death and permanent brain damage are common with use of many street drugs. However, the cause of this serious central nervous system morbidity and mortality is, in the vast majority of cases, inadvertent massive overdose, contaminants that are used to dilute the drug (particularly strychnine), or sepsis from contaminated syringes and needles. Another major problem in validly assessing the chronic effects of drug misuse concerns the population involved and the nature of drug abuse itself. Drug addicts tend to come from lower socioeconomic classes, have less education than the general population, frequently have character disorders or other personality and emotional problems, and have a high incidence of major head trauma. Most heavy drug users use a variety of drugs and the toxic effects of a single drug are impossible to define accurately. Accordingly, many studies group patients and discuss the resultant findings as the effect of polydrug abuse. The last, and one of the most difficult problems, is that of obtaining research subjects who have chronically used drugs but have subsequently stopped. Many studies have been carried out in which subjects have been studied after all signs of intoxication or withdrawal have subsided. However, the subjects have been totally free from drug use for no more than several days or, at the most, one or two weeks. Since some of the studies do show areas of impaired cognitive performance, it is important to determine if those performance deficits are temporary and would clear with an extended period of abstinence. The final answer to the question of permanent brain damage from drug abuse will have to wait until more individuals are studied carefully over a longer period of time.

A review of the recent literature reveals that, in general, chronic marijuana use does not result in any significant change in intellectual or emotional behavior.[9,18,37,38,44] The most impressive and well controlled study was performed in Costa Rica, a country that does not have the strong legal and social sanctions against marijuana present in the United States. This study evaluated a group of males who had smoked a mean of 9 marijuana cigarettes daily for an average of 17 years. No significant impairment was demonstrated on an extensive neuropsychologic battery.[37] The use of other drugs by the population was not extensive, thus the results seem to give a reasonable estimate of the long-term effects of heavy cannabis use.

Polydrug users, particularly those abusing heroin, sedatives, minor tranquilizers, and hallucinogens are not as fortunate as the marijuana smoker in escaping lasting toxic effects from their drug abuse. Significant impairment on neuropsychologic testing is shown by 35 to 65 percent of chronic polydrug users.[16–18,42] The cognitive functions that are affected most noticeably are those of high level reasoning, tasks involving conceptual shifting (e.g., Halstead category test), and overall intellectual functioning. These findings are not supported by all investigators, however. One group of 87 prisoners, who had been heavy multiple drug users, had no significant deficits when tested on a comprehensive psychologic test battery.[7] One of the reasons for the disparate results may have been that the prisoners had been drug-free for a much longer time than the typical subjects, and some of the effects seen in the nonincarcerated drug users may have been only temporary. Some support for this latter hypothesis is provided by a study of 66 heavy drug users who initially had a 46 percent incidence of cognitive impairment but on retest 5 months later had only a 27 percent[16] incidence. These results suggest an intermediate stage of encephalopathy much like that seen in the alcoholic. Whether improvement continues over a longer period of time is not yet known.

The problems involved in the study of the chronic use of hallucinogens are also complex. Seldom used in isolation, their specific long-term effects cannot be accurately judged. Some high level cognitive loss seems to be associated with heavy use,[17] but these data have not been satisfactorily corroborated.[18] The psychiatric effects are also poorly documented and much of the research in the field has not been scientifically rigorous. Some investigators hypothesize that the lasting psychiatric side effects are only seen in previously emotionally disturbed individuals who took the drugs in crisis situations or in unstable environments.[29] Others have observed serious psychiatric sequelae in perfectly normal individuals after minimal exposure to LSD or other such drugs.[1] No genetic predisposition toward schizophrenia has been reported in those who develop a psychosis secondary to hallucinogen use,[20] but some premorbid personality problems or constitutional factors such as childhood hyperactivity may be possible contributing factors.[40] The case is far from settled.

Several drugs seem to be particularly hazardous, with more consistent and objective demonstration of their deleterious side effects having been made. Drugs within the amphetamine class are one group. Both behavioral and physical effects can be catastrophic. With acute toxicity a full blown paranoid psychosis is often seen, and in some patients who consistently use high doses of these drugs, a marked disruption in the brain's normal microvasculature can occur. Venules as well as arterioles are involved and the resultant diffuse small vessel occlusions and petechial hemorrhage can lead to a profound encephalopathy.[35] Another devastating drug is phencyclidine (PCP or "angel dust"). During the acute intoxication stage, the patients are often extremely psychotic and violent. With large doses, excited or stuporous catatonia, mutism, and seizures can develop. Acute schizophrenic reactions lasting for several months have been reported.[11] Chronic abuse tends to result in organic cognitive problems, with memory and speech difficulties predominating.[11]

EVALUATION

The evaluation of the neurobehavioral side effects of toxic substances is the same as that for the evaluation of brain damage of any cause. Careful history taking, however, is extremely important in these cases. A complete occupational, environmental, and alcohol/drug history is necessary. In evaluating the drug or alcohol abuser, the accurate history often has to be obtained from a relative or friend rather than the patient. Therefore, it is prudent to interview the patient and family separately. After the history, a complete neurologic examination including mental status testing must be carried out. In any patient in whom there is any suggestion of cognitive or emotional change, a complete neuropsychologic battery should be administered. The objective data obtained from a test battery can be very valuable in documenting the patient's recovery, establishing the nature and degree of deficit for insurance and legal purposes, and planning the vocational rehabilitation program if this is necessary.

The particular laboratory studies chosen—drug screening, heavy metal analysis of urine and serum, or alcohol levels—will depend upon the suspected toxin. For purposes of assessing the degree of encephalopathy in chronic cases, the CT scan has become very useful, and the EEG is also occasionally of some help. In general, we find that the clinical data from mental status testing and neuropsychologic testing are the most helpful.

MANAGEMENT

Two basic aspects of the management of the patient with toxic exposure are important: (1) management of the toxic symptoms or residual effects in the individual and (2) identification and management of the toxic source itself. With industrial pollution or exposure, the problem is often a complex epidemiologic and environmental one. In some instances, simple safety precautions at a particular factory or shop will eliminate the problem. However, in other cases (e.g., the possible toxic effects of trace metals in drinking water in cities along the lower Mississippi), the solution is less obvious. One problem regarding toxic exposure which has not been dealt with sufficiently is the potential effect of combined exposure to toxic substances. Although the U.S. Department of Labor requires all companies producing volatile substances to file a "Material Safety Data Sheet" discussing the hazard potential and safe levels of exposure for each chemical and this information is vital to the safety officer in an individual plant where the substance is used, the effect of these substances in combination with other substances, whether industrial chemicals or environmental pollutants, is not known. Another problem that has not received adequate attention is the effect of toxic substances in the social drinker, diabetic, or hypertensive. These factors may make the hazard of exposure to a given substance greater and place certain individuals at greater risk of toxicity than is currently recognized.

The problem of medically managing the drug addict or the alcoholic is quite different. The toxin is usually known and prevention of side effects and sequelae is simple—abstinence. That is a simple solution but unfortunately very difficult to either impose or to enforce. The general emotional and social rehabilitation problems involved in alcoholism and drug addiction are great and beyond the scope of this book. They are well documented in numerous texts.

The actual medical management of the patient suffering from exposure to toxins is somewhat easier. First, the patient must be immediately removed from contact with the toxic agent and the acute symptoms treated. This acute treatment is dependent upon the specific toxin and the correct information is best obtained from standard medical and toxicology texts. After the acute effects have passed, the patient should be thoroughly examined by a physician and, if there has been any suggestion of encephalopathy, a neurologist and, in many cases, a psychologist. It is usually better to wait several weeks before undertaking extensive neuropsychologic testing because of the rather gradual recovery of full mental capacity in some of these patients. If significant cognitive impairment is present, the patient may require vocational assessment and retraining. As with patients with head injury or mild or moderate encephalopathy, family counseling and environmental manipulation may be necessary to help the patients cope with their limitations.

PATHOLOGY

Very little is known concerning the pathology of the mild encephalopathies seen with solvent exposure, alcohol, or drugs. There are reports of cortical atrophy in alcoholics, the degree of which is in direct proportion to their performance on psychologic tests. Therefore, it is fairly certain that brain damage is a gradual cytotoxic process in the alcoholic. The alcoholic dementia and Wernicke-Korsakoff syndrome have been discussed previously and the pathology of these states is well known. These syndromes are more completely discussed in Chapters 6 and 7.

In drug abuse (excluding the serious effects of anoxia from overdose and the reports of vasculitis in amphetamine abuse), there is almost no information about pathologic changes. An early report of cerebral atrophy secondary to chronic cannabis use has been much criticized in the literature and probably suffered from a sampling error.[8]

In general, toxic substances attack the metabolic processes of the neurons. With low levels of exposure, the neuron can withstand this challenge, whereas high doses or chronic medium-sized doses cause the cells to shrink and eventually to die. With sufficiently extensive cell death, irreversible mental changes and atrophy occur.

REFERENCES

1. Abruzzi, W.: Drug-induced psychoses. . . . or schizophrenia? Am. J. Psychoanal. 35:329, 1975.
2. American Psychiatric Association: Diagnostic and Statistic Manual III of Mental Disorders. Washington, 1980.
3. Banay, R.S.: Pathologic reaction to alcohol. Q. J. Stud. Alcohol 4:580, 1944.
4. Bennett, A.E.: Diagnosis of intermediate state of alcoholic brain disease. JAMA 172:1143, 1960.
5. Blusewicz, M.J., Dustman, R.E., Schenkenberg, T., and Beck, E.C.: Neuropsychological correlates of chronic alcoholism and aging. J. Nerv. Ment. Dis. 165:348, 1977.
6. Brecher, E.M.: Licit and Illicit Drugs. Little, Brown and Co. Boston, 1972.
7. Bruhn, P., and Maage, N.: Intellectual and neuropsychological functions in young men with heavy and long-term pattern of drug abuse. Am. J. Psychiatry 132:397, 1975.
8. Campbell, A., Evans, M., and Thompson, J.: Cerebral atrophy in young cannabis smokers. Lancet 1:1219, 1971.
9. Carlin, A.S., and Trupin, E.W.: The effect of long-term chronic marijuana use on neuropsychological functioning. Int. J. Addict. 12:617, 1977.
10. Clarke, J., and Haughton, H.: A study of intellectual impairment and recovery rates in heavy drinkers in Ireland. Br. J. Psychiatry 126:178, 1975.
11. Cohen, S.: Angel dust. JAMA 238:515, 1977.
12. Comstock, B.S.: A review of psychological measures relevant to central nervous system toxicity, with specific reference to solvent inhalation. Clin. Toxicol. 11:317, 1977.
13. Gerstenbrand, F., Hamdi, T., Kothbauer, P., Rustam, H., and AlBadri, M.: Apallic syndrome in chronic mercury poisoning. Eur. Neurol. 15:249, 1977.
14. Goodwin, D.W., and Hill, S.Y.: Chronic effects of alcohol and other psychoactive drugs on intellect, learning and memory, in Rankin, J.A.(ed.): Alcohol, Drugs and Brain Damage. Alcoholism and Drug Addiction Research Foundation of Ontario, Toronto, 1975, pp. 55–69.
15. Grandjean, E., Munchinger, R., Turrian, V., Haas, P.A., Knoepfel, H.K., and Rosenmund, H.: Investigations into the effects of exposure to trichlorethylene in mechanical engineering. Br. J. Ind. Med. 12:131, 1955.

16. Grant, I., and Judd, L.L.: Neuropsychological and EEG disturbances in polydrug users. Am. J. Psychiatry 133:1039, 1976.
17. Grant, I., Mohns, L., Miller, M., and Reitan, R.M.: A neuropsychological study of polydrug users. Arch. Gen. Psychiatry 33:973, 1976.
18. Grant, I., Adams, K.M., Carlin, A.S., and Rennick, P.M.: Neuropsychological deficit in polydrug users. Drug Alcohol Depend. 2:91, 1977.
19. Hanniner, H., Eskelinen, L., Husman, K., and Nurminen, M.: Behavioral effects of long-term exposure to a mixture of organic solvents. Scand. J. Work Environ. Health 4:240, 1976.
20. Hays, P., and Tilley, J.R.: The difference between LSD psychosis and schizophrenia. Can. Psychiatr. Assoc. J. 8:331, 1973.
21. Hofmann, F.G.: A Handbook on Drug and Alcohol Abuse. Oxford, New York, 1975.
22. Hollender, M.: Pathological intoxication—Is there such an entity? J. Clin. Psychiatry 40:424, 1979.
23. Inciardi, J.A., McBride, D.C., Pattieger, A.E., Russe, B.R., and Siegal, H.A.: Legal and Illicit Drug Use: Acute Reactions of Emergency Room Populations. Praeger, New York, 1978.
24. Knox, J.W., and Nelson, J.R.: Permanent encephalopathy from toluene inhalation. N. Engl. J. Med. 275:1494, 1966.
25. Kurland, L.T., Faro, S.N., and Siedler, H.: Minamata disease. The outbreak of a neurologic disorder in Minamata, Japan, and its relationship to the ingestion of seafood contaminated by mercuric compounds. World Neurology 1:370, 1960.
26. Lindström, K.: Psychological performances of workers exposed to various solvents. Scand. J. Work Environ. Health 10:151, 1973.
27. Long, A.J., and McLachlan, J.F.C.: Abstract reasoning and perceptual-motor efficiency in alcoholics. Q. J. Stud. Alcohol 35:1220, 1974.
28. Maghazaji, H.I.: Psychiatric aspects of methylmercury poisoning. J. Neurol. Neurosurg. Psychiatry 37:954, 1974.
29. McWilliams, S.A., and Tuttle, R.J.: Long-term psychological effects of LSD. Psychol. Bull. 79:341, 1973.
30. Page, R.D., and Linden, J.D.: "Reversible" organic brain syndrome in alcoholics. Quart. J. Stud. Alcohol 35:98, 1974.
31. Page, R.D., and Schaub, L.H.: Intellectual functioning in alcoholics during six months abstinence. J. Stud. Alcohol 38:1240, 1977.
32. Pradham, S.N. and Dutta, S.N. (eds): Drug Abuse: Clinical and Basic Aspects. Mosby, St. Louis, 1977.
33. Riding, A.: Derelict mexican boys sniff toxic chemicals. The New York Times, April 9, 1978, p. 21.
34. Ross, W.D., Gechman, A.S., Sholiton, M.C., and Paul, H.S.: Need for alertness to neuropsychiatric manifestations of inorganic mercury poisoning. Comp. Psychiat. 18:595, 1977.
35. Rumbaugh, C.L.: Small vessel cerebral vascular changes following chronic amphetamine intoxication, in Ellinwood, E.H., Jr., and Kilbey, M.M. (eds.): Cocaine and Other Stimulants, Plenum Press, New York, 1977, pp. 241–251.
36. Rustam, H., and Hamdi, T.: Methyl mercury poisoning in Iraq. Brain 97: 499, 1974.
37. Satz, P., Fletcher, J.M., and Sutker, L.S.: Neuropsychologic, intellectual and personality correlates of chronic marijuana use in native Costa Ricans. Ann. N. Y. Acad. Sci. 282:266, 1976.

38. Stefanis, C., Liakos, A., Boulougouris, J., Fink, M., and Freedman, A.M.: Chronic hashish use and mental disorder. Am. J. Psychiatry 133:225, 1976.
39. Sterner, J.H.: Study of hazards in spray painting with gasoline as a diluent. J. Indust. Hyg. Toxic. 23:437, 1941.
40. Stone, M.H.: Drug-related schizophrenic syndrome. Int. J. Psychiatry 11: 391, 1973.
41. Stopps, G.J., and McLaughlin, M.: Psychophysiological testing of human subjects exposed to solvent vapors. Am. Ind. Hyg. Assoc. J. 28:43, 1967.
42. Trites, R.: Neuropsychological deficits in 'primary' and 'secondary' non-medical drug users. Can. Psychiatr. Assoc. J. 20:351, 1975.
43. Victor, M., Adams, R.D., and Collins, G.H.: The Wernicke-Korsakoff Syndrome. F.A. Davis Co., Philadelphia, 1971.
44. Weckowicz, T.E., Collier, G., and Spreng, L.: Field dependence, cognitive functions, personality traits, and social values in heavy cannabis users and non-user controls. Psychol. Rep. 41:291, 1977.
45. Arlien-Søborg, P., Bruhn, P., Gyldensted, C., and Melgaard, B.: Chronic painters' syndrome. Acta Neurol. Scandinav. 60:149, 1979.
46. Prockop, L.: Neurotoxic volatile substances. Neurology 29:862, 1979.
47. Surawicz, F.G.: Alcoholic hallucinosis: a missed diagnosis. Can. J. Psychiatry, 25:57, 1980.
48. Blass, J.P., and Gibson, G.E.: Abnormality of a thiamine-requiring enzyme in patients with Wernicke-Korsakoff syndrome. N. Engl. J. Med. 297: 1367, 1977.
49. Butters, N. and Cermak, L.S.: Alcoholic Korsakoff's Syndrome: An information-processing Approach to Amnesia. Academic Press, Inc., New York, 1980.
50. Lee, K., Møller, L., Hardt, F., Haubek, A., and Jensen, F.: Alcohol-induced brain damage and liver damage in young males. Lancet 2:759, 1979.
51. Grant, I., Adams, K., and Reed, R.: Normal neuropsychological abilities of alcoholic men in their late thirties. Am. J. Psychiatry 136:1263, 1979.

314

10

INFECTIONS OF THE CENTRAL NERVOUS SYSTEM

J.R., a 52-year-old accountant, began to experience generalized headaches while at work on November 3, 1977. The patient lived alone and called a relative to tell her that he was not feeling well, was febrile, and stated that he would remain home from work the following day. On the next day, the relative telephoned the patient but received no answer. On the third day, she again tried to reach him by phone but he did not answer. Concerned, she went to his house, broke in, and found him in bed, virtually moribund. He was unresponsive, rigid, and covered with a petechial rash. He was immediately taken to a nearby hospital.

Initial examination in the emergency room revealed him to be stuporous, with grimacing and decorticate posturing in response to painful stimulation. His neck was extremely rigid, he was febrile (39.2°C.), had an extensive petechial and purpuric rash, and appeared to have a left hemiparesis. A spinal puncture was performed; the fluid was grossly purulent with an opening pressure of 300 mm. H_2O. It contained 27,200 leukocytes (all polymorphonuclear cells). The protein was 185 mg./100 ml. A gram stain of the spinal fluid and peripheral blood demonstrated intracellular gram negative diplococci and the diagnosis of meningococcal meningitis with meningococcemia was confirmed. He was immediately placed on high doses of intravenous penicillin (20 million units daily).

Within 48 hours, he began to show distinct improvement and by the third hospital day was awake and alert, yet mental status examination showed general confusional behavior. The left hemiparesis was still present and of a moderate degree. At this time, we first appreciated his neglect of his left side. He would never turn to his left when spoken to from that side and any examiner who approached him from the left was totally ignored. As his general medical condition improved, the neglect persisted, and he developed evidence of implicit denial. From his conversation, it was apparent that he thought he was in another hospital which was next door to his house and reported that he was only in the hospital "to see about a painful left knee" (he had developed joint pain during the acute stage of his illness and had an effusion of the left knee). This denial persisted for only several days and disappeared as his general orientation improved and his mental state cleared.

On November 30, 1977, 25 days after admission, the patient was ambulating well and was conversing normally, although there was a continued weakness of the left side. He was discharged from the hospital and went to stay with a relative. A CT scan done on the day of discharge was normal.

Re-evaluation on December 28, 1977, showed no motor deficit. The patient reported that he was again playing the piano and typing as proficiently as before his illness. It was his opinion that he was ready to return to work on a part-time basis. To enable us to advise him concerning any possible organic mental deficits secondary to the meningitis, we administered a full neuropsychologic battery. The evaluation demonstrated several clinically interesting problems. Throughout the testing, he was moderately anxious. He also had a substantial degree of denial which was judged to be of combined neurologic and psychologic origin.

On specific cognitive testing, there was considerable variability in performance. On the Wechsler Adult Intelligence Scale, he performed well on the information and comprehension subtests but significantly less adequately on verbal abstract reasoning as tested by the similarities subtest. He had great difficulty with all performance subtests, in particular the Digit Symbol Test and Block Designs. His Bender Gestalt protocol showed mild constructional difficulties and the Raven's Standard Progressive Matrices (a test of spatial analysis and nonverbal reasoning) was very severely impaired (less than the 5th percentile). The Trail-Making Test showed impairment on form B (less than the 15th percentile with two errors) in which conceptual-shifting is required. His Wechsler Memory quotient was significantly depressed, (MQ = 83) when compared with his Full Scale IQ (105). Memory for paragraphs showed the worst performance but visual memory was also significantly impaired.

In general, the testing showed well-retained verbal skills, with relative impairment of verbal and nonverbal memory, abstract reasoning, constructional ability, and the ability to make conceptual shifts. We were quite unsure about his ability to return to his demanding accounting job, but he, reinforced by a healthy amount of denial, stated that he "could do the job half asleep." Subsequent reports indicate that he was right; because 3 months after discharge he was back to work full time and living alone in his own house. A discussion with his employer raised no reservations concerning his performance. Accordingly, despite

316

his cognitive deficits, this patient has either been able to make the necessary adjustments to his disabilities or, more likely, he was fortunate in that his illness did not effect those cognitive skills necessary for his particular job.

The above case demonstrates one of the ways in which infections of the brain can produce behavioral sequelae in patients with no or only minor residual motor or sensory deficits. In this patient, the deficits fortunately did not interfere with his social and vocational reintegration. But, had he been an architect, engineer, or surgeon, his impaired perceptual motor skills could have significantly affected his work, or if he had been an independent business executive or lawyer, his memory, verbal reasoning, and conceptual deficits could have produced a substantial vocational disability.

In this chapter, we do not intend to make an extensive review of all infectious disease but rather will discuss in general those infectious entities that either present primarily with behavioral symptoms or, as in the case above, have behavioral sequelae which can be a significant factor in the patient's readjustment following illness.

There are various modes of presentation of infectious disease in the brain. Abscess, for instance, produces the picture of a focal lesion, whereas encephalitis frequently is manifested as a more generalized behavioral disturbance. Meningitis, conversely, may start with very innocuous generalized symptoms and subsequently develop into a severe encephalopathy with focal vascular lesions or hydrocephalus. In general, the behavioral abnormalities are determined more by the mode of presentation than by the specific agent responsible for the infection. For instance, a brain abscess caused by anaerobic Streptococcus, Nocardia, or Echinococcus may all produce the same focal behavioral changes although one infectious agent was bacterial, one fungal, and one parasitic. Despite the lack of specific correlation of the clinical syndrome with an individual infectious agent, classes of agents tend to act in a somewhat similar fashion: viruses usually produce encephalitis or meningitis and not an abscess, whereas bacteria, fungi, and parasites more frequently cause meningitis or abscess and rarely a diffuse encephalitis.

There are several recently recognized mechanisms in infections of the brain that have relevance to neurobehavior. The first is the discovery, by Dr. Gajdusek and his coworkers, of unconventional viruses and their ability to produce a transmissible dementia (e.g., kuru and Creutzfeldt-Jakob disease). The second is a special sensitivity to generally nonpathogenic agents in patients who have suppression of their normal immune mechanisms. In these patients (e.g., those with myeloproliferative disease, immunosuppression for transplantation, and

317

other conditions treated with high dose steroids), a variety of diseases either become reactivated, such as toxoplasmosis, or allow normally nonpathogenic agents, such as Cryptococcus, to become opportunistic. These infections frequently present with new behavioral abnormalities in an already ill patient. Unfortunately, these new behavioral abnormalities are all too frequently ascribed to the primary disease and are not recognized as being a suprainfection by one of the uncommon agents. A third interesting type of condition is that in which a dormant infection becomes virulently reactivated for no apparent reason. This is the case with measles virus in subacute sclerosing panencephalitis, a tragic disease of childhood that is classically heralded by a gradual change in the child's behavior.

In any field of medicine, an early diagnosis with early treatment affords the patient the most favorable prognosis. This is particularly true for infectious disease. Bacterial and fungal diseases respond well to medication, and we are now seeing encouraging responses to medication with some viral illnesses (e.g., papovavirus in progressive multifocal leukoencephalopathy). Accordingly, early clinical recognition of these conditions is becoming of increasing importance.

BRAIN ABSCESS

By its nature, the brain abscess presents as a focal mass lesion and produces symptoms relative both to its location and to the general effects of increased intracranial pressure. Confusional behavior, headache, papilledema, and seizures are the most prominent features, with focal neurologic and behavioral signs being less common. The source of the infection in brain abscess is usually the middle ear or paranasal sinuses (predominately the frontal sinuses[29]) but in some reported series metastatic abscesses from congenital heart disease and pulmonary infection form the majority of cases.[47] Dental abscess is an uncommon yet important source to consider, particularly with frontal abscess.[26]

Since the infection often enters the brain by direct extension from a purulent infection in the frontal sinuses or the middle ear and the mastoid processes, there is a much higher than expected incidence of both frontal lobe and inferior temporal lobe abscesses. Patients with frontal abscesses have an increased tendency to present with confusional behavior, while a frontal lobe syndrome is not common unless both frontal lobes are involved. With an inferior temporal lobe abscess in the language dominant hemisphere, a remarkable anomic aphasia or a fluent aphasia with poor comprehension are frequently the presenting signs. In patients with systemic infection, most commonly originating in the lung, there is a random distribution of the abscesses with approximately half of such cases having multiple lesions.

318

The evaluation and treatment of brain abscess has improved dramatically since the introduction of the CT scan.[47] With this procedure, it is now much easier to diagnose, localize, and follow the course of an abscess, this is particularly true when multiple or loculated abscesses are present.

Treatment usually involves a combined approach of aggressive antibiotic treatment and surgical extirpation or aspiration.[9] Antibiotic treatment should be tailored to the specific organism grown on culture. Although culture of peripheral tissues is often negative, cultures of material aspirated from the abscess itself and immediately placed on culture media are almost always positive.[14] A high percentage of the cases are caused by Streptococcus so penicillin is still the mainstay of treatment,[13] this is particularly true of lesions resulting from sinus infection. With otic or metastatic infection a mixture of gram positive and gram negative organisms is found and a broad spectrum antibiotic such as chloramphenicol should also be used.[13] In traumatic cases, staph infection is more probable and fusidic acid or other such agent must be used.[13]

Prompt and aggressive medical plus surgical treatment has helped to greatly reduce the mortality from brain abscess to about 20 percent,[14,50] a vast improvement from the untreated mortality figure of 60 percent reported in 1950.[57] Use of the CT scan has resulted in even more favorable statistics, with a recent report of 0 percent mortality in 20 consecutive cases diagnosed with the aid of CT scanning.[47]

MENINGITIS

Virus, bacteria, mycobacteria, fungus, and some parasites can all produce an inflammatory disease of the meninges and, except for the more insidious onset of the fungal diseases, the behavioral symptoms are remarkably similar. An alteration in level of consciousness with or without confusion is the primary behavioral symptom and when present with fever and headache should always alert the physician to the possibility of meningitis. As discussed in Chapter 6, the chronic meningitides due to fungus, tuberculosis, or Cryptococcus can sometimes manifest as a rather rapid (several weeks) dementing illness but rarely, if ever, without the associated signs of fever, headache, and stiff neck.

Early diagnosis is very important since many of the diseases can be very destructive if not rapidly arrested. Some agents are more pathogenic than others, but all nonviral meningitis results in very high mortality and morbidity if not treated. Probably the agent most infamous for producing extensive brain damage, seizures, and cranial nerve (especially the auditory nerve) damage is Hemophilus influenza. Seen primarily in children, this infection can leave its host with mental retardation, seizures, deafness, hemiplegia, blindness, or a variety of lesser physical and mental symptoms. In the adult, of the purulent meningitides, pneumococcus is most likely to leave the patient with significant mental sequelae. Meningococcus, by contrast, is relatively benign once the initial infection is controlled. Tuberculosis and fungal meningitis often give focal brain and cranial nerve damage but in general are less devastating than the Hemophilus bacteria.

There are two main types of sequelae in nonviral meningitis: (1) communicating hydrocephalus from scar tissue formation around the base of the brain and over the convexities and (2) focal lesions of the cortex. Hydrocephalus must always be considered when a patient's infection is apparently responding to medication yet his mental status and neurologic examination either fails to improve or worsens. The clinical features of the hydrocephalus are similar to those discussed in Chapter 6: gait disturbance, urinary incontinence, and signs of mental change.

There are many mechanisms by which meningitis can cause focal lesions and often more than one mechanism may be operating in any individual case. Local invasion of brain parenchyma by toxic products or the agents themselves will cause an area of cerebritis (cortical infection). These areas are often unstable electrically and serve as a nidus for seizures. Eventually these areas will show actual cell loss and focal damage. The other principal problem in meningitis is invasion of the walls of both veins and arteries by the infection with subsequent venous and arterial occlusion. When major arteries or the venous sinuses are occluded in this way, a stroke-like picture evolves and the patient suffers a substantial brain infarction. Unfortunately, in many patients, particularly those infected with Hemophilus, pneumococcus, or tuberculosis, multiple infarction frequently occurs. In these cases, a severe encephalopathy and attendant dementia results. Meningitis is further complicated by the effects of massive cerebral edema and congestion. This then compromises the cerebral circulation and metabolism and produces brain herniation in many cases.

SYPHILIS

Syphilis is discussed separately, as it has various manifestations at different stages of the illness. In the earlier stages, the neurologic symptoms result from meningeal and vascular inflammation, whereas in the later stages, parenchymatous involvment is the most prevalent. It is impossible to classify all cases, since features of meningeal, vascular, and parenchymatous disease can all exist in a single patient.[40] The meningitis seen with syphilis is similar to any subacute meningitis. We saw one man in his 50s who came to the emergency room with a history of having suffered a seizure while at work. On examination, he was quite confusional, febrile, and had early papilledema. A spinal fluid examination demonstrated 250 cells (50 percent polymorphonuclear, 50 percent lymphocytes) and a strongly positive Kolmer reaction. With prompt treatment, his meningitis cleared and he escaped without any vascular or cranial nerve lesions.

On occasion, a focal meningeal granulomatous lesion will occur (gumma) and produce a picture of a slowly progressive mass lesion. The more common focal lesion is of vascular origin and is due to a specific endarteritis. These lesions have an acute onset and resemble a typical stroke.

In the chronic stage of syphilis, parenchymatous degeneration occurs, with the classic behavioral syndrome being that of general paresis. This condition has been more fully discussed in Chapter 6 as one of the progressive dementias.

ENCEPHALITIS

Encephalitis is a generalized infection of the brain which is usually caused by the viral invasion of neuronal or glial cell bodies. In some instances, other infectious agents can present as encephalitis because of their widespread involvement of brain tissue; Toxoplasma gondii is one such agent. Although often producing a generalized infection with diffuse mental symptoms, some forms of encephalitis manifest as focal or multifocal disease; herpes simplex encephalitis, progressive multifocal leukoencephalopathy, and toxoplasmosis are three such conditions. Many of the clinical and behavioral characteristics of these diseases allow early diagnosis.

Toxoplasmosis

The protozoa Toxoplasma gondii produces several different clinical syndromes of the central nervous system: (1) a focal or multifocal infection, (2) a widespread inflammatory disease which can be rightfully called an encephalitis, and (3) a meningoencephalitis.[55] Seventy percent of the cases present with a picture of focal or multifocal lesions, but in 20 percent, the general signs of confusion and lethargy usually associated with encephalitis are all that are evident on examination.[55] The disease is progressive and, depending upon its mode of presentation, will be indistinguishable clinically from expanding mass lesions, progressive multifocal leukoencephalopathy, cryptococcal or other chronic meningitis, or viral encephalitis. As with many of the conditions mentioned above, toxoplasmosis of the central nervous system in adults is seen much more frequently in patients who have been treated by immunosuppressive drugs. The largest single group of patients acquiring toxoplasmosis is that of patients treated for myeloproliferative illness. Given this fact, when treating the immunosupressed patient who developes focal or general cerebral symptoms, it is critical to consider the possibility of a treatable infectious agent rather than to assume that the CNS symptoms are secondary to the spread of the primary disease.

The diagnosis is fairly easily made using modern immunologic techniques. The Sabin-Feldman fluorescent antibody dye test, though difficult to perform, is diagnostic if either a rising titer is demonstrated or if a very high titer (1:32,000) is found on the initial reading. Although 30 percent of the normal population has a positive test, in such cases it is usually of low order and stable.[17] Immunodiffusion tests on serum are also important, as the patient with active toxoplasmosis will have a greatly reduced IgM and an elevated IgA and IgG.[49] The combination of a markedly positive dye test and an equally markedly reduced IgM is virtually diagnostic. The decreased IgM is more specific for acute infection than the IgG, because the latter can stay elevated for years, whereas the IgM is only depressed during active infection.

Treatment is usually very successful. A combination of sulfadiazine and pyrimethamine (Daraprim) are administered for a period of at least one month. This treatment is efficacious even in the face of immunosuppression and should be intiated as soon as the diagnosis is made. These drugs eradicate only the tachyzoite form of the protozoa and will not eliminate the encysted forms. Therefore, the patient should be treated until an adequate degree of immunocompetence is restored, which allows the patient to combat any tachyzoite forms that spill from lysed cysts.[19]

The pathophysiology of adult toxoplasmosis is far from determined. Feldman's data show clearly that the percentage of individuals in the society with positive fluorscent antibodies to toxoplasma rises steadily with age.[17] This suggests that individuals are continually exposed to the agent throughout their lives and raises the possibility that the full-blown infection in the compromised patient represents an unfortunate recent infection by the opportunistic agent. Equally persuasive, however, is the argument that the acute infection is the recrudescence of a previously asymptomatic infection in which the host's defenses did not allow the agent full expression but forced it into a dormant cystic stage.[19] The mechanism leading to activation of the dormant infection is not yet known, but a compromise of the host's defenses is certainly one important factor.

322

Viral Encephalitis

GENERAL COMMENTS

Many conventional viruses can produce a clinical picture of encephalitis with a wide range of manifestations. Certain viruses, such as mumps virus, often produce a mild encephalitis with lethargy, headache, and irritability as the principal features. In these cases, behavioral and neurologic sequelae are rare and the entire disease is usually quite benign and can go unrecognized. Other agents, cat-scratch virus for instance, may produce a rapidly evolving devastating, yet completely reversible encephalopathy as the following case reveals:[54]

A young psychiatric house officer was neurologically intact on morning rounds but by afternoon was grossly confusional and paranoid. By early evening he was mute, suspicious, combative, and increasingly difficult to arouse. Within hours he became comatose and decerebrate. He was sustained on a respirator for two days and thereafter recovered rapidly. A diagnosis of cat-scratch encephalitis was made immunologically and two months after onset, he had returned to work with no residual problems noted on an extensive neuropsychologic battery.

However, other viral agents result not only in severe behavioral and neurologic symptoms during the acute phase but are also known to produce very serious residual behavioral deficits. Among the most frequent are the arbor viruses and the herpes simplex virus. Since herpes simplex encephalitis is such an interesting condition from a behavioral standpoint and also because early diagnosis holds some promise for treatment and prevention of sequelae, we will discuss its clinical picture more fully.

HERPES SIMPLEX ENCEPHALITIS

The most common of the serious viral encephalitides, herpes simplex presents with a rather short prodromal phase (3 to 5 days) of fever and headache.[5] Rapidly thereafter, a fulminant encephalitis develops with either acute delirium or focal, usually temporal lobe, signs[60] (i.e., aphasia, apraxia, agnosia, memory disturbance, and emotional change). A decreased level of consciousness, seizures, memory problems, and focal neurologic and behavioral signs are very common.[42] The signs are often asymmetric and can quite easily be mistaken for a mass lesion rather than encephalitis.

The diagnosis can certainly be suspected clinically, but it is important to establish the etiologic diagnosis before beginning treatment. A spinal fluid examination, though frequently the first study obtained in a febrile illness involving the central nervous system, is sometimes unrewarding unless special antibody studies are available. Twenty-five percent of cases of herpes simplex encephalitis have normal spinal fluid,[42] while the remaining 75 percent will usually have some evidence of blood from the hemorrhagic destruction of brain tissue and a few lymptocytes (< 500). It is almost impossible to retrieve the virus from the spinal fluid, but specific immunofluorescent antibody studies on the cerebrospinal fluid leukocytes are positive, even when cultures are negative.[51] These studies are currently the best test, if available, because accurate determination can be made in 3 to 4 hours without a brain biopsy.

Ancillary neurodiagnostic tests can be used. These are not specific for herpes infection but can be suggestive. The EEG will show slowing that is typically focal. Temporal spikes and sharp waves are also seen, a feature not common with other encephalitides.[8,16] Nucleotide brain scan usually demonstrates a temporal mass[31,44] and CT scan characteristically shows a wedge-shaped area of edema in the temporal lobe.[32,53]

In most clinical settings, the most satisfactory available method of establishing the diagnosis is a brain biopsy. The needle biopsy has been shown to be effective and is certainly much less traumatic than an open biopsy.[2] The biopsy material should be handled as follows: One piece should be smeared for microscopic analysis, this can be done in a few minutes and will verify the diagnosis of an infectious process in almost 80 percent of the cases. The second piece should be examined for immunofluorescent antibodies, a process which takes several hours and will establish a correct diagnosis in 75 to 80 percent of cases. The final piece must be cultured for virus, this requires approximately 3 days but is the most accurate method of diagnosis.[2]

Treatment has thus far been discouraging yet not hopeless.[61] Three factors are critical: (1) treatment must be initiated before the patient becomes comatose if there is to be any chance for a decent quality of survival,[59] (2) cerebral edema must be controlled by high doses of steroids, mannitol, or decompression, as brain swelling and herniation is the primary cause of death,[36] and (3) anti-DNA drugs should be used; adenine arabinoside has proved to be the most efficacious and is remarkably free of toxic side effects.[35,52,59] With the above aggressive diagnostic and treatment plan, the mortality from herpes simplex encephalitis can be reduced from 75 to 30 percent.[36,52,59] Unfortunately, at least half of the survivors will have some sequelae, severe in 30 percent and moderate in 20 percent.[59]

Pathologically, herpes simplex infection has a predilection for the medial temporal lobes and the orbital surface of the frontal lobes. This unusual distribution suggests that the infection spreads to the brain from structures in or around the base of the brain rather than via the

324

blood stream, unless there is a specific selective cell vulnerability in these regions. Microscopic examination shows that all cell types (neurons and glia) are involved in the inflammatory process. This observation adds support to the theory that the infection spreads from and through contiguous tissues rather than in specific vulnerable cell populations. For some time it was felt that the infection reached the brain through the nose and olfactory system, but recent evidence strongly suggests that the virus either spreads from the trigeminal ganglion or is activated from latency in the brain itself.[12] Since many individuals harbor herpes virus in a latent state in their trigeminal ganglion, this is an appealing hypothesis. This theory leaves only the question as to why some individuals develop encephalitis yet most do not.

SUBACUTE SCLEROSING PANENCEPHALITIS (SSPE)

Of the various encephalitides that are caused by the recrudescence of a latent central nervous system virus, subacute sclerosing panencephalitis is a very important one. The condition, caused by the reactivation of latent measles virus, is seen primarily in older children (ages 4 to 10) or in young adolescents (90% of cases occurs between age 4 and 16).[24] In the first stage of the illness, almost all of the symptoms are those of behavioral change. The following case is a typical example:

The patient was a 16-year-old boy who had been a well liked, social young man who was not a superior student but was a good musician and had his own rock band. Approximately a year before we saw him, his family began to notice that he would occasionally have difficulty expressing himself and tended to use words out of context. Concurrently, he became withdrawn, depressed, and lost both skill and interest in his guitar playing. He did not display any inappropriate social behavior but often became lost in the school halls and could not find his room. In the three months prior to our seeing him, he developed a distinct stutter, had progressive memory loss, and began to display facial grimaces and a stumbling gait.

On initial examination, the patient was neat, well behaved, and seemed quite concerned about his problem. His speech was fluent yet slurred and contained grammatical errors and frequent word finding pauses. Comprehension, naming, reading, and writing were all impaired. There was evidence of ideomotor apraxia, dyscalculia, and constructional difficulty. The patient had occasional subtle choreiform and myoclonic movements of the face, arms, and legs and also had a mild snout reflex and prominent palmomental reflexes.

Cerebral dysfunction with behavioral abnormalities such as decreased school performance, withdrawal, aggressiveness, inappropriate nonchalance, and a variety of other intellectual and emotional changes characterize the first stage of the disease.[27,30] In this initial phase, there is little, if any, motor or sensory abnormality. In the second stage, motor findings begin to appear, including choreiform movements, myoclonus, ataxia, and various early extrapyramidal signs. The motor findings are initially subtle, as in the case above, but can progress to be disabling. We saw one 10-year-old boy who had developed significant myoclonic movements in his legs quite early in the course of his illness and was hospitalized primarily because of this. This patient had such massive lower extremity myoclonus that he would actually be thrown to the floor whenever the contractions occurred.

The third and fourth stages of SSPE involve progressive intellectual deterioration to the point of mutism. Neurologically, seizures develop as does spasticity, brainstem dysfunction, and hypothalamic dysfunction. In the fourth stage, the myoclonus decreases and the patients become comatose and often opisthotonic.

The diagnosis is usually quite easy to make clinically by the time myoclonus is present, but there are two laboratory examinations that are very useful in establishing a firm diagnosis: the EEG and the immunoglobulin levels in serum and spinal fluid. The EEG shows periodic diphasic or triphasic delta bursts that occur every 5 to 7 seconds (Fig. 10-1)[37] and frequently persist into the sleeping state.[28,58] This characteristic pattern is not always present in the first stage of the illness[48] but inevitably appears as the disease progresses.

The second, and by far the most specific, test is the IgG level in cerebrospinal fluid. In SSPE, the level of spinal fluid IgG is very high, and 25 to 75 percent of that IgG is measles specific antibody.[39] A comparison of IgG in serum to IgG in cerebrospinal fluid shows that the cerebrospinal fluid level is considerably elevated, giving strong evi-

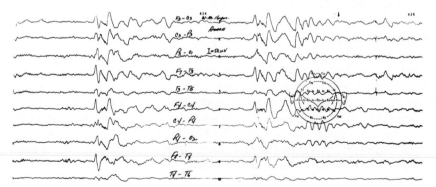

FIGURE 10–1. Electrocardiogram of patient with subacute sclerosing panencephalitis.

dence that the antibodies are being produced in the central nervous system and are not transferred from serum.[33,45]

Once the diagnosis has been made, the treatment of choice is adenine arabinoside, an anti-DNA substance that has been shown to arrest the condition and improve survival rate but tends to stabilize rather than reverse the condition.[56] The prognosis in untreated SSPE is grim: 50 percent die in the first year; the range of survival is from 6 weeks to 8 years.[24] Many of the survivors have severe encephalopathies and only 1 in 100 is normal mentally. Hopefully, early detection and early treatment will alter these statistics.

The pathogenesis of these so-called slow or latent viruses is not yet known. In SSPE, the dormant virus has virtually been proved to be measles virus. Children who develop SSPE usually have had a rather severe primary measles infection early in life (less than 2 years of age).[30] In some fashion, the measles virus remains dormant until years later. It has been hypothesized that the later panencephalitis is caused by a transformation of the RNA measles virus to a DNA form by a concommitant second viral infection. This new DNA virus is believed to become the pathogenic agent in SSPE.[1]

The virus attacks the deep layers of cortex and adjacent white matter causing a subacute inflammatory reaction. All brain areas except the cerebellum are affected. Demyelination, necrosis, and gliosis occur with the eventual pathologic picture being one of diffuse severe destruction.

PROGRESSIVE MULTIFOCAL LEUKOENCEPHALOPATHY (PML)

Progressive multifocal leukoencephalopathy is another central nervous system inflammatory disease caused by the activation or reactivation of a latent virus. Like toxoplasmosis, PML most commonly afflicts those individuals with compromised cellular immunity. Patients with myeloproliferative and lymphoproliferative diseases, sarcoid, tuberculosis, polycythemia, cancer, and artificially induced immunosuppression from cytotoxic drugs and steroids are all at risk for the development of this type of leukoencephalopathy. Because of the availability of new drugs to treat this condition, it is important that all physicians become acquainted with PML and consider it in their differential diagnosis in immunosuppressed patients who develop central nervous system symptoms.

The clinical picture is one of a rather rapidly progressive encephalopathy (2 to 4 months from first symptoms to death) that frequently begins with confusional behavior, alterations in language function, and other neurologic signs and symptoms, particularly visual field defects, seizures, and pyramidal findings.[18,46] On many occasions, the initial signs are focal and, in the case of the cancer patient, simulate those of a metastasis. Most lesions occur in the cerebral hemispheres and have a distinct predilection for the posterior quadrants. Brainstem and cerebellum are sometimes involved but less frequently.

The diagnosis can certainly be suspected clinically from history and examination, but the CT scan can be very helpful in differentiating PML from a variety of other lesions, especially metastatic tumor. The lesions in PML as visualized on the CT scan are low density, found in the central and convolutional white matter, and have scalloped lateral borders. They produce no mass effect, do not enhance with the infusion of contrast, and are more commonly seen posteriorly.[7,11] Most routine laboratory studies are much less diagnostic: the EEG may be slow and the arteriogram and brain scan abnormal, but none of these is as specific as the CT scan.[34,46]

Treatment with cytosine arabinoside has been encouraging in some individual cases, but a substantial treatment experience has not yet been obtained.[3,6,10,38]

The etiology and pathology of this condition are very interesting. The basic pathogens causing this syndrome of progressive multifocal white matter degeneration are a small group of viruses, mostly papovaviruses.[41,43,46] These viruses are usually not pathogenic unless a patient has a defect in immunologic competence. Under such conditions of immunosuppression, the host is then either vulnerable to attack by these opportunistic viruses from the environment or is unable to continue to suppress the activity of the virus which may have lain dormant for years in the host tissue.[20,25] Irrespective of the mechanism, these viruses attack the oligodendroglial cells (the myelin producing cells of the central nervous system), causing them to first swell and then degenerate.[46] Subsequent to the damage of the oligodendrocytes, the myelin dies and patches of demyelination appear. There is a paucity of inflammatory changes with the exception of some perivascular infiltrate of lymphocytes, plasma cells, and macrophages. Astrocytes are also affected, becoming very large and developing bizarre form. On electron microscopic study, the cell nuclei, particularly the oligodendroglia, are packed with viral particles.

TRANSMISSIBLE VIRAL DEMENTIA

In the past two decades, largely due to the investigative efforts of Gajdusek, a completely different type of slow or latent infection of the brain has been discovered. Called the subacute spongiform virus encephalopathies, these conditions are caused by an unconventional virus that is transmitted by the direct inocculation of infected tissue in the recipient host. This mode of transmission and the nature of these diseases were first understood through the study of kuru in the cannibalistic Fore tribe in New Guinea.[21] In that group, the eating of fresh human brain caused contamination by infected tissue either through the conjuntiva or open cuts. The resultant encephalopathy was a slowly progressive disease that did not respond to any treatment efforts.

It was soon recognized that the familiar presenile dementia, Creutzfeldt-Jakob disease, was a similar type of encephalopathy and its transmission to monkeys was experimentally achieved via direct tissue inoculation. The clinical picture of Creutzfeldt-Jakob disease has been described in Chapter 6 but, in brief, it is a progressive encephalopathy that has a variety of neurologic signs, the most prominent being confusion, dementia, pyramidal and extrapyramidal motor signs, and myoclonus. The mode of transmission of this disease in humans is still not known, but the recent reports of transmission to patients undergoing corneal transplantation,[15] to neurosurgeons via direct inoculation from contaminated brain during surgery or autopsy of infected specimens,[23] and to patients undergoing surgery for epilepsy via depth electrodes[4] suggest that many cases may have actually been inoculated in some way by infected tissues. In addition to these reports, it has been observed that a large percentage of Creutzfeldt-Jakob patients had undergone previous brain surgery.[22] This, again, suggests the possibility of some direct contamination of the host tissues.

It is known that simple person-to-person contact is not involved in transmission, so isolation of patients is not necessary. However, because of the possibility of tissue contamination, great care must be exercised in handling both the tissues of patients with Creutzfeldt-Jakob disease and also any instruments that have been used to cut or probe their tissues. Unfortunately, the unconventional virus that causes this disease is resistant to the usual methods of sterilization by heat and formalin. Autoclaving for one hour at 121°C. and 20 psi is necessary. Phenol, iodine, 0.03 percent permanganate, and 5 percent hypochlorite solutions are also satisfactory disinfectants.[22]

In an effort to persue the study of transmissible unconventional viruses, brain tissue from a large variety of diseases has been inoculated into monkey brains. One additional disease, to date, has been demonstrated as transmissible by this method; that is the familial form of Alzheimer's disease.[21,62] Why the familial form of this condition is transmissible and not the sporadic form is not known, but the answers to such questions may soon change our entire perspective on the study of dementia.

The pathophysiology of these slow viruses, particularly the unconventional transmissible viruses, is much different than that of normal viral infection. Incubation periods are very long, there are none of the usual inflammatory changes seen in conventional viral disease, resistance to chemical and physical agents is quite different, and these viral agents act in a very different fashion biologically.[21]

The expanding contribution of these recent developments in the field of virology has provided an entirely new direction for the study of infectious disease and will undoubtedly have ultimate clinical significance.

REFERENCES

1. Adams, D.H., and Bell, T.M.: The relationship between measles virus infection and subacute sclerosing panencephalitis (SSPE) Med. Hypotheses 2:55, 1976.
2. Adams, J.H., and Urquhart, G.E.D.: Early diagnosis of herpes encephalitis. N. Engl. J. Med. 297:1288, 1977.
3. Baver, W.R., Turel, A.P., and Johnson, K.P.: Progressive multifocal leukoencephalopathy and cytarabine. JAMA 226:174, 1973.
4. Bernoulli, C., Siegfried, J., Baumgartner, G., Regli, F., Rabinowicz, T., Gajdusek, D.C., and Gibbs, C.J., Jr.: Danger of accidental person-to-person transmission of Creutzfeldt-Jakob disease by surgery. Lancet 1:478, 1977.
5. Boyle, R.S., and Landy, P.J.: Herpes simplex encephalitis. Aust. N. Z. J. Med. 7:408, 1977.
6. Buckman, R., and Wiltshaw, E.: Progressive multifocal leukoencephalopathy successfully treated with cytosine arabinoside. Br. J. Haematol. 34:153, 1976.
7. Carroll, B.A., Lane, B., Norman, D., and Enzmann, D.: Diagnosis of progressive multifocal leukoencephalopathy by computed tomography. Radiology 122:137, 1977.
8. Chien, LT., Boehm, R.M., Robinson, H., Liu, C., and Frenkel, L.D.: Characteristic early electroencephalographic changes in herpes simplex encephalitis. Arch. Neurol. 34:361, 1977.
9. Choudhury, A.R., Taylor, J.C., and Whitaker, R.: Primary excision of brain abscess. Br. Med. J. 2:1119, 1977.
10. Conomy, J.P., Beard, N.S., Matsumoto, H., and Roessmann, U.: Cytarabine treatment of progressive multifocal leukoencephalopathy. JAMA 229:1313, 1974.
11. Conomy, J.P., Weinstein, M.A., Agamanolis, D., and Holt, W.S.: Computed tomography in progressive multifocal leukoencephalopathy. Radiology 127:663, 1976.
12. Davis, L.E., and Johnson, R.T.: An explanation for the localization of herpes simplex encephalitis? Ann. Neurol. 5:2, 1979.
13. DeLouvois, J.: The bacteriology and chemotherapy of brain abscess. J. Antimicrob. Chemother. 4:395, 1978.
14. DeLouvois, J., Gortvai, P., and Hurley, R.: Bacteriology of abscesses of the central nervous systems: a multicentre prospective study. Br. Med. J. 2:981, 1977.
15. Duffy, P., Wolf, J., Collins, G., DeVoe, A.G., Streeten, B., and Cowen, D.: Possible person-to-person transmission of Creutzfeldt-Jakob disease. N. Engl. J. Med. 299:693, 1974.
16. Elian, M.: Herpes simplex encephalitis. Arch. Neurol. 32:39, 1975.
17. Feldman, H.A.: Toxoplasma and toxoplasmosis. Hosp. Pract. 4:64, 1969.

18. Fermaglich, J., Hardman, J.M., and Earl, K.M.: Spontaneous progressive multifocal leukoencephalopathy. Neurology 20:479, 1970.
19. Frenkel, J.K., Nelson, B.M., and Arias-Stella, J.: Immunosuppression and toxoplasmic encephalitis. Hum. Pathol. 6:97, 1975.
20. Gajdusek, D.C.: Slow virus disease of the central nervous system. Am. J. Clin. Pathol. 56:320, 1971.
21. Gajdusek, D.C.: Unconventional viruses and the origin and disappearance of kuru. Science 197:943, 1977.
22. Gajdusek, D.C., Gibbs, C.J., Jr., Asher, D.M., Brown, P., Diwan, A., Hoffman, P., Nemo, G., Rohwer, R., and White, L.: Precautions in medical care of, and handling materials from patients with transmissible virus dementia (Creutzfeldt-Jakob disease). N. Engl. J. Med. 297:1253, 1977.
23. Gajdusek, D.C., Gibbs, C.J., Jr., Earle, K., Dammin, C.J., Schoene, W., and Tyler, H.R.: Transmission of subacute spongiform encephalopathy to the chimpanzee and squirrel monkey from a patient with papulosis atrophicans maligna of Kohnmeier-Doegs, in Neurology, Proceedings of the Tenth International Congress of Neurology, Barcelona, September 8–15, 1973.
24. Haddad, F.S., Risk, W.S., and Jabbour, J.T.: Subacute sclerosing panencephalitis in the Middle East: report of 99 cases. Ann. Neurol. 1:211, 1977.
25. Ho, M.: Virus infections after transplantation in man. Arch. Virol. 55:1, 1977.
26. Ingham, H.R., High, A.S., Kalbag, R.M., Sengupta, R.P., Tharagonnet, D., and Selkon, J.B.: Abscesses of the frontal lobe of the brain secondary to covert dental sepsis. Lancet 2:497, 1978.
27. Jabbour, J.T., Duenan, D.A., and Modlin, J.: SSPE: Clinical staging, course and frequency. Arch. Neurol 32:493, 1975.
28. Jabbour, J.T., Garcia, J.H., Lemmi, H., Ragland, J., Duenas, D.A., and Sever, J.L.: Subacute sclerosing panencephalitis. JAMA 207:2248, 1969.
29. Jefferson, A.A., and Keogh, A.J.: Intracranial abscesses: a review of treated patients over 20 years. Q. J. Med. 46:389, 1977.
30. Johnson, K.P., Byington, D.P., and Goddis, L.: Subacute sclerosing panencephalitis. Adv. Neurol. 6:77, 1974.
31. Karlin, C.A., Robinson, R.G., Hinthorn, D.R., and Liu, C.: Radionuclide imaging in herpes simplex encephalitis. Radiology 126:181, 1978.
32. Kaufman, D.M., Zimmerman, R.D., and Leeds, N.E.: Computed tomography in herpes simplex encephalitis. Neurology 29:1392, 1979.
33. Kiessling, W.R., Hall, W.W., Yung, L.L., and TerMeulen, V.: Measles-virus-specific immunoglobulin-M response in subacute sclerosing panencephalitis. Lancet 1:324, 1977.
34. Kirsh, J., Rosenthall, L., Finlayson, M.H., and Wee, R.: Progressive multifocal leukoencephalopathy. Radiology 119:399, 1976.
35. Liversedge, L.A.: Herpes simplex encephalitis: current ideas and treatment plans for the future. Proc. R. Soc. Med. 69:193, 1976.
36. Longson, M.: The treatment of herpes encephalitis. J. Antimicrob. Chemother. 3 (supp A): 115, 1977.
37. Markand, O.N., and Panszl, J.G.: The electroencephalogram in subacute sclerosing panencephalitis. Arch. Neurol. 32:719, 1975
38. Marriott, P.J., O'Brien, M.D., MacKenzie, I.C., and Janota, I.: Progressive multifocal leukoencephalopathy: remission with cytarabine. J. Neurol. Neurosurg. Psychiatry 38:205, 1975.

39. Mehta, P.D., Kane, A., and Thormar, H.: Quantitation of measles virus—specific immunoglobulins in serum, C.S.F. and brain extract from patients with subacute sclerosing panencephalitis. J. Immunol. 118:2254, 1977.

40. Merritt, H.H., Adams, R.D., and Solomon, H.C.: Neurosyphilis. Oxford University Press, New York, 1946.

41. Narayan, O., Penney, J.B., Jr., Johnson, R.T., Herndon, R.M., and Weiner, L.P.: Etiology of progressive multifocal leukoencephalopathy. N. Engl. J. Med. 289:1278, 1973.

42. Oxbury, J.M., and MacCallum, F.O.: Herpes simplex encephalitis: clinical features and residual damage. Postgrad. Med. J. 49:387, 1973.

43. Padgett, B.L., Walker, D.L., ZuRhein, G.M., Hodach, A.E., and Chou, S.M.: JC papovavirus in progressive multifocal leukoencephalopathy. J. Infect. Dis. 133:686, 1976.

44. Pexman, K.H.W.: The angiographic and brain scan features of acute herpes simplex encephalitis. Br. J. Radiol. 47:179, 1974.

45. Polna, I., and Cendrowski, W.: Serological studies on the etiological role of measles-like virus in subacute sclerosing panencephalitis. J. Neurol. 216:301, 1977.

46. Richardson, E.P.: Our evolving understanding of progressive multifocal leukoencephalopathy. Ann. N.Y. Acad. Sci. 230:358, 1974.

47. Rosenblum, M.L., Hoff, J.T., Norman, D., Weinstein, P.R., and Pitts, L.: Decreased mortality from brain abscesses since advent of computerized tomography. J. Neurosurg. 49:658, 1978.

48. Sisk, M., and Griffith, J.F.: Normal electroencephalograms in subacute sclerosing panencephalitis. Arch. Neurol. 32:575, 1975.

49. Slavick, H.E., and Lipman, I.J.: Brainstem toxoplasmosis complicating Hodgkin's disease. Arch. Neurol. 34:636, 1977.

50. Snell, G.E.: Sinogenic and otogenic brain abscesses—a review of 63 cases occurring at Toronto General Hospital, 1956–75. J. Otolaryngol. 7:289, 1978.

51. Taber, L.H., Brasier, F., Couch, R.B., Greenberg, S.B., Jones, D., and Knight, V.: Diagnosis of herpes simplex virus infection by immunofluorescence. J. Clin. Microbiol. 3:309, 1976.

52. Taber, L.H., Greenberg, S.B., Perez, F.I., and Couch, R.B.: Herpes simplex encephalitis treated with Vidarabine (adenine arabinoside). Arch. Neurol. 34:608, 1977.

53. Thomson, J.L.C.: The computed axial tomograph in acute herpes simplex encephalitis. Br. J. Radiol. 49:86, 1976.

54. Torres, J.R., Sanders, C.V., Strub, R.L., and Black, F.W.: Cat-scratch disease causing reversible encephalopathy. JAMA 240:1628, 1978.

55. Townsend, J.J., Wolinsky, J.S., Baringer, J.R., and Johnson, P.C.: Acquired toxoplasmosis. A neglected cause of treatable nervous system disease. Arch. Neurol. 32:335, 1975.

56. Webb, H.E., Kelly, R.E., Adams, D.H.: Intravenous and intrathecal adenine arabinoside phosphate in a child with subacute sclerosing panencephalitis. Lancet 2:978, 1977.

57. Webster, J.E., and Gurdjian, E.S.: The surgical management of intracranial suppuration. Int. Abst. Surg. 90:209, 1950.

58. Westmoreland, B.F., Gomez, M.R., and Blume, W.T.: Activation of periodic complexes of subacute sclerosing panencephalitis by sleep. Ann. Neurol. 1:185, 1977.

59. Whitley, R.J., Soong, S., Dolin, R., Galasso, G.J., Chien, L.T., and Alford, C.A.: Adenine arabinoside therapy of biopsy proved herpes simplex encephalitis. N. Engl. J. Med. 297:289, 1977.
60. Wilson, L.G.: Viral encephalitis mimicking functional psychosis. Am. J. Psychiatry, 133:165, 1976.
61. Editorial: Antiviral treatment of varicella zoster and herpes simplex. Lancet 1:1337, 1980.
62. Goudsmit, J., Morrow, C.H., Asher, D.M., Yanagihara, R.T., Masters, C.L., Gibbs, C.J., and Gajdusek, D.C.: Evidence for and against the transmissibility of Alzheimer disease. Neurology 30:945, 1980.

11

EPILEPSY

M.B. is a 65-year-old female with onset of seizures at age 61. She came to medical attention because of an initial, generalized seizure of tonic-clonic type (grand mal). However, the family described a two month period preceding the seizure during which the patient had begun to exhibit progressively bizarre behavior. Following the grand mal seizure, the patient was treated with phenobarbital. The seizures ceased as did the abnormal behavior. She discontinued the medication after 6 months.

A year later she became very "foggy" in conversation and would frequently stop talking in the middle of a conversation. Occasionally during these arrests of conversation, she would display restless automatic movements of her hands and mouth but no true adversive movements. She was often drowsy and could not remember common personal details. The patient had always led a rather structured and compulsive existence, but at this time she began to show very ritualized behavior such as very rigid dieting, sleeping on the floor with exactly 14 Reader's Digest *magazines under her head, and constantly expressed dissatisfaction about how the house looked and with her personal appearance.*

The patient was again brought to the hospital. On examination, she appeared very dazed and responded most laconically, answering only a few questions and staring into space most of the time. The neurologic exam was completely normal. An EEG revealed bursts of irregular sharp waves in the frontal region. She was again treated with phenobarbital and her mental functioning improved. As she became more communicative and natural in her behavior, the EEG became normal. However, she still displayed some abnormal behavior and demonstrated a significant thought disorder. The patient was hospitalized in the psychiatric unit for further treatment of what was diagnosed as paranoid schizophrenia. A complete mental status examination for organic disease was normal except for concreteness in proverb interpretation. This was attributed to the thought disorder and not to organicity. A CT scan of the brain was normal as were skull x-rays. The patient was discharged in a month.

During the past few years the patient has been maintained on both phenobarbital and phenothiazines. She has had no further seizures or "foggy spells" but continues to show evidence of an intermittent thought disorder.

This case demonstrates some of the puzzling behavioral changes that can occur in patients with epilepsy. This individual always had a "strange personality" according to her family but compensated well until the onset of the seizures. The first symptoms she exhibited were reminiscent of the type of chronic confusional behavior seen in petit mal status, but her EEG showed only episodic trains of frontal sharp activity. We assume, since her behavior ameliorated considerably after the control of the abnormal discharges, that this subclinical seizure activity was responsible both for producing the confusional behavior and unmasking or exacerbating an underlying psychiatric disorder. Her behavior prior to the onset of seizures had been obsessive and somewhat paranoid, but with the onset of the seizures she became clinically schizophrenic. It is possible that her EEG had been abnormal for many years and that her odd life-long behavior reflected this physiologic disturbance. However, this is only a speculation.

Although it is far beyond the scope of this book to present a comprehensive overview of the epidemiology, description, medical treatment, and social rehabilitation of the myriad forms of epilepsy; the importance of these syndromes to the practicing clinician cannot be overestimated. Epilepsy is a common disease and one that is frequently associated with significant behavioral change. The social, vocational, and emotional impact that epilepsy has upon the patient, his family, and society in general is considerable. In this chapter we will provide a relatively brief description of the various types of epilepsy and their incidence. The behavioral changes which are seen either in association with the seizures themselves or as chronic interictal phenomena will be emphasized. More comprehensive reviews of both the medical and social/rehabilitative aspects are readily available to the interested reader.[88,92,110,112,127]

Epilepsy, is among the most common of the chronic neurologic disorders. Although it varies with the particular study and the sample studied; generally 4 to 5 cases per 1000 population is given as the incidence.[72,73,76,112] These figures indicate that there are approximately 1.7 million persons in the United States alone with a diagnosis of epilepsy. The great social and economic impact of this problem and the likelihood that the practicing clinician will have frequent contact with epileptic patients is obvious.

The term "epilepsy," as used by most physicians, implies a recurrent paroxysmal uncontrolled discharge of cerebral neurons resulting in clinical signs and symptoms that interfere with normal levels and quality of the individual's functioning.[112] In most cases there is impaired thinking, awareness of and/or observable convulsive movements or repetitive behaviors (automatisms).[30] During attacks in which the seizure discharge remains well localized without spread, there may be no loss of consciousness. In other cases with a deeper locus or bilateral spread, lapses in consciousness can be a very prominent feature of the disorder. One of the most striking clinical features of epilepsy is the intermittent nature of the disorder and the almost total lack of overt symptoms between the actual seizures. Some patients may experience multiple seizures daily, while most patients have intervals between attacks of many months or years.

Because of the complex nature of epilepsy and the wide spectrum of its clinical manifestations, a simple definition and a universal concise description is impossible. Nor is it possible to provide an all encompassing discussion of the treatment of this complicated medical problem. Therefore, this chapter will provide only a framework for the clinical classification of epilepsy and definitions of basic relevant terms. Traditionally, proposed schemes for classification of epilepsy have tended to fall into one or a combination of several categories. In an excellent historical review and critique Masland,[84] has grouped the major classification systems as classification by: (1) symptomatology, (2) physiology (including EEG), (3) anatomy, (4) etiology, and (5) response to therapy.

The most widely disseminated and currently utilized classification schema is that proposed by Gastaut[44] which groups patients by symptomatology. This system has been adopted by the International League Against Epilepsy and the World Federation of Neurology. This classification (Table 11-1) provides a standardized and uniform system which is internationally recognized and has greatly aided communication among epileptologists.

It may be of value to briefly review several of the terms most frequently used in describing epilepsy. *Grand mal* is a generalized convulsion with accompanying loss of consciousness and a sequence of tonic-clonic motor movements. *Petit mal* refers to a seizure characterized by brief absences, occurring predominantly in children, and with an EEG pattern of paroxysmal three per second spike and wave bursts. The seizure may be accompanied by a rhythmic blinking of the eyes, automatisms, and at times by a myoclonic jerking of the extremities.

TABLE 11–1. International Classification of Epileptic Seizures

I. Partial Seizures (seizures beginning locally)
  A. Partial seizures with elementary symptomatology (generally without impairment of consciousness)
    1. With motor symptoms
      a. Focal motor
      b. Jacksonian
      c. Versive (generally contraversive)
      d. Postural
      e. Somatic inhibitory (?)
      f. Aphasic
      g. Phonatory (vocalization and arrest of speech)
    2. With special sensory or somatosensory symptoms
      a. Somatosensory
      b. Visual
      c. Auditory
      d. Olfactory
      e. Gustatory
      f. Vertiginous
    3. With autonomic symptoms
    4. Compound forms
  B. Partial seizures with complex symptomatology (generally with impairment of consciousness)
    1. With impaired consciousness only
    2. With cognitive symptomatology
      a. With dysmnesic disturbances
      b. With ideational disturbances
    3. With affective symptomatology
    4. With "psychosensory" symptomatology
      a. Illusions
      b. Hallucinations
    5. With "psychomotor" symptomatology (automatisms)
    6. Compound forms
  C. Partial seizures secondarily generalized
II. Generalized Seizures (bilaterally symmetrical and without local onset)
  A. Absences (petit mal)
    1. Simple absences, with impairment of consciousness only
    2. Complex absences with other associated phenomena
      a. With mild clonic components (myoclonic)
      b. With increase of postural tone (retropulsive)
      c. With diminution or abolition of postural tone (atonic)
      d. With automatisms
      e. With automatic phenomena (e.g., enuresis)
      f. Mixed forms
  B. Bilateral massive epileptic myoclonus (myoclonic jerks)
  C. Infantile spasms
  D. Clonic seizures
  E. Tonic seizures
  F. Tonic-clonic seizures ("grand mal" seizures)
  G. Atonic seizures
    1. Of very brief duration (drop attacks)
    2. Of longer duration (including atonic absences)
  H. Akinetic seizures (loss of movement without atonia)
III. Unilateral or Predominantly Unilateral Seizures
IV. Unclassified Epileptic Seizures (Includes all seizures which cannot be classified because of inadequate or incomplete data).

Previously, the term was used to refer to any minor seizure attack. *Temporal lobe seizures* or *psychomotor attacks* are partial seizures with complex symptomatology.

Aura is the consciously recalled experience (often sensory) that heralds the actual onset of the seizure and is recognized as a component of the seizure itself.[108,112] This behavioral component is clinically relevant, as the nature of its manifestation can be useful in localizing the seizure focus. Formerly, this term referred to the patient's subjective warning of an incipient seizure or the last remembered experience or sensation of the patient prior to the onset of a seizure.

The *prodrome* is the behavioral or mood change that may precede the actual onset of a seizure by as many as several days. Such symptoms are more difficult to directly relate to the seizure itself and may reflect either alterations in basic physiologic processes such as premenstrual water retention or the gradual accentuation of unstable electrochemical activity which interferes with normal central nervous system functioning.[108]

Ictal refers to the actual seizure itself. The *postictal* period is that time immediately following the seizure and is typically characterized by changes in behavior including drowsiness, confusion, poorly directed activity, and at times abnormal motor movement. *Interictal* denotes the time between actual seizures in which the patient is not experiencing any direct effects of the seizure itself. Interictal changes in behavior and personality in patients with epilepsy have been reported for centuries and are one of the most interesting aspects of the interaction between epilepsy and behavior. There is little doubt that the behavioral and emotional concomitants or sequelae of epilepsy are virtually as diverse as the manifestations of the seizures themselves. On the other hand, the etiology and precise nature of these behavioral disorders have been the source of considerable, often conflicting, speculations for centuries.[82,96] Tizard[121] has reviewed the major contributions to this area and subsequently categorized the theories into five basic groups: (1) all or most epileptics have a characteristic personality pattern, (2) there is no characteristic epileptic personality and an identical range and combination of personality traits are found among epileptics and nonepileptics, (3) there is no characteristic personality type or disturbance, but the epileptic population does demonstrate a higher incidence of neurotic disturbance than the nonepileptic, (4) there is no characteristic epileptic personality, but epileptic patients do tend to have a personality resembling that of individuals with demonstrable organic lesions which differs from that of normal individuals, and (5) there is no personality pattern common to all or even most epileptics, but different types of epilepsy do have associated different types of personality. Tizard's review of the world's literature and the conclusions of most workers in this field provide little support for the long-held theory that a characteristic "epileptic personality" exists. However, the data do suggest: (1) that the incidence of a wide range of personality disturbances may be higher than expected in the epileptic population, particularly in certain groups such as temporal lobe epileptics, and (2) that different types of personality disorders may be associated with different types of epilepsy.[93,108,121]

Accurate statistics concerning the actual incidence of clinically significant behavioral changes associated with epilepsy are difficult to obtain because of problems in the comparability of the various studies in this area and the nature of many such reports (e.g., case studies, anecdotal reports, studies of a particular problem associated with a discrete form of epilepsy). However, the consensus of these investigations is that a far higher than expected incidence of problems in intellectual, emotional, and social functioning does exist within the epileptic population, with estimates of the frequency of such problems ranging from 10 to 70 percent in the various samples under study.[33,55,96] Such disorders in all probability result from a complex interaction of personality structure, environment, brain pathophysiology, and the effects of anticonvulsant medication.[27,28,96]

The frequency and variety of emotional and behavioral changes seen in epileptic patients are sufficiently high and the psychologic and social impact of such disorders can be so great that the clinician must be thoroughly prepared to recognize their presence, make the appropriate neurobehavioral diagnosis, and provide efficacious treatment and/or referral as he deals with his epileptic patient. The rest of this chapter provides one conceptual framework for classifying these behavioral changes and descriptions of the most frequently encountered clinical syndromes.

To help in the categorization and understanding of the wide range of behavioral changes seen in patients with epilepsy, we propose the use of the following classification schema which has largely been adapted from Pond.[96] This system has the advantage of attempting to relate a particular behavioral disturbance to an underlying neurophysiologic dysfunction rather than being merely a tedious compilation of each clinical symptom which has been reported in association with epilepsy. We will use this framework in our discussion.

Personality Disorders and Epilepsy

    I. Personality disorders directly related to clinical seizures
        A. Preictal: Events preceding or leading to overt seizures
            1. Prodromal states
            2. Psychophysiologic precursors

340

B. Ictal: Disorders directly related to ongoing epileptic discharges.
1. Disturbances in consciousness
2. Psychomotor expressions of discharge
C. Postictal: Disturbances following overt seizures
1. Alterations in consciousness
a. Focal paralyses
b. Automatism with amnesia
2. Violent behavior
D. Emotional reactions to ictal experiences
II. Personality disorders not clearly related to clinical seizures (i.e.,
nonictal, anictal, or interictal psychologic disorders occurring in
proven epileptics)
A. Cognitive dysfunction
B. Personality changes
1. Neurotic-like disorders
2. Psychotic-like disorders
3. Characterologic disorders
4. Special problems of temporal lobe epilepsy

DESCRIPTION OF THE CLINICAL SYNDROMES

As the reader may assume from glancing over the classification
schema, a wide variety of emotional, behavioral, and cognitive changes
have been reported to be associated with epilepsy. These changes range
from increased anxiety and irritability levels to episodic violent behavior, characterologic-like disorders, and the schizophreniform psychosis
seen in some poorly controlled chronic temporal lobe epileptics. Those
which have been most frequently reported or which have a rate of
incidence sufficiently high to be clinically important will be described
in some detail, while certain more uncommon behavioral changes will
be briefly reviewed.

Personality Disorders Directly Related to Clinical Seizures

PREICTAL BEHAVIORAL CHANGES

Prodromal States/Psychophysiologic Precursors

Within the category of prodromal states, we include both the presei-
zure aura, which is a patient-perceived and consciously remembered
(usually sensory, but sometimes purely emotional) experience which
marks the onset of a seizure, and premonitory or prodromal symptoms
which are more generalized and are often primarily psychologic in

manifestation (including depression, irritability, and hypomania).[76,96] Theoretically, auras may be differentiated from the prodromal states, as the former have clear neuropathophysiologic bases (i.e., a focal epileptic discharge which may be documented by electroencephalogram [EEG] before the onset of an overt seizure). In contrast, the prodromal states are not associated with a worsening of the EEG during the days or hours preceding a seizure[96] and may or may not be related to a variety of physiologic states (e.g., premenstrual hormonal changes or water retention). Certain patients or their close associates are able to accurately predict an impending seizure before its onset on the basis of a change in behavior (e.g., increased anxiety, irritability, mental dullness, depression, or social withdrawal).[108]

The etiology of these generalized emotional changes is as yet uncertain, but it is probable that they are physiologically related to the seizure disorder (i.e., a build-up of epileptic interference with brain function) and represent a type of premonitory emotional response by the patient to the imminent seizure. The patient's conscious perception of and response to either the aura (e.g., inopportune sensory perception or fear) or the prodrome (e.g., gradually increasing anxious irritability) constitute one common type of epilepsy-associated behavioral change. It is quite easy to understand how the naive patient, after years of experiencing fleeting episodes of subconscious emotion (e.g., fear, pleasure, uneasiness) which are generated spontaneously by the epileptogenic discharges and are unrelated to environmental circumstances, might well become anxious, irritable, and even paranoid.

In some cases, the patient's actual behavior precipitates an overt seizure. This has been categorized as self-induced reflex epilepsy and has been well covered in the literature.[87,96] Environmental stress, photic stimulation (either environmentally or personally induced), reading, listening to music (in some cases, even specific types of music), repetitive motoric activity, acute startle as well as other similar stimuli have been well known to precipitate a seizure in the electrophysiologically susceptible individual.

ICTAL BEHAVIORAL CHANGES

Disturbances in Consciousness

The significant self-sustained electrical discharge that characterizes the overt ictal phase of an epileptic seizure can result in a wide variety of both physiologic and psychologic changes. The most obvious and most physiologically based behavioral changes involve varying degrees of disturbed levels of consciousness. The alterations range from the deep coma-like state of the grand mal seizure to the transitory lapse of awareness in the absence (petit mal) seizure or the complex dream-like states which are typical of some seizures originating deep within the temporal lobes.[96] Accordingly, the patient with a history of intermittent lapses in awareness or consciousness should be fully evaluated to assess the possibility of epilepsy.

Mental and behavioral changes have been reported as manifestations of petit mal epilepsy since the first description of this disorder.[75] Such manifestations have received a variety of labels including "prolonged twilight state," "prolonged behavioral disturbance," "ictal psychosis," and "acute prolonged confusion."[32,35,106,125] Clinical manifestations include a spectrum of altered consciousness which embraces: (1) normal or subjective impairment of awareness, (2) deep stupor, (3) impaired motivation and initiative, (4) deficits in planning, (5) aphasic-like language disorders including paraphasia and perseveration, (6) confusion and disorientation, (7) infantile behavior (primarily in children), (8) incontinence, (9) amnesic periods, (10) fugue-like states, (11) hallucinations, paranoia, (12) delusional ideation, (13) manic-depressive affectual changes, and (14) apraxia.[5,32] Although petit mal status has primarily been reported in children and patients with an early onset, the onset in middle-age of petit mal status with its attendant behavioral features has been described.[47] Ellis and Lee[32] reported on a series of six patients between the ages of 42 and 69 with no past history of seizures who initially presented with an acute behavioral change characterized by the abrupt unprovoked onset of fluctuating confusion, memory dysfunction, and psychotic-like symptomatology, associated with continuous generalized 1 to 1½ Hz. multiple spike and wave EEG activity.

Transient psychotic-like episodes which may mimic depressive, hysterical, and schizophrenic reactions unaccompanied by clinically observable seizures are relatively uncommon among patients with epilepsy but have been reported to occur.[125] Such states may so dominate the clinical picture that the patient may be repeatedly admitted to a psychiatric unit before the true nature of the patient's condition is accurately diagnosed.[1] Any patient who presents with (1) a history of previous seizures, (2) intellectual deterioration, and (3) intermittent periods of confusion, mental dullness, or schizophreniform behavior, with periods of complete (or almost complete) resolution should strongly alert the clinician to suspect petit mal status.[109]

Psychomotor Expressions of Seizure Discharge

The characteristic behavioral changes associated with temporal lobe seizure foci have been among the most widely reported and certainly the most readily noticed behavioral changes in the field of epilepsy. In the late 1880s, John Hughlings Jackson[64] described a man with a glioma of the frontotemporal area whose overt seizures were preceded by an aura consisting of a "dreadful disagreeable smell" which was than followed by "chewing movements of the jaws and spitting of saliva." Although this particular manifestation is certainly not common,[60] the combination of a psychic aura and unprovoked automatic behavior is representative of this category of ictal behavioral change. The term "psychomotor attacks" was traditionally utilized to categorize and describe this form of seizure,[49] while in the more recently adopted nomenclature[44] this form of seizure is included in the category of partial seizures with complex symptomatology. Classically, the ictal automatism is defined as a seizure resulting in a period of altered behavior for which the patient is amnesic and during which he responds to the environment in a limited, often stereotyped, fashion as if only partially conscious.[108] In most patients, the seizure begins with a recognizable aura which may be olfactory, gustatory, visceral, autonomic, or a sense of unexplained pleasure or anxiety, or a sense of intense environmental recognition (déjà vu). The most characteristic feature of the partial seizure with complex symptomatology is the actual ictal automatism. This typically includes stereotyped motor movements (e.g., lip smacking, leg kicking, picking at clothing, chewing movements) which may be repeated in similar form from attack to attack.[112] At times, partial seizures may be so brief and discreet that they are not noticed by the casual observer; while in other cases it is difficult, if not impossible, to fail to recognize the prolonged and bizarre repetitive behavior of the seemingly dazed or "wide-eyed" patient (e.g., the stereotyped "sniffing" of the air followed by shouting of "hallelujah" observed by one of us [FWB] in a patient with a rather significant penetrating missile wound of the right temporal lobe).

In addition to sensory aura and psychomotor automatisms experienced by the patient with temporal lobe involvement, alterations in higher cognitive and emotional function are often seen. Such alterations in behavior may include: illusory and hallucinatory experiences, sexual arousal, feelings of prescience or familiarity (the déjà vu phenomenon previously mentioned), feelings of strangeness or unreality, ictal pleasure, violence, fear, depression, and cognitive dysfunction.[12,15,42,103,108] Subsequent to the period of altered behavior associated with the active seizure, the patient is typically amnesic for the episode, often confused, and drowsy. Although rare, it is usually only during this latter stage of the seizure that ictal rage reactions and aggressive behavior occur (particularly if attempts are made to restrain the patient).[51,103] The actual reported incidence of violent or aggressive behavior in patients with temporal lobe dysfunction, including epilepsy, is decidedly low despite the popularization of this aspect of psychomotor epilepsy in the lay and even some professional literature.[108] Violence as a subclinical expression of ictal behavior is a special situation and will be discussed later in this chapter.

From both a theoretic, psysiologic, and clinical viewpoint, the basis of the ictal emotional and behavioral phenomena is important. It is generally conceded that such focal abnormalities are related to dysfunction of the limbic portions of the temporal lobe. Temporolimbic structures are of considerable importance in the development and expression of emotions and emotional behavior, although it is quite apparent that the precise association between emotions and behavior and the structures within the temporolimbic system have yet to be fully elucidated.

Those readers desiring a more comprehensive review of this complex area are referred to the several excellent overviews dealing with the behavioral manifestations of temporal lobe epilepsy.[12,14,22,61,92,118]

POSTICTAL BEHAVIORAL CHANGE

The postictal period is that time which immediately follows an active seizure and is characterized by behavioral changes including drowsiness, confusion, abnormal motor movement, and semipurposeful activity.[112] There is a gradual transition from the ictal to the postictal phase of the seizure and there is some overlap in the behavioral manifestations during each stage. Hypothetical etiologies for postictal behavioral changes include a metabolic derangement of cells secondary to the hypoxia associated with the active seizure,[88] an active inhibitory state,[31] and cellular metabolic exhaustion.[34] Whatever the precise etiology of the dysfunction at the cellular level, pathologic measurement of the metabolism of single Betz's cells from animals with experimentally produced status epilepticus demonstrate that postictally the cells are unable to metabolize oxygen and are thus either markedly deranged metabolically or dead. Such disruption of neural function obviously can result in alterations in all aspects of brain function.

Disturbances in Consciousness

The most frequent of the postictal behavioral disturbances are those associated with an alteration of both level and content of consciousness. Those behavioral changes which are of primary psychiatric importance occur when the electrical discharge involves the cortex that serves as a substrate for consciousness (particularly deep temporal areas).[96] Some investigators[66] feel that automatisms with amnesia for the event result only when the previous seizure has involved at least all of one hemisphere and the contralateral temporal lobe (i.e., relatively bilateral generalized epileptic activity). During the postictal phase, the patient is typically confused initially (although this may be imperceptible in some patients) and then gradually interacts with the environment in an increasingly more organized fashion. Conversation becomes possible and behavior appears reasonably coherent, although the patient is often unable to recall the events which transpired during the latter stage of the postictal phase.[12] The duration of this postictus is variable, but it typically lasts from two to ten minutes[65] with an outside range of a few seconds to several hours. Prolonged confusional or delirious states lasting from hours to days may follow generalized seizures. If there has been a series of seizures, the altered state of consciousness may persist for as long as a few weeks.[12] The severity of the disorder as well as its clinical manifestations may well fluctuate both during a given day and over the course of several days. In this regard, the postictal confusional state is analogous to confusion of any etiology as discussed in Chapter 4. Acts committed during this confusional state vary widely in the degree to which they are coherently organized and overtly or inadvertently directed towards people or objects in the environment. Psychogenic factors including basic personality make-up, preexisting modes of reacting in given situations, and particular environmental stress play a major role in the manifestation of acts committed during the confusional state. Theoretically, during the state of clouded consciousness, there is a diminution of the highest levels of emotional and behavioral control, allowing expression of more basic highly emotionally charged impulses.[2] On a more pragmatic level, the behavior exhibited during this postictal state and its underlying dynamics are akin to a state of alcoholic or drug intoxication in which behavior that is usually under relatively adequate control (e.g., aggression, sexuality, dysinhibition, or even psychosis) may be expressed with minimal provocation, much to the detriment of the individual and the environment.

The behavioral changes associated with altered levels of consciousness have often been termed "psychotic" and both a classification system and descriptions of the various states are widely disseminated in the literature.[17] Although certainly some of the behaviors exhibited by patients during the postictal stage meet the American Psychiatric Association's[3,4] criteria for psychosis (i.e., mental functioning sufficiently impaired to interfere grossly with the capacity to meet the ordinary demands of life), we feel it to be more in keeping with the total clinical picture of these patients to classify such behavioral changes as components or associates of the altered level of consciousness rather than to categorize the behavior on the basis of one psychiatric clinical feature.

Violence

Increased irritability and overtly violent behavior, although infrequent in most patients, is a sufficiently common feature of the postictal stage that it deserves special mention here. Aggression, irritability, and at times outbursts of extreme violence reaching forensic significance have been reported in patients during the confusional amnesic postictal stage.[12,61,67,96] Criminal attacks including homicide are not unknown during such states and accordingly this aspect of epileptic behavioral change frequently has medicolegal significance.[56,70] The two primary points that the clinician should keep in mind are: (1) such dramatic behavioral changes do occur and must be recognized and (2) genuine postictal violent behavior takes place during a confusional period and the patient's amnesia for the event is genuine not feigned. The complex medicolegal ramifications implicit in such cases are far beyond the scope of this text. The interested reader is referred to Jüül-Jensen[67] and Knox[70] for more thorough reviews of this subject.

EMOTIONAL REACTIONS TO ICTAL EXPERIENCES

Both the ictal and postictal direct effects of an epileptic discharge are, by their electrophysiologic nature, paroxysmal and transitory. However, the ways in which patients respond to their perception and experience of the ictal phenomena are of major significance in the development of longstanding behavioral changes. The perception of an ictal sensation, emotion, or motor behavior is basically a passive experience and generally felt as something alien to the individual.[96] The intermittent and unexpected imposition of any ictal phenomenon (e.g., feeling of fear) without appropriate environmental stimuli is usually disquieting at the very least (although some individuals actually enjoy and self induce their seizures). In most patients, the repeated occurrence of unpredicable events such as prodromes, auras, and seizures understandably leads to the development of anxiety, paranoia, anger, and other emotional reactions. Compounding this basic process of ictal stimulus and emotional response are the reactions of others to the overt manifestations of the patient's seizures.[92] The epileptic convulsion or petit mal ictal features involve aspects which are often strange, frankly bizarre, and frightening to the patient's family as well as the naive observer. It represents a total lack of control to the patient and, usually, to those around him.[54] The long history of negative social reaction to epilepsy and its sufferers has been well documented in the world's literature and needs no reiteration here. Suffice it to say that many of the emotional and social problems experienced by the epileptic patient are not directly related to preictal, ictal, or postictal phenomena but are associated with a complex interplay among (1) the ictal experience, (2) the patient's emotional and behavioral response to the ictal experience, and (3) emotional and social responses by individuals within the patient's environment to his epilepsy per se and to its overt (or covert) manifestations.

Personality Disorders Not Clearly Related to Clinical Seizures

The personality disorders which fall within this category are the interictal psychologic changes which occur in patients with documented epilepsy but which are not directly related to the physiologically induced preictal, ictal, or postictal phenomena. Included are changes in cognitive functioning, the controversial "epileptic personality," and the wide range of psychologic disorders which have been reported in proven epileptics. Literature on this topic strongly suggests that the majority of the numerous psychologic disturbances noted in epileptic patients cannot be directly related to the actual epileptic discharge. Much of the pioneer work in this area involved an attempt to delineate an "epileptic personality" characteristic of all or most epileptics. This included rather specific psychopathologic changes that were considered an integral part of the epileptic syndrome. In marked constrast has been the contention of some writers that the basic personality of the epileptic is normal and that the only observable emotional differences between the epileptic and others are secondary to the unusual anxieties generated by recurrent unpredictable seizures and exclusion from the opportunities of a normal life by public attitude.[6] As previously mentioned, probably the best review of this controversy is that of Tizard.[121] The concept of a universal characteristic epileptic personality has, with relatively few recent revivals,[55,117] been largely discounted in the current literature. It is apparent that there is a greater incidence of cognitive, emotional, and social disturbances interictally in patients with epilepsy than would be expected in the general population.[55,96] This is also true of patients with temporal lobe seizures when compared with patients with equally severe, but different types of epilepsy.[8,12,93,108]

COGNITIVE DYSFUNCTION

The incidence of mental retardation among epileptic patients is higher than among the normal population, and although most noninstitutionalized epileptics do have intelligence quotients within the normal range, their scores tend to cluster at the lower end of this range.[102] The prevalence of seizures among mentally retarded individuals increases proportionately with the degree of retardation. Tredgold[122] found that more than 50 percent of institutionalized individuals with IQs within the most severe category of retardation had epilepsy, while only a small proportion of epileptics in the community are of significantly subnormal intelligence.[96] The correlation between epilepsy and increasing degrees of mental retardation undoubtedly has cultural and environmental associations as well as neuropathologic factors. Institutionalized patients with severe mental retardation very often have brain damage of some type,[107] thereby increasing the chance of epilepsy. Concomitantly, patients with severe uncontrolled and often deteriorating seizure disorders are more apt to be institutionalized, to be unable to learn at the rate expected for increases in chronological age, and to fail to benefit from normal environmental stimulation. The clinician should be mindful that epilepsy does not imply mental retardation and that the vast majority of patients with idiopathic epilepsy achieve adequate seizure control with anticonvulsant medication and suffer no subsequent cognitive effects.[112] The age of onset of major motor seizures[25] as well as the frequency of such seizures[26] have been demonstrated to be associated with greater psychologic impairment in adults as assessed by both IQ functioning and a broad range of tests of adaptive abilities. The results of these studies, however, indicate a degree of cognitive dysfunction in epileptic adults, even when the seizures are of relatively recent onset and low frequency. Severe impairment of intellectual and adaptive abilities is correlated with a seizure history of long duration, high seizure frequency, and an early age of seizure onset.[26] This association does, of course, depend to a great extent on the type of seizure (e.g., a patient having dozens of petit mal seizures daily may have very adequate cognitive functioning).

Two factors concerning cognitive functioning deserve special attention: (1) the specific effects of focal epileptogenic foci, particularly within the temporal lobe and (2) the question of intellectual deterioration in patients with chronic, less than perfectly controlled epilepsy. Dennerll,[24] after reviewing the literature pertaining to the effects of lateralized epileptic loci, reported significant differences in specific test performances relating to laterality. Patients with left hemisphere lesions, particularly temporal, demonstrated deficits on tests of verbal abilities, while those with right hemisphere lesions showed the expected deficits in perceptual motor and visual spatial skills. Relatively poorer performance in tests of short term memory has been reported by Glowinski in unilateral temporal lobe epileptics when compared with a similar group of centrencephalic epileptic patients[52] although the study was unable to demonstrate any consistent effects of laterality. Glowinski explained his findings by postulating an impairment in verbal encoding which interfers with the consolidation stage of the memory process and produces the chronic interictal memory deficit. Other studies also provide evidence that differences in performance on specific tests may well be related to either the diffuse or focal nature of the epileptic process. Accordingly, attention and more generalized cognitive performance may be depressed in diffuse or petit mal seizures,[90,115] while more specific aspects of intellect (e.g., memory) are impaired with localized foci.[89]

349

No definitive studies have been done to support the generally held contention that intellectual deterioration is seen in chronic epileptics. Satisfactory delineation of this factor will require long-term longitudinal studies with adequate control of the complicating variables of age, seizure onset, duration of epilepsy, forms of the seizure disorder (to include etiology and presence or absence of frank brain damage), patient's socioeconomic status and intellectual level prior to the onset of seizures, anticonvulsant medication used and both its dosage and serum levels, seizure frequency, and elapsed time between the last seizure and examination.[93] Although there has been some evidence of intellectual deterioration with poorly controlled seizures,[102] the consensus is that deterioration is by no means universal and, if present, may well not be permanent but rather a reflection of drug effects or the state of the patient at the time of testing. By their demonstration of the positive effect of carbamazepine upon the neuropsychologic performance of epileptics in comparison to phenytoin, Dodrill and Troupin[28] have shown the importance of drugs as a factor.

In summary, the research on the cognitive performance of epileptics generally has found that (1) epileptics as a group have slightly lower average IQ scores than nonepileptic controls,[85] (2) the lower IQ scores may be related to age of seizure onset,[25] (3) poorer cognitive performance appears to be associated with the frequency of seizures,[26] (4) patients in whom the etiology of the seizures is known perform less adequately than those in whom the cause is not apparent,[68] (5) institutionalized patients routinely show lower test scores than do epileptics being treated at public clinics, who in turn have lower IQ scores than patients in private care,[108] and (6) specific cognitive deficits (as opposed to full scale IQ scores) may correlate to a degree with the laterality or localization of the epileptic focus.[24] For a more complete review of the effects of epilepsy upon psychologic test performance and adaptive abilities, see Reitan.[98]

PERSONALITY CHANGE

There is general agreement that the frequency of clinically recognizable, relatively stable chronic personality disorders is higher in the population of epileptics than in that of normal individuals. This increased frequency is particularly true for patients with temporal lobe foci. The personality change referred to here is not the transient emotional and behavioral change directly related to ictal discharges, but rather a more generalized change in personality which is interictal and unrelated to the actual seizure. Discounting the now generally discredited "epileptic personality," these conditions can be broadly grouped as follows: (1) disturbances resembling neuroses, (2) disorders resembling psychoses or schizophreniform disorders, and (3) those conditions including aggressive and/or violent behavior, hypersexuality or hyposexuality, and the wide range of symptoms seen with temporal lobe or psychomotor seizures.

Disorders Resembling Neuroses

A wide variety of personality changes resembling neuroses have been reported in epileptic patients. These occur with far higher incidence than that expected within the general population.[95,96] A number of conditions resembling neuroses manifesting as interictal phenomena probably result from a combination of the effects of (1) long-term exposure to the abnormal behavioral and emotional experiences (e.g., fear, disagreeable sensory perceptions, confusion) which are related to physiologic factors (i.e., active spike discharges without seizure), (2) environmental response to the patient's seizure disorder (e.g., misunderstanding, anxiety, overprotection), and (3) the patient's emotional response to both the seizure disorder itself and its social and environmental implications and ramifications. Given this complex of factors, it is not unexpected that the epileptic patient who is without strong emotional and social support may develop some or many "neurotic" symptoms.

The association between the functional syndrome of neurotic hysteria and epilepsy has been the focus of centuries of philosophizing and research. The problem is of clinical importance as: (1) some epileptic patients demonstrate hysteriform personality traits, (2) hysterical or psychogenic seizures must be differentiated from actual epileptic attacks, and (3) some epileptics demonstrate a complex combination of both syndromes. Differentiating hysterical from genuine epileptic seizures is not always easy, particularly if one has only the patient's report of the event. The situation is somewhat improved if the episode has been observed, but this too can be discouragingly inadequate in many instances. The most useful approach is to ask the patient or observer to describe the attack in detail and see if there are any inconsistencies between the report and what is expected in a real seizure. Hysterical patients often report a significant degree of awareness during their seizure, a feature uncommon in epilepsy except for certain focal seizures. The hysterical patient also may evidence uncharacteristic movements such as arching of the back, flailing from side to side, or on occasion purposeful movements such as striking at people around him. The hysterical seizure frequently contains a wide and varying repertoire of movements, whereas the movements of a true epileptic seizure are rather stereotyped. Urinary incontinence and tongue biting are usually not seen other than in genuine seizures, but, of course, their absence does not rule out epilepsy, particularly of temporal lobe origin. The postictal period in true epilepsy is usually one of confusion, depression, and lethargy; features not often seen in the hysterical patient.

The diagnosis is made much easier with use of the EEG as: (1) in true seizures epileptic features may be present, (2) if used shortly after the seizure, postictal slowing may be seen in true seizures, (3) hysterical patients are often suggestible and a seizure can sometimes be precipitated by careful encouragement while the EEG is being performed. In most instances, a skilled electroencephalographer can separate true seizure discharges from muscle artifact and correctly diagnose a hysterical seizure. However, as mentioned in the previous section many patients will have both true and hysterical seizures; in such cases, control is difficult and the physician often finds himself very unsure about the patient's actual seizure frequency.

Psychologic precipitating factors may also result in a so-called "stress induced" genuine seizure. Suffice it to say that during the diagnostic process, the possible role of psychogenic factors, including hysteroid seizures, must be considered. Additionally, when managing the patient with documented epilepsy, psychologic variables are also important either as behavioral concomitants of the seizure disorder itself or as functional precipitators of a seizure. Glaser[50] has recently provided an interesting review of the historical consideration of hysteria and epilepsy.

Disorders Resembling Psychoses

A state resembling a psychosis can be observed as either a component or the sole manifestation of the ictal or immediate postictal phase of a seizure. In addition, a schizophreniform psychosis has been reported in epileptic patients (most frequently those with temporal lobe seizures)[9,15,17,120] whose seizures are poorly controlled for an extended period of time,[9,50] or a schizophreniform psychosis may develop as the overt seizures are decreasing in frequency.[94,100] The psychosis seen with psychomotor seizures will be discussed in greater detail in the section regarding temporal lobe personality changes.

Dongier,[29] in a study of psychotic episodes occurring in 516 epileptic patients, reported that a high proportion of the episodes in patients with nontemporal lobe epilepsy tend to be relatively brief and characterized primarily by confusional behavior or delirium. These conditions, then, are similar if not identical to the psychotic states associated with disturbances of consciousness which have been previously described. In contrast, those psychotic periods occurring in temporal lobe epileptics are more commonly longer lasting and associated with disorders of affect and fluctuating mood but without confusion or alterations in the level of consciousness.[29] The brief, at times periodic, psychosis not associated with overt temporal lobe seizures tends to have a duration ranging from days to weeks and to be difficult to differentiate from the "twilight states" because of problems in ascertaining the patient's level of consciousness.[17]

Psychotic-like episodes manifesting as dysphoric states (i.e., transient changes in mood which occur and then gradually diminish in intensity),[74,79] hypomanic states,[29] and depressive states[23,124] as well as the more common schizophreniform psychosis have been reported in patients with both generalized and temporal lobe seizures. Other conditions of psychotic proportions described in epileptics include prolonged or even chronic psychosis, paranoid syndromes, marked regressive psychosis, and manic-depressive psychosis.[17] The incidence of such disorders appears to be higher in epileptics than normally expected in the general population. Among patients with seizures, the frequency is highest among those with temporal lobe foci.

Any consideration of the general topic of psychosis and epilepsy must at least briefly touch upon the many etiologic theories. The reader is cautioned that, although a variety of hypotheses have been advanced, none have yet received definitive support. The major etiologic theories which have been adapted from Bruens[17] are as follows:

I. Epilepsy and psychosis are not directly related as there is a limited chance occurrence of two relatively common diseases. This chance combination theory has been largely discounted on the basis of epidemiologic data which suggests a higher than chance incidence of psychosis among epileptics.[16,110]

II. There is a direct causal relationship between epilepsy and psychosis which can be further subdivided into the following categories:

A. Psychosis is precipitated by seizures (usually chronic) in patients who are genetically predisposed to the development of a particular psychotic state (e.g., schizophrenia). As with the chance combination theory, epidemiologic studies do not provide strong support for this hypothesis as there tends to be very little evidence of hereditary predisposition in most cases of epilepsy related psychosis.[16,110]

B. The psychosis can be directly related to the epilepsy, in which case the following possibilities must be considered: (1) The psychosis results from an organic brain lesion which was caused by long-term poorly controlled seizures (i.e., overt seizures cause brain damage which in turn can result in psychosis). (2) The psychosis is a nonspecific organic condition which results from the underlying organic disorder which also underlies the epilepsy. (3) The psychosis is a behavioral manifestation of subcortical seizures which are not overtly apparent or demonstrated on the routine surface electrode EEG. (4) The psychosis is an emotional reaction to the seizure disorder and to its social ramifications.

A number of researchers have reported an inverse relationship between seizure frequency and degree of psychosis. Flor-Henry,[41] Standage and Fenton,[114] and Taylor[119] found that there was a higher incidence of psychosis in epileptic patients with destructive lesions when compared to a similar group with mesial sclerotic lesions (scars resulting from anoxia). These data do not provide strong support for theories 1 and 2 and, in fact, suggest that severity of epilepsy, at least as expressed by the frequency of seizures, is not related to psychosis. Some authors have suggested that the psychosis manifested by some epileptics, especially those with discharges in the deep temporal structures, is a reflection of subclinical seizures which are not overt and cannot be demonstrated with standard scalp EEG electrodes.[41] As the association between limbic structures and behavior and emotion have been well documented, it seems quite possible that the development of a schizophreniform psychosis does result from chronic subictal electrical discharges within the limbic system occurring over years. With our current lack of knowledge regarding the electrical status of deep brain structures both with psychosis and during a seizure, the theory that psychosis is a manifestation of undetected seizures remains speculative and in need of further investigation.

The early literature regarding the association of psychosis and epilepsy considered the psychiatric syndrome to be a functional emotional reaction to the physical and social stresses engendered by the seizures.[19] The basis of this theory seems sufficiently apparent that further elaboration here is unnecessary. More recently, researchers have taken a more organically oriented position and postulated that the psychosis associated with epilepsy is a psychogenic reaction to many years of experiencing the abnormal emotional phenomena, sensations, and clouded consciousness which are precipitated by seizure activity and unrelated to environmental reality.[16] Although this mechanism may well operate in some epileptic patients, the hypothesis cannot be universally applied as not all psychotic epileptics have this type of seizure (i.e., psychomotor with distinct aura) and not all temporal lobe epileptics develop psychosis.[93] Functional or psychogenic factors cannot be discounted in the explanation of any psychotic-like state in epileptics, but they do not appear to be the sole etiologic variable in all cases.

III. The psychosis results from anticonvulsant medication. There are two main theories regarding this hypothesis: (1) the theory that psychosis becomes more frequent and apparent upon "forced normalization" of the EEG with medication and (2) the theory that chronic anticonvulsant therapy itself may cause psychosis either through metabolic interference or a toxic effect upon mental functioning. The results of those studies which have concentrated on the "forced normalization" hypothesis[37,100,114] are in considerable disagreement and cannot be considered strong support for this theory. Reynolds[99,100] has suggested that anticonvulsant medication itself may lead to psychosis. His research has indicated a diminution of folic acid levels in the serum, red blood cells, and spinal fluid in treated epileptic patients, and he then suggested that the behavioral changes seen in epileptic psychosis might result from a similar depression of folate and B_{12} in brain tissue. Other researchers have been unable to replicate Reynold's observation that an improvement in emotional status associated with an increase in seizure frequency followed administration of folic acid.[113] There is currently no evidence that brain tissue levels of these substances are lower in psychotic epileptics than in similar nonpsychotic patients, and it appears quite improbable that metabolism of folic acid or B_{12} plays a direct role in the development of psychosis.[21,91,113]

It seems unlikely that actual drug toxicity is a significant factor in producing psychosis because of the lack of association between medication dosage and the incidence or severity of the psychosis[93] (although the potential toxicity of anticonvulsant drugs has been well documented and an occasional toxic psychosis undoubtedly occurs). Untreated epileptics also develop psychoses at least as frequently as treated patients.[7] Interestingly, there has been some limited evidence from the work of Reynolds and Travers that those patients treated with diphenylhydantoin and/or phenobarbital who demonstrated marked behavioral abnormalities tended to have higher serum phenytoin levels than did those without such symptoms.[101] Accordingly, this line of research should be pursued with replication and extension of the research design of Reynolds and Travers.

In summary, as would be expected in this complex neurologic-psychiatric disorder, no single hypothesized etiology has been consistently demonstrated to hold true for all cases and all conditions. It should be emphasized that several of the theories are consistent with the experimental data as we currently understand it and many of the theories are by no means mutually exclusive. In reviewing the literature, it is apparent that when studying the patient with epilepsy and psychosis, there is very frequently a history of prolonged anticonvulsant use and a less than completely controlled seizure disorder (often involving the temporal lobe limbic structures).[93] Secondly, one cannot discount the role played by the patient's environment and his psychologic reactions to both the epilepsy and its social limitations. It seems then, that the etiology of the psychosis in epileptic patients is a complex, multifaceted series of variables of both organic and psychogenic origin. The complicated interplay of physiologic, social, and psychologic factors undoubtedly varies from patient to patient and helps to explain both why some epileptics become psychotic and others do not and the disparate manifestations of the behavioral disturbance among patients with similar seizure and treatment histories. For more thorough reviews of this very interesting topic, see Bruens[17] and Pincus and Tucker.[93]

Characterologic Disorders

Among the traits most commonly ascribed to the "epileptic personality" previously mentioned were perseveration, excessive religiosity, paranoia, egocentric selfishness, impulsivity, mental slowness, emotional viscosity, circumstantiality, irritability, and mood fluctuations. There may be some agreement that such traits have a higher incidence among epileptics than among normal individuals; however, there are indications that these behavioral features are as common in other brain damaged individuals as in epileptic patients. There is now general consensus that these and similar traits do not constitute a symptom cluster deserving of the label "epileptic personality"[121] and that, in fact, there is no single characterologic disorder that is either typically found only among epileptics or is characteristic of epileptics as a group. The range of personality changes observed in epileptic patients appears to be as wide (and in many cases as variable) as that seen in either other neurologically impaired populations or among those with no discernible central nervous system disease.

Violence and/or impulsive behavior as well as sexual deviations, both often considered characterologic disorders, will be discussed in the section dealing with temporal lobe disorders because these changes are seen most commonly, if not almost exclusively, in those patients with temporal lobe or psychomotor seizure disorders.

Personality Changes Associated with Temporal Lobe Epilepsy

The nature and incidence of the behavioral changes associated with seizures localized within the temporal lobe and its limbic projection areas (hereafter referred to interchangeably by the terms temporal lobe or psychomotor seizures) are sufficiently interesting and frequent that this topic deserves special mention. On both theoretical and clinical grounds, the importance of the investigation of temporal lobe behavioral changes has been succinctly pointed out by Geschwind who refers to the use of temporal lobe epilepsy as a probe for research of the neurophysiology of human emotion.[46] The personality changes associated with temporal lobe seizures are of major medical importance as an investigative model and an introduction to the borderland between neurology and psychiatry.[8] Accordingly, in this section we will briefly review three behavioral changes commonly reported to occur in patients with temporal lobe epilepsy: (1) an increased incidence and severity of all emotional and behavioral changes, (2) alterations in sexuality, and (3) violent behavior.

General Behavioral and Personality Changes. As mentioned throughout this chapter, the incidence of virtually all behavioral and personality changes is higher among those patients with temporal lobe seizures than any other seizure group. Historically, researchers and clinicians have noted a relatively high incidence of a wide variety of psychiatric disorders among psychomotor epileptics, ranging from schizophrenic-like psychosis to characterologic and neurosis-like changes.[42,48,118,129] But there are also statistical comparisons of psychomotor and nonpsychomotor epileptics that have failed to find significant behavioral differences between the two groups.[86,111] Recent work by Blumer[12,13] and Rodin[104] suggests that these apparent contradictions may be accounted for by the high incidence of behavioral change seen in temporal lobe patients who have more than one type of seizure, whereas there are few significant differences when only one seizure type is present. Prominent among the behavioral changes noted both clinically and statistically are: (1) increased emotionality, (2) elation or euphoria, (3) depression, (4) anger and irritability, (5) hostility and aggressive behavior, (6) altered and compulsive behavior, (10) circumstantiality, (11) viscosity (i.e., stickiness in general mode of behavior), (12) hypergraphia, (13) religiosity, (14) overconcern with philosophy, (15) dependence and passivity, (16) lack of humor, and (17) paranoia.[129] Baer[8] in a study of patients with unilateral temporal lobe epilepsy found a lateralized distinction in behavior within the samples, with right temporal lobe patients being more overtly or externally emotional (i.e., aggressive, depressed, and labile), while patients with left temporal foci developed a characteristic ideational pattern of behavioral traits including religiosity, philosophical interest, belief in personal destiny, and hypergraphia. These findings provide support for the suggestion of previous studies[10,43] that distinctive behavioral and emotional changes are associated with focal right hemisphere lesions while language functions are affected with left hemisphere lesions.

Perhaps the most interesting and certainly the most clinically noteworthy behavioral change associated with temporal lobe epilepsy is the development in some patients of chronic paranoid hallucinatory states resembling schizophrenia which are often termed "schizophreniform psychosis."[9,61,94,120] Although this disorder is relatively rare, there is little doubt that it does occur.[12,96] The symptoms tend to resemble those of simple or paranoid schizophrenia. A careful history almost always reveals the onset of epileptic attacks many years prior to the appearance of the psychotic symptoms and the clinical examination demonstrates a relatively warm and basically appropriate affect in such patients, in contrast to "true" schizophrenia.[9] In addition, the hallucinations, when present in patients with temporal lobe epilepsy, tend to be visual or auditory in the form of noises or music, contrary to the voices and verbal comments on personal behavior more common in schizophrenics.[120] Accordingly, although the temporal lobe schizophreniform psychosis may overtly mimic true schizophrenia, the two conditions can usually be differentiated on the basis of the history and the nature of the symptoms elicited during examination.

Violence. Increased irritability, aggressiveness, and occasional violent outbursts are among the most common of the behavioral changes reported in patients with temporal lobe epilepsy. "Pathological aggressiveness" was noted in 38 percent of the psychomotor epileptics studied by Falconer,[37] while others have reported somewhat lower but still high incidence rates.[83] As previously described, this tendency has been found to be particularly characteristic of patients with seizure foci in the right hemisphere[8] and is also reported in other patients with right hemisphere lesions.[59] Like other epilepsy-related behavioral changes, impulsive-irritable behavior whether manifested as generalized irritability or as outbursts of abusive or even physically aggressive behavior develops gradually over a period of years.[12] Such episodes are characteristically noted during the confusional ictal and postictal phases, particularly in the patient who is restrained. Aggressive-irritable behavior, though observed, is distinctly less common during the later phase of the postictal stage.[70] In general, the typical episodic impulsive-irritable behavior pattern is a phenomenon of the interictal stage. This aggressiveness tends to occur on provocation, is directed toward the environment, is not associated with overt seizure phenomena, and tends to be recalled by the patient.[12]

Two primary lines of research have been followed in attempts to investigate this complicated sociomedical problem: one has been the study of increased frequency and levels of violence among temporal lobe epileptics, while the second involves a review of the frequency of EEG abnormalities (especially of the temporal lobe) among individuals known to be violent. Despite numerous controversies which have been well described by Pincus and Tucker,[93] the consensus of the literature does support the clinical impression that when social factors and the operational definition of "violence" are held relatively constant, there is an increase in aggressive and violent behavior among temporal lobe epileptics. The study of temporal lobe EEG abnormalities in violent individuals has been fraught with problems of patient selection and definition and the difficulty in establishing the diagnosis of temporal lobe seizures using routine scalp EEG. There have been some reports of a high incidence of epilepsy in prison populations and, despite some reservations, the theory that interictal episodes of violence do appear more frequently than expected in prisoners with temporal lobe epilepsy should not be ruled out.

Other researchers have noted an increased incidence of either temporal lobe epilepsy or evidence of cerebral dysfunction in known violent or aggressive individuals.[77,81,83] Such studies do support the hypothesis that some, but certainly not all, violent behavior may well have basic neuropsychologic determinants. The limbic structures are most readily implicated because of their known association with emotions and behavior. This also is consistent with the experimental evidence provided by neurologic and electroencephalographic studies. The reader must be cautioned that, as with all other behavioral changes associated with epilepsy, a unitary physiologic theory is untenable and careful attention must be given to the roles played by social and psychogenic factors.[58,103] Personality development, family dynamics, and socioeconomic factors undoubtedly exert a strong predisposing or supressing influence upon the exhibition of aggressive and violent behavior, whatever its basic etiology. Another example of abnormal aggressiveness, often termed the "episodic dyscontrol syndrome," will be discussed in detail in Chapter 14. For more comprehensive reviews of the possible etiologies of aggressive and violent behavior, see Mark and Erwin,[83] Valenstein,[123] and Fields and Sweet.[40]

Alterations in Sexual Behavior. Disturbances in sexual function have been described in epileptic patients, especially those with temporal lobe seizure foci. Both hyposexuality and hypersexuality have been described as well as a variety of odd, if not bizarre, sexual manifestations of ictal discharge. Global hyposexuality, at times to the point of total sexual disinterest and even impotence, has been considered as the most frequent sexual behavioral change associated with temporal lobe seizures.[14,45,62] The most significant feature of this problem is that it most typically represents a lack of development of normal sexual arousal and drive (hyposexuality), despite normal development of appropriate secondary sexual characteristics, and is not usually a true impotence.[15] Males and females appear to be equally affected. The onset of the sexual dysfunction seems to parallel the onset of the overt seizures and intervention, either with the use of medication or neurosurgery, may result in normal sexual interest and performance.

Though relatively less common, frank impotence (in contrast to a lack of sexual interest) has been described in temporal lobe epileptics.[62,63] Hierons[62] has postulated a reflex arc between the temporal lobe and the septum and hypothalamic structures which are known to be related to penile erection as a mechanism to explain this phenomenon physiologically. Experimental animal studies relating the amygdala to sexual arousal[69] and limbic structures to erection[80] provide support for this theory.

Other research has suggested a higher than expected incidence of a variety of sexual deviations among temporal lobe epileptics.[11,71] Among the disorders reported have been homosexuality, hypersexuality, transvestism, exhibitionism, and fetishism. In addition to these more stable interictal changes, perictal sexual auras, ictal sexual arousal (at times to the point of overt behavior including transvestism), and postictal sexuality have been recorded in the literature.

The presence of brain centers (particularly the septal area, anterior cingulate gyrus, hypothalamus, temporal lobe, and paracentral cortex) known to be associated with sexual behavior and their involvement in temporal lobe epilepsy undoubtedly explains the range of altered sexual behaviors seen in some temporal lobe patients. Blumer[15] provides a thorough overview of the neural bases of sexual behavior and further description of the range of behaviors seen.

EVALUATION

The medical evaluation of the patient with suspected or known epilepsy is very similar to the evaluation of any patient with brain dysfunction. A careful family and medical history is necessary to obtain information regarding the seizure or behaviors suggestive of seizure activity (e.g., lapses in awareness, periods of eye blinking) both from the patient himself and from members of his family. Specific attention should be given to objective and subjective events occurring before (i.e., aura and prodrome), during (i.e., ictal phenomonon), and after (e.g., postictal confusion) the seizure. Seizure type, frequency, and possible precipitating events or stresses should be investigated. Similarly, the possible association between the seizures and drug ingestion (including alcohol) must be thoroughly evaluated.

The neurologic evaluation of the epileptic is relatively routine. However, as epilepsy is a specialized disorder, few primary care physicians are experienced with its many and oftentimes complex presentations. Because of the rapidly changing recent advances in medical treatment,[39] neurologic consultation may be very valuable. The neurologist can be of great assistance in the initial evaluation, differential diagnosis, and institution of the appropriate medication regimen.

The electroencephalogram is, of course, the neurodiagnostic test of choice in evaluating the epileptic patient. The routine EEG should include recording periods during which the patient is awake but calm, drowsy, asleep, hyperventilating, and photically stimulated. These latter activation procedures may precipitate abnormalities in the resting or sleeping EEG which are absent in the waking record. The sleep EEG is very important in evaluating temporal lobe epilepsy because a significantly higher incidence of abnormalities are seen during sleep. If abnormal activity is strongly suspected, specialized EEG procedures such as the use of nasopharygeal leads or, in extreme cases, Metrazol activation may be necessary to elicite abnormal electrical activity which is not apparent on routine studies. Repeat EEGs are also of value when the spike focus in a known epileptic cannot be demonstrated on the initial recording by any of the above procedures.

In addition to the EEG, routine skull x-rays, CT scan of the brain, serum electrolyte determinations including calcium level, and complete blood count should be obtained. In some cases, spinal puncture and more invasive radiologic tests (e.g., arteriogram) are indicated.

This is obviously a very sketchy overview of the medical evaluation of the epileptic; it can and should be augmented by reference to standard neurologic texts.

As we have repeated throughout this chapter, behavioral factors are critically important in epilepsy, as they may (1) serve as precipitants of seizures, (2) mimic a "true" seizure disorder (i.e., hysterical seizures), (3) be a partial or even the sole manifestation of a seizure, or (4) serve as significant obstacles to successful emotional, social, and vocational adjustment. Accordingly, the neurobehavioral evaluation is essential in all patients with epilepsy. The minimal evaluation should consist of the complete mental status examination as outlined in Chapter 3 and elsewhere.[116] In more complex cases or in situations in which psychogenic variables are obvious factors, consultation for a more thorough neuropsychologic and psychiatric evaluation is valuable. This evaluation can be of considerable aid in: (1) contributing to the differential diagnosis, (2) assessment and description of the behavioral aspects of the seizure disorder, (3) documenting the degree of the role of psychogenic and organic factors in the patient's seizures and life adjustment, (4) evaluation of emotional and cognitive abilities and deficits for use in rehabilitation measures, and (5) documenting by repeated testing the effects of medical (anticonvulsant medication) or surgical (excision of seizure foci in intractable seizures) treatment of the seizure disorder. Full description of the neuropsychologic evaluation and its clinical and research uses is available.[53,78,98,116]

MANAGEMENT

As with most of the neurologic conditions discussed in this volume, the two components of the management of the epileptic patient are: (1) medical control of the actual seizure disorder and (2) psychosocial management of the psychologic, social, and vocational problems experienced by many such patients. All too often, the sole emphasis in treatment is upon the first category of management, much to the detriment of the patient's overall adjustment. The complex often multifaceted nature of the problems experienced by the epileptic patient must be carefully considered in the organization of the total management program and all necessary specialists and treatment modalities should be consulted and instituted as early as is feasible.

It is not our intent to provide more than a cursory introduction to both medical and psychosocial treatment of the epilepsies. Complete information is readily available in all medical school curricula and in numerous standard texts.[39,92,104,105,112,127] Some patients will respond well to a single medication (often with dosage manipulation to maximize seizure control and minimize side effects), while others will require a careful combination of two or more anticonvulsant drugs with changes over time. Some patients will appear relatively intractable until careful observation (at times in the hospital) and monitoring of drug compliance and serum drug levels and manipulation of medication dose levels and social factors result in adequate control. It should be emphasized that the majority of seizure patients obtain complete or good control with medication; only a small number (5 to 10%) of patients fail to receive significant benefit.

Patients with a high frequency of seizures which are intractable to medication and result in a significant disruption of social and vocational adjustment may, after careful study, be candidates for neurosurgical intervention. Two basic approaches have been utilized: (1) the excision of a well localized seizure focus (often temporal lobe)[36,37,97] and (2) cerebral commissurotomy to limit the spread of electrical discharge from an epileptogenic hemisphere to the contralateral one.[126] Another relatively recent neurosurgical approach has been that of cerebellar stimulation in an effort to augment the brain's innate mechanisms of seizure inhibition. The long-term efficacy of this procedure remains uncertain[18] despite encouraging results in some patients.[20] It should be apparent that these procedures are extreme, include risk of both morbidity and mortality to the patients, and are not universally effective even when all precautions are taken. They must be considered only for those patients who (1) have failed to respond to long-term concerted efforts to control the seizures through all other available modalities and (2) are unable to live satisfactory lives because of the severity of their seizure disorders.

The psychosocial management of the epileptic patient has been directed toward: (1) attempts to reduce seizure frequency through behavior modification and alleviating possibly precipitant stress factors by environmental manipulation (or eliminating seizures entirely as in the case of "hysterical seizures"), (2) helping the patient to deal with the psychogenic associations and ramifications of the seizure disorder by the use of various modes of psychotherapy, and (3) planning comprehensive social, educational, vocational and rehabilitation programs for patients in need of such services. The adjunctive use of behavior modification has shown some early encouraging results in reducing the frequency of stress-induced and reflex epilepsy but has not yet proven efficacious in all seizure types or patients. An excellent current review of this approach has been provided by Feldman and Ricks.[38] The methods of ancillary psychotherapy and rehabilitation programs are very similar to those described in previous sections of this volume and comprehensive resource material covering this essential component of the total management of the epileptic patient is readily available.[96,103,116,128]

REFERENCES

1. Adebimpe, V.R.: Complex partial seizures simulating schizophrenia. JAMA 237:1339, 1977.
2. Aggernaes, M.: The differential diagnosis between hysterical and epileptic disturbances of consciousness or twilight states. Acta Psychiatr. Scand. [Suppl.] 185:9, 1965.
3. American Psychiatric Association: Diagnostic and Statistical Manual of Mental Disorders (DSM II). American Psychiatric Association, Washington, 1968.
4. American Psychiatric Association: Diagnostic and Statistical Manual of Mental Disorders (DSM III). American Psychiatric Association, Washington, 1980.
5. Andermann, F., and Robb, M.P.: Absence status. Epilepsia 13:177, 1971.
6. Angers, W.P.: Patterns of abilities and capacities in the epileptic. J. Genet. Psychol. 103:59, 1963.
7. Asuni, T., and Pillutla, U.S.: Schizophrenia-like psychosis in Nigerian epileptics. Br. J. Psychiatry 113:1375, 1967.
8. Bear, D.: The significance of behavior change in temporal lobe epilepsy. McLean Hospital Journal (Special Issue). 1977, pp. 9–21.
9. Beard, A.W., and Slater, E.: The schizophrenic-like psychosis of epilepsy. Proc. R. Soc. Med. 55:311, 1962.
10. Black, F.W.: Unilateral brain lesions and MMPI performances: A preliminary study. Percept. Mot. Skills 40:87, 1975.
11. Blumer, D.: Transsexualism, and sexual dysfunction, and temporal lobe disorder, in Green, R, and Money, J. (eds.): Transexualism and Sexual Reassignment. John Hopkins Press, Baltimore, 1969.
12. Blumer, D.: Temporal lobe epilepsy and its psychiatric significance, in Benson, D.F., and Blumer, D. (eds.): Psychiatric Aspects of Neurologic Disease. Grune & Stratton, New York, 1975, pp. 171–198.
13. Blumer, D.: Treatment of patients with seizure disorder referred because of psychiatric complication. McLean Hospital Journal (Special Issue) 1977, pp. 53–73.
14. Blumer, D., and Levin, K.: Psychiatric complications in the epilepsies: Current research and treatment. McLean Hospital Journal (Special Issue) 1977, pp. 4–103.
15. Blumer, D., and Walker, A.E.: The neural basis of sexual behavior, in Benson, D.F., and Blumer, D. (eds.): Psychiatric Aspects of Neurologic Disease. Grune & Stratton, New York, 1975, pp. 199–217.
16. Bruens, J.H.: Psychosis in epilepsy. Psychiatr. Neurol. Neurosurg. 74:175, 1971.
17. Bruens, J.H.: Psychosis in epilepsy, in Vinken, P.J., and Bruyn, G.W.: The Epilepsies, Vol. 15 in Handbook of Clinical Neurology. Elsevier-North Holland Publishing Co., New York, 1974, pp. 593–610.

18. Check, W.: Brain stimulation for seizures, spasticity needs better evaluation. JAMA 239:915, 1978.
19. Clark, R.A., and Lesko, J.M.: Psychoses associated with epilepsy. Am. J. Psychiatry 96:595, 1939.
20. Cooper, L.S., Amin, I., Gilman, S, and Waltz, J.M.: The effects of chronic stimulation of cerebellar cortex in man, in Cooper, I.S., Riklam, M., and Snider, R.S. (eds.): The cerebellum, epilepsy and behavior. Plenum Press, New York, 1974, pp. 119–171.
21. Cramer, J.A., Mattson, R.H., and Brillman, J.: Folinic acid therapy in epilepsy. Fed. Proc. 35:582, 1976.
22. Daly, D.D.: Ictal clinical manifestations of complex partial seizures, in Penry, J.K., and Daly, D.D. (eds.): Complex Partial Seizures and Their Treatment, Vol. 11 in Advances in Neurology. Raven Press, New York, 1975.
23. Delay, J., Deniker, P., and Baraude, R.: Lesuicide des epileptiques. Encephale 46:401, 1957.
24. Dennerll, R.D.: Cognitive deficits and lateral brain dysfunction in temporal lobe epilepsy. Epilepsia 5:177, 1964.
25. Dikmen, S., and Matthews, C.G.: Effect of major motor seizure frequency upon cognitive-intellectual functions in adults. Epilepsia 18:21, 1977.
26. Dikmen, S., Matthews, C.G., and Harley, J.P.: The effect of early versus late onset of major motor epilepsy upon cognitive-intellectual performances. Epilepsia 16:73, 1975.
27. Dodrill, C. B.: Diphenylhydantoin serum levels, toxicity and neuropsychological performance in patients with epilepsy. Epilepsia 16:593, 1975.
28. Dodrill, C. B., and Troupin, A. S.: Psychotropic effects of carbamazepine in epilepsy: A double-blind comparison with phenytoin. Neurology 27:1023, 1977.
29. Dongier, S.: Statistical study of clinical and electroencephalographic manifestations of 536 psychiatric episodes occurring in 516 epileptics between clinical seizures. Epilepsia 1:117, 1959.
30. Dreifuss, F.E.: The nature of epilepsy, in Wright, G.N. (ed.): Epilepsy Rehabilitation. Little, Brown and Company, Boston, 1975, pp. 8–27.
31. Efron, R.: Post-epileptic paralysis: Theoretical critique and report of a case. Brain 84:381, 1961.
32. Ellis, J.M., and Lee, S.I.: Acute prolonged confusion in later life as an ictal state. Epilepsia 19:119, 1977.
33. Epilepsy Foundation of America: Basic Statistics on the Epilepsies. F.A. Davis Company, Philadelphia, 1975.
34. Epstein, M.H., and O'Connor, J.S.: Destructive effects of prolonged status epilepticus. J. Neurol. Neurosurg. Psychiatry 29:251, 1966.
35. Escueta, A.V., Boxley, J., Stubbs, N., Waddel, G., and Wilson, W.A.: Prolonged twilight state and automatisms: A case report. Neurology 24:331, 1974.
36. Falconer, M.A.: Clinical, radiological and EEG correlations with pathological changes in temporal lobe epilepsy and their significance in surgical treatment, in Baldwin, M., and Bailey, P. (eds.): Temporal Lobe Epilepsy. Charles C Thomas, Springfield, Illinois, 1958, p. 396.
37. Falconer, M.A., and Taylor, D.C.: Surgical treatment of drug resistant epilepsy due to mesial temporal sclerosis. Arch. Neurol. 18:353, 1968.
38. Feldman, R.G., and Ricks, N.L.: Neuropharmacologic and behavioral methods, in Ferris, G.W. (ed.): The Treatment of Epilepsy Today. Medical Economics Co., Oradell, New Jersey, 1978, pp. 89–111.

39. Ferris, G.W.: Treatment of Epilepsy Today. Medical Economics Co., Oradell, N.J., 1978.
40. Fields, W.S., and Sweet, W.H.: The neural basis for violence and aggression. Warren H. Green, Inc., Saint Louis, 1975.
41. Flor-Henry, P.: Psychosis and temporal lobe epilepsy. Epilepsia 10:363, 1969.
42. Flor-Henry, P.: Ictal and interictal psychiatric manifestations in epilepsy: Specific or non-specific? Epilepsia 13:773, 1972.
43. Gainotti, G.: Emotional behavior and hemispheric side of the lesion. Cortex 8:41, 1972.
44. Gastaut, H.: Clinical and electroencephalographical classification of epileptic seizures. Epilepsia 11:102, 1970.
45. Gastaut, H., and Colomb, H.: Étude du comportement sexual chez les epileptiques psychomoteurs. Ann. Med. Psychol. (Paris) 112:657, 1954.
46. Geschwind, N.: Current research: Introduction. McLean Hospital Journal (Special Issue), 1977, pp. 6–8.
47. Gibberd, F.B.: Petit mal status presenting in middle age. Lancet 1:269, 1972.
48. Gibbs, F.A.: Ictal and nonictal psychiatric disorders in temporal lobe epilepsy. J. Nerv. Ment. Dis. 113:522, 1951.
49. Gibbs, F.A., Gibbs, E.L., and Lennox, W.G.: Likeness of cortical dysrhythmias of schizophrenia and psychomotor epilepsy. Am. J. Psychiatry 95:255, 1938.
50. Glasser, G.H.: Epilepsy, hysteria and possession. J. Nerv. Ment. Dis. 166: 268, 1978.
51. Gloor, P., and Feindel, W.: Affective behavior and the temporal lobe, in Monnier, M. (ed.): Physiologie und Pathophysiologie des Vegetativen Nervensystems. Pathophysiologie, Hippokrates-Verlag, Stuttgart, 1963, pp. 685–716.
52. Glowinski, H.: Cognitive deficits in temporal lobe epilepsy. J. Nerv. Ment. Dis. 153:129, 1973.
53. Golden, C.J.: Diagnosis and Rehabilitation in Clinical Neuropsychology. Charles C Thomas, Springfield, Illinois, 1978.
54. Goldin, G.J., and Margolin, R.J.: The psychosocial aspects of epilepsy, in Wright, G.N. (ed.): Epilepsy Rehabilitation. Little Brown and Company, Boston, 1975, pp. 66–80.
55. Gudmandsson, G.: Epilepsy in Iceland. Acta Neurol. Scand. [Suppl.] 25:43, 1966.
56. Gunn, J.: Epileptic homicide: A case report. Br. J. Psychiatry 132:510, 1978.
57. Gunn, J.: Evaluation of violence. Proc. R. Soc. Med. 66:1133, 1973.
58. Harbin, H.T.: Episodic dyscontrol and family dynamics. Am. J. Psychiatry 134:1113, 1977.
59. Hecaen, H.: Clinical symptomatology in right and left hemisphere lesions, in Mountcastle, V. (ed.): Interhemispheric Relations and Cerebral Dominance. Johns Hopkins Press, Baltimore, 1962, pp. 215–243.
60. Hecker, A, Andermann, F, and Rodin, E.A.: Spitting automatism in temporal lobe seizures. Epilepsia 13:767, 1972.
61. Herrington, R.N. (ed.): Schizophrenia, epilepsy, the temporal lobe. Current problems in neuropsychiatry. Br. J. Psychiatry Special publication No. 4, 1969.
62. Hierons, R.: Impotence in temporal lobe lesions. J. Neuro-Visceral Relations Suppl X, 1971, pp. 477–481.

63. Hierons, R., and Saunders, M.: Impotence in patients with temporal lobe lesions. Lancet 2:761, 1966.
64. Jackson, J.H.: Selected writings of John Hughlings Jackson (Taylor, J., ed.), Vol. 1. Basic Books, New York, 1958, p. 500.
65. Janz, D.: Die Epilepsien. G. Thieme, Stuttgart, 1969.
66. Jasper, H.H.: Some physiological mechanisms involved in epileptic automatisms. Epilepsia 5:1, 1964.
67. Jüül-Jensen, P.: Social prognosis, in Vinken, P.J., and Bruyn, G.W. (eds.): The Epilepsies, Vol. 15 in Handbook of Clinical Neurology. Elsevier-North Holland Publishing Company, New York, 1974, pp. 800–814.
68. Kløve, H., and Matthews, C.G.: Psychometric and adaptive abilities in epilepsy with differential etiology. Epilepsia 7:330, 1966.
69. Klüver, H., and Bucy, P.C.: Preliminary analysis of functions of the temporal lobes in monkeys. Arch. Neurol. Psychiatry 42:979, 1939.
70. Knox, S.J.: Epileptic automatism and violence. Med. Sci. Law 8:96, 1968.
71. Kolorsky, A., Freund, K., Machek, J., and Polak, O.: Male sexual deviation. Arch. Gen. Psychiatry 17:735, 1967.
72. Kurland, L.T.: The incidence and prevalence of convulsive disorders in a small urban community. Epilepsia 1:143, 1959.
73. Kurtzke, J.F., Kurland, L.T., Goldberg, I.D., Choi, N.W., and Reeder, F.A.: Convulsive disorders, in Kurland, L.T., Kurtzke, J.F., and Goldberg, I.D. (eds.): Epidemiology of Neurologic and Sense Organ Disorders (American Public Health Association Monograph) Harvard University Press, Cambridge, Massachusetts, 1973.
74. Landolt, H.: Serial-EEG investigation during psychotic episodes in epileptic patients and during schizophrenic attacks, in Lorentz de Haas, A.M. (ed.): Lectures on Epilepsy. Elsevier-North Holland Publishing Co., New York, 1958, pp. 91–133.
75. Lennox, W.G.: The treatment of epilepsy. Med. Clin. North Am. 29:1114, 1945.
76. Lennox, W.G.: Epilepsy and Related Disorders, Vol. 2. Little, Brown and Company, Boston, 1960.
77. Lewis, D.O.: Delinquency, psychomotor epileptic symptomatology and paranoid symptomatology: A triad. Am. J. Psychiatry 133:1395, 1976.
78. Lezak, M.D.: Neuropsychological Assessment. Oxford University Press, New York, 1976.
79. Lorentz de Haas, A.M., and Magnus, O.: Clinical and electro-encephalographic findings in epileptic patients with episodic mental disorders, in Lorentz de Haas, A.M. (ed.): Lectures on Epilepsy. Elsevier-North Holland Publishing Co., New York, 1958, pp. 134–167.
80. MacLean, P.D., and Ploog, D.W.: Cerebral representation of penile erection. J. Neurophysiol. 25:29, 1962.
81. Maletzky, B.M.: The episodic dyscontrol syndrome. Dis. Nerv. Sys. 34:178, 1973.
82. Marchand, L., and DeAjuriaguerra, J.: Epilepsies, leurs formes cliniques ex leurs traitements. Desclee de Brouwer et Cie, Paris, 1948.
83. Mark, V.H., and Ervin, F.R.: Violence and the Brain. Harper and Row, New York, 1970.
84. Masland, R.L.: The classification of the epilepsies, in Vinken, P.J., and Bruyn, G.W. (eds.): The Epilepsies, Vol. 15 in Handbook of Clinical Neurology. Elsevier-North Holland Publishing Co., New York, 1974, pp. 1–29.

85. Matthews, C.G., and Kløve, H.: Differential psychological performances in major motor, psychomotor, and mixed seizure classifications of known and unknown etiology. Epilepsia 8:117, 1967.

86. Matthews, C.G., and Kløve, H.: MMPI performances in major motor, psychomotor and mixed seizure classifications of known and unknown etiology. Epilepsia 9:43, 1968.

87. Merlis, J.K.: Reflex epilepsy, in Vinken, P.J., and Bruyn, G.W. (eds.): The Epilepsies, Vol. 15 in Handbook of Clinical Neurology. Elsevier-North Holland Publishing Company, New York, 1974, pp. 440–456.

88. Meyer, J.S., and Portnoy, H.D.: Post-epileptic paralysis. Brain 82:162, 1959.

89. Milner, B.: Psychological defect produced by temporal lobe excision. Res. Publ. Assoc. Res. Nerv. Ment. Dis. 36:244, 1956.

90. Mirsky, A.F., Primac, D.W., Marsan, C.C., Rosvold, H.E., and Stevens, J.R.: A comparison of the psychological test performance of patients with focal and nonfocal epilepsy. Exp. Neurol. 2:75, 1960.

91. Norris, J.W., and Pratt, R.F.: A controlled study of folic acid in epilepsy. Neurology 21:659, 1971.

92. Penry, J.K., and Daly, D.D. (eds.): Complex Partial Seizures and their Treatment. Adv. Neurol. 11: 1975.

93. Pincus, J.H., and Tucker, G.J.: Behavioral Neurology. Oxford University Press, New York, 1978.

94. Pond, D.A.: Psychiatric aspects of epilepsy. J. Indian Med. Prof. 3:1401, 1957.

95. Pond, D.A.: The influence of psychophysiological factors on epilepsy. J. Psychosom. Res. 9:15, 1965.

96. Pond, D.A.: Epilepsy and personality disorders, in Vinken, P.J., and Bruyn, G.W. (eds.): The Epilepsies, Vol. 15 in Handbook of Clinical Neurology. Elsevier-North Holland Publishing Co., New York, 1974, pp. 576–592.

97. Rasmussen, T.: Surgical treatment of patients with complex partial seizures. Adv. Neurol. 11:415, 1975.

98. Reitan, R.M.: Psychological testing of epileptic patients, in Vinken P.J., and Bruyn, G.W. (eds.): The Epilepsies, Vol. 15 in Handbook of Clinical Neurology. Elsevier-North Holland Publishing Co., New York, 1974, pp. 559–575.

99. Reynolds, E.H.: Schizophrenia-like psychoses of epilepsy and disturbances of folate and vitamin B_{12} metabolism induced by anticonvulsant medication. Br. J. Psychiatry 113:911, 1967.

100. Reynolds, E.H.: Anticonvulsant drugs, folic acid metabolism, fit frequency and psychiatric illness. Psychit. Neurol. Neurochirg. 76:167, 1971.

101. Reynolds, E.H., and Travers, R.D.: Serum anticonvulsant concentrations in epileptic patients with mental symptoms. Br. J. Psychiatry 124:440, 1974.

102. Rodin, E.A.: The Prognosis of Patients with Epilepsy. Charles C Thomas, Springfield, Illinois, 1968.

103. Rodin, E.A.: Psychomotor epilepsy and aggressive behavior. Arch. Gen. Psychiatry 28:210, 1973.

104. Rodin, E.A.: Psychosocial management of patients with complex partial seizures. Adv. Neurol. 11:383, 1975.

105. Rodin, E.A.: Psychosocial management of patients with seizure disorders. McLean Hospital Journal (Special Issue), 1977, pp. 74–84.

106. Roger, J., Lob, H., and Tassinari, C.A.: Generalized status epilepticus expressed as a confusional state (petit mal status or absence status epilepticus), in Vinken, P.J., and Bruyn, G.W. (eds.): The Epilepsies, Vol. 15 in Handbook of Clinical Neurology. Elsevier-North Holland Publishing Company, New York, 1974, pp. 167–175.

107. Sarason, S.B., and Doris, J.: Psychological Problems in Mental Deficiency. Harper & Row, New York, 1969.

108. Schmidt, R.P., and Wilder, B.J.: Epilepsy. F.A. Davis, Philadelphia, 1968.

109. Shev, E.E.: Syndrome of petit mal status in the adult. Electroencephalogr. Clin. Neurophysiol. 17:466, 1964.

110. Slater, E., Beard, A., and Glithero, E.: The schizophrenia-like psychoses in epilepsy. Br. J. Psychiatry 109:95, 1963.

111. Small, J.G., Small, L.F., and Hayden, M.P.: Further psychiatric investigations of patients with temporal and nontemporal lobe epilepsy. Am. J. Psychiatry 123:303, 1966.

112. Solomon, G.E., and Plum, F.: Clinical Management of Seizures. W.B. Saunders, Co., Philadelphia, 1976.

113. Spaans, F.: Epilepsie en foliamzuur. Thesis, Amsterdam, 1970.

114. Standage, K.F., and Fenton, G.W.: Psychiatric symptom profiles of patients with epilepsy. Psychol. Med. 5:152, 1975.

115. Stores, G., Hart, J., and Piran, N.: Inattentiveness in school children with epilepsy. Epilepsia 19:169, 1978.

116. Strub, R.L., and Black, F.W.: The Mental Status Examination in Neurology, F.A. Davis Co., Philadelphia, 1977.

117. Szondi, L.: Schicksalsanalytische, Therapie. Huber, Bern, 1963.

118. Taylor, D.C.: Mental state and temporal lobe epilepsy. Epilepsia 13:727, 1972.

119. Taylor, D.C.: Facts influencing the occurrance of schizophrenia-like psychosis in patients with temporal lobe epilepsy. Psychol. Med. 5:249, 1975.

120. Taylor, D.C.: Epileptic experience, schizophrenia and the temporal lobe. McLean Hospital Journal (Special Issue), 1977, pp. 22–39.

121. Tizard, B.: The personality of epileptics: A discussion of the evidence. Psychol. Bull. 59:196, 1962.

122. Tregold, A.F., and Soddy, K. (eds.): Textbook of Mental Deficiency. Bailliere, Tindall and Cox, London, 1963.

123. Valenstein, E.S.: Brain Control. John Wiley and Sons, New York, 1973.

124. Weil, A.: Ictal depression and anxiety in temporal lobe disorders. Am. J. Psychiatry 113:149, 1956.

125. Wells, C.E.: Transient ictal psychosis. Arch. Gen. Psychiatry 32:1201, 1975.

126. Wilson, D.H., Reeves, A., Gazzaniga, M., and Culver, C.: Cerebral commissurotomy for control of intractable seizures. Neurology 27:708, 1977.

127. Wright, G.N. (ed.): Epilepsy Rehabilitation. Little, Brown and Company, Boston, 1975.

128. Wright, G.N.: Rehabilitation and the problem of epilepsy, in Wright, G.N. (ed.): Epilepsy Rehabilitation. Little, Brown, and Company, Boston, 1975, pp. 1–7.

129. Bear, D.M.: Temporal lobe epilepsy—a syndrome of sensory-limbic hyperconnection. Cortex 15:357, 1979.

12

CEREBROVASCULAR DISEASE

C.H., a 63-year-old hypertensive woman, was admitted to the Charity Hospital in New Orleans because of the recent abrupt appearance of paranoid and abusive behavior. Her husband reported that they often fought but that on the day of admission she was totally irrational and believed that he was trying to kill her. In response to this false belief, she attacked her husband with a knife. The police were called and she was admitted to the hospital in a most agitated state.

On initial examination, she was raving incoherently yet was also intermittently lethargic. Her paranoid delusions persisted and on occasion she claimed she saw her husband lurking in the hall outside her ward despite numerous assurances that he had returned home. The initial diagnostic impression of the admitting psychiatrist was a confusional state due either to a metabolic imbalance or a toxic effect from medication. Subsequent laboratory and toxicology screenings proved negative and accordingly we were consulted.

When we first saw her, she had calmed considerably. She was still quite lethargic but was more attentive than she had been on admission. Her speech was fluent and had lost much of its paranoid content, but she had definite word finding difficulty and produced several rather garbled words that sounded paraphasic. Comprehension was intact for general conversational questions. However, she did not understand more exacting questions such as "Is a fork good for eating soup?" or "Is a hammer good for chopping wood?" She also could not point accurately on command to objects in the room. Repetition was marked by hesitation and paraphasias, particularly when the sentence contained many nouns and transitive verbs. Naming was grossly paraphasic. Visual memory was good, drawings were impaired, and most other cortical testing was invalid because of the patient's aphasia.

Because of the rather clear-cut aphasia, we strongly suspected that the patient had an infarction or hemorrhage in the left temporoparietal area. A brain scan was obtained which showed a wedge-shaped infarct in the appropriate area. The confusional state and paranoia cleared quickly over the following few days and the patient was left with only a mild anomic aphasia.

The above case demonstrates the rather typical organic behavioral change seen in occlusive cerebrovascular disease. The patients are often confusional at the onset and may be misdiagnosed as having a metabolic or toxic encephalopathy unless outstanding neurologic findings such as a hemiplegia are present. Frequently, a careful mental status examination of the confusional patient will reveal focal behavioral findings (e.g., aphasia, neglect, or denial) that are out of proportion to the changes seen with confusional behavior alone. The elucidation of such focal symptoms changes the entire diagnostic approach.

This case demonstrates one of the myriad ways in which cerebrovascular disease can produce behavioral symptoms. For a comprehensive discussion of the behavioral changes seen in cerebrovascular disease, see Benton's fine text.[4] The primary purpose of this chapter is to emphasize the fact that such behavioral changes are a common presenting symptom in vascular disease and must be appreciated for their importance both in diagnosis and patient management. Since cerebrovascular disease ranks third among the most frequent causes of death from medical disease in America, every physician will encounter its effects regularly. The possibility of a cerebrovascular accident or transient ischemic attack (TIA) is high in any patient as he ages but particularly in patients with hypertension, heart disease, diabetes, gout, and peripheral vascular disease. As seen in the case above, the symptoms of a stroke may be manifested solely as a radical change in the patient's behavior, without the usual "hard" neurologic findings.

Each year in the United States, over 150,000 people die of various types of stroke, and a significant number of new cases are reported.[11] A clearer picture of the true significance of this problem is gained when the general mortality figure is broken down according to age, sex, race, and type of stroke. In deaths per million, Caucasian males have a mortality rate of 811 while females have 713. Nonwhites show a ratio of 1300 males to 1311 females per million.[20] The incidence of new cases of stroke per year has an expected direct relationship to age, with 2,500 to 7,200 strokes per million population occurring in the 55 to 65 year age range, 6,000 to 12,000 per million in the 65 to 75 year range, and 15,000 to 25,000 per million in individuals over the age of 75.[19] There are many types of stroke and the incidence figures always suffer from the combining of subgroups, however some breakdown has been made to separate cases into the major categories: 65 to 80 percent of all strokes are caused by thromboembolic disease, 10 to 15 percent by intracerebral hemorrhage, 5 to 10 percent by subarachnoid hemorrhage, and 5 to 10 percent by other less common disorders.[11,19]

Another very important aspect of cerebrovascular disease is the tremendous social impact which it has on its victims and their families. The patient is frequently left mentally as well as physically compromised.[1] Employment may no longer be possible. The patient's family and the community at large (as tax payers) are asked to share in the major financial burden of rehabilitation and maintenance. It should be the goal of every physician to learn to recognize the warning signals and risk factors in cerebrovascular disease and to identify and treat these conditions before irreversible brain damage occurs.

DESCRIPTION OF THE CLINICAL SYNDROMES

There are many types of cerebrovascular disease but by far the most common are thromboembolic disease secondary to atherosclerosis and hypertensive cerebrovascular disease with intracerebral hemorrhage. With increased age, fatty deposits collect on the endothelium of major blood vessels throughout the vascular system. These deposits occur at any point along the major vessels but are particularly likely to occur at points of bifurcation. Atheromatous plaques are commonly found in the carotid and vertebral vessels and these are important locations of narrowing, thrombosis, and subsequent stroke. In the region of the bifurcation of the common carotid in the neck, large plaques often form and become ulcerated. Within the cavities of these ulcers, platelets commonly aggregate and often embolize to the brain causing an acute cerebral infarct. A second source of cerebral embolism is the heart. Patients with recent myocardial infarction often form mural thrombi over the area of infarction; pieces of these clots frequently embolize to the brain. By the above mechanisms, most of the focal cortical stroke syndromes occur.

Hypertensive vascular disease with cerebral hemorrhage is somewhat different since the hemorrhages usually occur deep in the brain, most commonly in the corpus striatum, thalamus, cerebellum, or pons. The syndrome resulting from these lesions is usually more devastating neurologically than it is behaviorally since the cortex is relatively spared. The major behavioral feature of deep cerebral hemorrhage is a decrease in the level of alertness of the patient with associated confusion.

Vascular disease can present as any of the primary clinical behavioral syndromes and must always be considered in the differential diagnosis in any patient presenting with confusional behavior, dementia, or focal symptomatology. In previous chapters, we have discussed some of the behavioral aspects of many of the vascular diseases commonly seen in clinical practice and we will not reiterate them here other than to identify them in tabular form (Table 12-1).

Two very important specific clinical features of vascular disease are (1) its frequent sudden onset and (2) the common occurrence of warning symptoms (transient ischemic attacks) that precede the ictus and mimic the actual attack. Transient ischemic attacks (TIA) are often the harbinger of a major cerebrovascular accident and quite frequently the TIA is characterized by behavioral symptoms alone. Transient aphasia, agraphia, amnesia, geographic disorientation, and confusion are all well described in the literature and frequently seen clinically.[9,12] Such symptoms should always be taken seriously and the patient investigated fully. Although TIAs are most common in older patients with atheromatous disease of their major cerebral vessels, identical symptoms can be seen in younger patients with arteriovenous malformations, aneurysms which have leaked causing vascular spasm, collagen vascular disease, and migraine. We saw one 18-year-old girl with a migraine attack that presented with a clinical picture similar to that of the case described at the beginning of this chapter. She became acutely confusional and could only scream, hold her head, and mumble incoherently. Within several hours, her confusion began to clear and

TABLE 12–1. Behavioral Syndromes and Symptoms Seen with Cerebrovascular Disease

Symptoms	Causes
Confusional states and/or delirium	1. Acute vascular occlusion 2. Transient ischemia: Focal, particularly limbic, or whole brain secondary to bilateral carotid stenosis 3. Subarachnoid hemorrhage 4. Acute systemic lupus erythematosus 5. Subdural hematoma 6. Intracerebral hemorrhage 7. Hypoxia during surgery or arteriography
Dementia	1. Multiple infarcts 2. Borderzone atrophy (granular atrophy) 3. Rare cases of bilateral severe extracranial vessel stenosis 4. Binswanger's disease 5. Systemic lupus erythematosus 6. Subdural hematoma
Focal symptomatology	1. Infarct: Extracranial or intracranial occlusion, embolus, vasculitis 2. Intracerebral hemorrhage 3. Subdural or epidural hemorrhage 4. Hemorrhage from aneurysm or arteriovenous malformation

she demonstrated significantly paraphasic speech and poor comprehension. Ten hours after the onset, she had recovered and the mental status examination was completely normal.

Another vascular condition which can result in either transient or permanent vascular symptoms is systemic lupus erythematosus (SLE). The most common mental symptom associated with SLE is a confusional state or delirium.[7,10,16] This can appear concurrently with other symptoms of SLE or may be the sole initial manifestation in a small percentage of the cases. As mentioned in Chapter 6, some patients with longstanding disease will develop dementia. One aspect of SLE not covered previously is the spectrum of psychiatric manifestations that can mimic functional psychiatric disease and constitute as much as 50 percent of all the mental changes reported in some SLE series.[10,13,16] The most common clinical syndrome encountered is depression, but anxiety reactions, asocial behavior, paranoid schizophrenia, and mania have all been described. In one large series (140 patients), 15 percent of the patients were considered to have definable psychiatric symptoms, but the authors deduced that all but 1 percent had evidence of organicity on careful mental status examination.[7] There are cases in which the onset of psychiatric problems preceded the neurologic or systemic features of the illness by as many as 10 years. In other cases, the psychiatric features sufficiently overshadowed the medical problems that the diagnosis was delayed.

A 20-year-old woman was first seen at Charity Hospital in 1966 with a clinical picture of catatonic schizophrenia. On the review of systems at admission, she had given a history of joint pain, however this was not persued because of the pressing matter of her severe catatonia. She subsequently developed a low grade fever which was then felt to be secondary to hypostatic pneumonia. She was discharged after remission of the overt psychosis. In 1969, she was again admitted because of exacerbation of the schizophrenic reaction. A fever was again noted, but at that time, she had a perirectal abscess which was considered to be the etiology of the fever. An RA factor was positive but again was not persued. In 1973, she was again admitted with schizophrenia and a fever of undetermined origin; on this admission, she also had wrist drop on the right. During this hospitalization, a full evaluation was carried out and a positive diagnosis of SLE was made. On a later admission (January 1976) she still showed evidence of schizophrenia, yet showed no signs of organic mental change on a full mental status examination.

One could question whether both the functional schizophrenia and SLE or the lupus alone was the origin of her psychosis. We suspect the latter is the case, since the patient had had some symptoms of SLE (although they went unrecognized) when her initial and subsequent psychotic episodes occurred.

The exact pathophysiology of both the transient and permanent behavioral changes has become quite elusive. It was long thought that the vasculitis per se, with its associated vascular occlusions and ischemia, resulted in the mental symptoms.[10] This is certainly true in many cases of SLE related dementia, but it has been recently demonstrated that very different mechanisms may be responsible for producing the acute psychotic episodes. One theory hypothesizes that the psychiatric symptoms are caused by a generalized membrane failure in the endothelial cells of the cerebral capillaries. This membrane failure or lysis is caused by active biogenic amines that are produced during the complement cascade seen during the acute exacerbation of the disease.[14] IgG levels are low in the cerebrospinal fluid, and it has been shown that antibodies are attached to capillary membranes; it is this immune complex that then sets off the complement cascade.[3] A second theory, and the most recent in this field, proposes that the cryoprecipitates from the serum of SLE patients actually contain a lymphotoxic antibody that also attacks neurons.[5] If true, the central nervous system forms of SLE may not represent just a collagen vascular process but also a direct effect of antibodies on the nerve cells themselves. Whatever the mechanism, it is readily apparent why the anti-immune effects of steroids can so quickly reverse the mental symptoms when treatment is begun promptly.

Another type of behavioral syndrome that can be seen in cases of cerebrovascular disease is that of akinetic mutism. The clinical picture is very facinating, as the following case demonstrates.

A 35-year-old hypertensive woman entered the hospital with a 6 hour history of rapidly progressive headache and leg weakness. Within several hours after admission, she had a very stiff neck and was stuporous. A spinal puncture revealed grossly bloody spinal fluid and a subsequent CT scan and arteriogram demonstrated an anterior communicating artery aneurysm with an interhemispheric clot between the frontal lobes. As her level of consciousness improved, she lay in the bed and regarded her surroundings with sentient intensity. She offered no speech or spontaneous movement yet would eat when fed and seemed to be observing the activity around her. When spoken to, she would turn and look at the examiner and with great encouragement, she would follow complicated commands such as "Wiggle one finger on your right hand and two on the left." She never spoke but occasionally would cough audibly to command. She had good arm movement control but a flaccid

374

paraparesis. Repeat CT scan showed resolution of her clot and no evidence of hydrocephalus.

This type of akinetic mutism, often called a "coma vigil," is caused by a destruction of the deep structures in the frontal lobe: septal nuclei; anterior cingulate gyrus, and many reticulocortical fibers in their course to the frontal lobes. This can be caused by destruction of tissue as in the case above or the effects of hydrocephalus developing secondary to subarachnoid hemorrhage. Such patients are intellectually intact, yet are totally unable to muster adequate reticular energy to stimulate the cortex to action. The sensory receiving system is passive and does not require extensive effort to merely observe the environment; therefore, the patients seem to be quite cognizant of the activity around them. The alert appearance is quite uncanny at times, and we have had families come to us very distraught as they felt that the patient was consciously refusing to speak to them for some psychologic rather than organic reason.

Another state, almost indistinguishable from the above, can be seen when an occlusion of the small perforating vessels at the distal end of the basilar artery causes an infarct in the subthalamic region.[17] These patients have the same picture of akinetic mutism described above with the frontal lesion, but they tend to be more apathetic. They also can have a variety of signs of midbrain dysfunction (convergence difficulty, oculomotor nerve dysfunction, up gaze paralysis, reflex changes, and occasionally Babinski's toe signs) from damage to contiguous structures. The basic lesion causing the syndrome is a butterfly shaped infarct which disconnects the mesencephalic reticular formation from the midline reticular structures.[17] The effect is the same as that in the frontal lesion; reticular innervation to higher structures is impaired, and the patients cannot adequately stimulate the motor cortex to initiate action. Additional mechanisms are also impaired and the patients cannot sustain attention for more than short intervals.

These mute states, while not common, are clinically interesting examples of the correlation of basic behavioral phenomona and neuroanatomic structure. Mutism, as a symptom, can be seen in a variety of diseases and not strictly in vascular disease. The original description of the clinical state was of a patient with an epidermoid cyst of the third ventricle[6] and subsequent reviews have described akinetic mutism in hydrocephalus, basal ganglion tumors and diseases, viral encephalitis, central pontine myelinolysis, and basilar artery occlusion.[18] Psychiatric disease, particularly catatonic schizophrenia, psychotic depression,[2] and hysterical coma or psychiatric unresponsiveness[15] must also be considered in the differential diagnosis. Psychiatric states are usually quite easily differentiated from organic conditions because of the dearth of concomitant positive medical or neurologic signs.

EVALUATION

The extensive topic of evaluating the medical and neurologic aspects of vascular disease is far beyond the scope or intention of this chapter. We wish only to point out some specific factors of significance with respect to behavioral change and to mention the general principles involved in evaluation.

The first important point is that vascular disease should be suspected whenever a patient presents with a history of a sudden behavioral change. As a corollary to this, the patient with known vascular disease must be watched or questioned concerning the onset of any acute behavioral change, since this is quite common in such patients.

A second point is the frequent history of similar, but transient, episodes of behavioral change occurring in the past. The transient ischemic attack is well known to cause behavioral symptoms; therefore, the history of such events must be assiduously persued. A history of TIAs makes the diagnosis of a thrombotic or embolic vascular accident more certain.

Of the neurobehavioral symptoms of vascular disease, focal symptoms are by far the most common. Because of this, a full mental status exam should be performed ensuring that specific symptoms will stand out. In addition, however, there are frequently other general medical and neurologic symptoms and signs (e.g., headache [particularly in hemorrhagic disease], dizziness, weakness, visual sensory change).

To fully evaluate the patient with a vascular insult to the brain, it is important to obtain history and physical examination information concerning the following areas:

1. Age
2. Handedness
3. Blood pressure
4. Heart disease
5. Diabetes
6. Smoking
7. Use of medications, particularly birth control pills
8. Peripheral vascular disease
9. Carotid artery examination—palpation (internal and extracranial vessels[8]) and auscultation.

Laboratory examinations should include a hematocrit, lipid screen, blood sugar, uric acid, blood urea nitrogen, EEG, and rhythm monitoring for the first several days after a thrombo-embolic stroke. The CT scan has become indispensable in differentiating hypertensive hemorrhage, infarct, tumor, and hemorrhagic infarct. We see little advantage in also obtaining a nucleotide scan, but we do routinely obtain an isotope flow study. Arteriography is frequently necessary but should only be ordered after a consulting internist, vascular surgeon, neurologist, or neurosurgeon has evaluated the case.

MANAGEMENT

As with the evaluation of vascular disease, a comprehensive review of the medical and surgical treatment of all vascular disease would be out of place in this volume. The general treatment modalities are summarized in Table 12-2.

After the patient's medical condition has stabilized and the acute phase of the vascular event is over, it is important to conduct a comprehensive neuropsychologic and rehabilitation evaluation and initiate a management program. This process is similar to that outlined in previous chapters and must take into full account the patient's strengths and weaknesses in the formulation of a final plan. Since patients sustaining vascular accidents are generally in the older age range, the plan is often directed toward activities of daily living rather than vocational rehabilitation. These are no less important to the patient, his family, and society, however, since achieving independence for a stroke

TABLE 12–2. Treatment Modalities in Cerebrovascular Disease

Disease Process	Treatment Available
Systemic lupus erythematosus	1. Steroids
Hypertensive and arteriosclerotic vascular disease (general)	1. Blood pressure control 2. Control of blood lipids 3. Control of diabetes mellitus 4. Control of hyperuricemia 5. Termination of smoking 6. Correction of cardiac arrhythmias 7. Possibly control of hematocrit below 42
Transient ischemic attacks	1. Carotid artery surgery if an ulcerated or significantly stenotic plaque is found 2. Extracranial/middle cerebral artery shunts for high stenosis or occlusion of internal carotid arteries 3. Anticoagulants 4. Aspirin

patient can be the difference between a meaningful social life and custodial care.

REFERENCES

1. Adams, G.F., and Hurwitz, L.J.: Mental barriers to recovery from strokes. Lancet 2:533, 1963.
2. Akhtar, S., and Buckman, J.: The differential diagnosis of mutism: A review and a report of three unusual cases. Dis. Nerv. Syst. 38:558, 1977.
3. Bennahum, D.A., and Messner, R.P.: Recent observations on central nervous system lupus erythematosus. Semin. Arthritis Rheum. 4:253, 1975.
4. Benton, A.L. (ed.): Behavioral Change in Cerebrovascular Disease. Harper and Row, New York, 1970.
5. Bluestein, H.G.: Heterogeneous neurocytotoxic antibodies in systemic lupus erythematosus. Clin. Exp. Immunol. 35:210, 1979.
6. Cairns, H., Oldfield, R.C., Pennybacker, J.B., and Whitteridge, D.: Akinetic mutism with an epidermoid cyst of the 3rd ventricle. Brain 64:273, 1941.
7. Feinglass, E.J., Arnett, F.C., Dorsch, G.A., Zizic, I.M., and Stevens, M.B.: Neuropsychiatric manifestations of systemic lupus erythematosus: Diagnosis, clinical spectrum, and relationship to other features of the disease. Medicine 55:323, 1976.
8. Fisher, C.M.: Facial pulses in internal carotid artery occlusion. Neurology 20:476, 1970.
9. Futty, D.E., Conneally, P.M., Dyken, M.L., Price, T.R., Haerer, A.F., Poskanzer, D.C., Swanson, P.D., Calanchini, P.R., and Gotshall, R.A.: Cooperative study of hospital frequency and character of transient ischemic attacks. V. Symptom analysis. JAMA 238:2386, 1977.
10. Johnson, R.T., and Richardson, E.P.: The neurological manifestations of systemic lupus erythematosus. Medicine 47:337, 1968.
11. Kurtzke, J.F.: An introduction to the epidemiology of cerebrovascular disease, in Scheinberg, P. (ed.): Cerebrovascular Disease. Tenth Princeton Conference. Raven Press, New York, 1976, pp. 239–254.
12. Lishman, W.A.: Organic Psychiatry. Blackwell Scientific Publications, London, 1978, pp. 450–526.
13. O'Conner, J.F.: Psychosis associated with systemic lupus erythematosus. Ann. Intern. Med. 51:526, 1959.
14. Petz, L.D., Sharp, G.C., Cooper, N.R., and Irvin, W.S.: Serum and CSF complement. Medicine 50:259, 1971.
15. Plum, F., and Posner, J.: Diagnosis of Stupor and Coma. F.A. Davis Company, Philadelphia, 1972.
16. Sargent, J.S., Lockshin, M.D., Klempner, M.S., and Lipsky, B.A.: Central nervous system disease in systemic lupus erythematosus. Am. J. Med. 58:644, 1975.
17. Segarra, J., and Angelo, J.: Anatomical determinants of behavior change, in Benton, A. (ed.): Behavioral Change in Cerebrovascular Disease. Harper and Row, New York, 1970, pp. 3–14.
18. Skultety, F.M.: Clinical and experimental aspects of akinetic mutism. Arch. Neurol. 19:1, 1968.
19. Stallones, R.A., Dyken, M.L., Fang, H.C.H., Heyman, A., Seltser, R., and Stamler, J.: Epidemiology for stroke facilities planning, in Sahs, A.L.,

and Hartman, E.C.: Fundamentals of Stroke Care. U.S. Department of Health, Education, and Welfare Publication, No. (HRA) 76-14016, 1976, pp. 5–13.

20. Wylie, C.M.: Epidemiology of cerebrovascular disease, in Vinken, P.J., and Bruyn, G.W. (eds.): Vascular Diseases of the Nervous System, Vol. 11 in Handbook of Clinical Neurology, Elsevier-North Holland Publishing Co., New York, 1972, pp. 183–207.

13

BRAIN TUMOR

E. M. is a 73-year-old retired dock worker who had enjoyed good health until 3 weeks prior to his hospital admission. At that time, he began to have word finding difficulty in spontaneous speech, and his family felt that he was easily confused. During the 3 weeks preceding his admission, his symptoms gradually became more prominent and he also developed chronic, dull, early morning headaches.

On admission, the patient was alert and attentive to the examiner, but this tended to flucuate throughout the day. His spontaneous speech was fluent, and he could carry on a relatively adequate superficial conversation, but word searching and paraphasic errors marred his language production. Comprehension was relatively intact for general conversation, but he was able to point accurately to only 2 items in succession. Repetition was normal, but naming to confrontation was very poor. Naming was characterized by perseveration, paraphasia, and total inability to name some items. He was fully oriented and his memory for recent events was good. His drawings showed only minimal organic features (loss of three dimensionality). Proverb interpretation, however, was concrete. His motor, sensory, and cranial nerve examinations were all normal. The CT scan demonstrated a left frontal mass which at surgery proved to be a glioblastoma.

This case demonstrates some of the many behavioral symptoms which can be produced by a tumor of the cerebral hemispheres. Tumors, because they are focal expanding lesions, can produce one or a combination of several general types of behavioral symptoms: focal symptoms such as the aphasia seen in the case above, confusional behavior from the increased intracranial pressure, simple dementia, and, finally, purely psychiatric symptoms primarily with tumors of the frontal or temporal lobes. Since tumors are focally destructive lesions, motor, sensory, and other general neurologic features will also frequently accompany or even dominate the clinical picture. Seizures, for instance, are quite common and have been described in as many as 20 to 30 percent of all tumor cases.[7,10] They can be generalized in type but more typically are focal; this is particularly true when the tumor is located in the temporal lobe. Headaches and dizziness are variably present, with headache alone being reported in over 85 percent of the cases in one series.[10] Papilledema is also quite common (in 45 to 65%) and must always be sought if brain tumor is suspected.[7,10] Incontinence, while uncommon during the early stages of tumor growth, is a very strong indicator of organic disease when present.

Although these general neurologic features are extremely important, we will concentrate our discussion on the behavioral aspects of the clinical picture not only to highlight these aspects of the problem but also because behavioral symptoms are very common with cerebral neoplasm and are frequently the only initial symptom of the disease. In a large series of brain tumors reported upon from the Ochsner Clinic, over 50 percent of the cases demonstrated mental symptoms when first admitted to the hospital.[12] The mode of presentation and clinical course varies considerably but, in general, the symptoms evolve slowly over a period of several months. Due to the general nature of tumors, the symptoms may fluctuate over time, and anything causing the tumor or surrounding tissue to accumulate or lose edema fluid will produce a change in clinical symptoms. An acute stroke-like presentation is uncommon, however, unless a hemorrhage has occurred into the substance of the tumor or there is an acute increase in intracranial pressure, such as that accompanying a sneeze or cough.

Various features of the tumor, such as type, growth characteristics, and location are important in determining the nature of the particular behavioral symptoms displayed. With slowly growing hemispheric masses, gradual focal deficits usually develop. In tumors located in the limbic structures of the frontal or temporal lobes, psychiatric rather than cognitive behavioral change is more likely to occur.[8] On occasion, a slowly growing tumor can produce a clinical picture which resembles simple dementia; however, this is not common.

In contrast, tumors that are very large, rapidly growing, or associated with considerable edema (primarily metastatic), produce a rapid rise in intracranial pressure and an attendant acute confusional state. In these patients, one of the earliest signs has been a general decrease in level of alertness and a slowing of mental processes. We saw one woman with a large meningioma who came into the emergency room complaining only of general fatigue, but it took her at least five minutes to laboriously tell us of this chief complaint.

Another factor influencing the nature of the symptoms produced is the type of tumor. Meningiomas, for example, are extrinsic to the brain, slow growing, and produce pressure on a specific area of cortex. Such tumors, most frequently cause focal symptoms until they become very large; whereas gliomas grow through the white matter of the brain and more frequently give a picture of generalized mental deterioration.

By and large most patients with tumors present with a combination of behavioral features though one clinical symptom may predominate. The most remarkable aspect is the brain's phenomenal ability to adapt to the encroachment of the mass lesion without producing any neurologic or neurobehavioral symptoms or signs. We are always impressed by the paucity of findings demonstrated by patients with immense tumors, irrespective of their type, growth pattern, or location. Because of this, it is often impossible to diagnose these lesions when they are small and easily resectable.

In the 1870s, John Hughlings Jackson, wrote that the effects of all brain tumors started both with an almost imperceptible decline in delicate intellectual processes and a loss of finer emotions.[3] He felt that such patients suffered a "limitation in intellectual field" that was not sufficient to attract the notice of the casual observer and was certainly not apparent in their day to day routine. As the tumor grew, Jackson stated that these subtle changes became accentuated, memory failed, and a general dementia developed. Today we realize that whereas this clinical course is seen in some patients, it is far from universal. A diagnosis of mental disease is made initially in 18 to 50 percent of all patients with brain tumors, [2,6,10,14] but the mode of presentation varies considerably and no single behavioral syndrome due to brain tumor exists. Some patients develop a gradual dementia as described by Jackson but far more present with other behavioral symptoms, both cognitive and emotional.

Owing to the focal nature of tumors, focal behavioral symptoms are commonly seen: aphasia; geographic disorientation; reading, writing, and calculating difficulties; and frontal lobe symptoms. Since the focal syndromes have been discussed in Chapter 7, only several specific points referable to brain tumors need to be made here. The first is that the relationship between lesion size and the magnitude of symptoms is usually far less with tumor than with destructive lesions such as cerebral infarction. Tumors push and infiltrate brain tissue rather than devastate it, and the resultant lesions are often surprisingly large when compared with their neurobehavioral effects. Secondly, focal symptoms tend to be slowly progressive with tumors, a very important point in differentiating tumor from stroke. Thirdly, as stated in the last section, with rapidly growing lesions, the focal symptoms are soon accompanied by signs of confusional behavior, particularly decreased alertness and clouding of all mental processes.

Acute confusion with or without the symptoms of focal disease is a very important organic behavioral change to recognize since it is seen in approximately 50 to 67 percent of those tumor cases who have mental symptoms.[7,14] The patient's behavior is clinically the same as that seen in any acute confusional state and differs only if outstanding focal symptoms such as aphasia are found concurrently. Confusional behavior is usually seen when the brain substance can no longer accommodate to the expanding mass and increases in intracranial pressure occur. This is most frequently found in rapidly growing tumors, very large lesions, or tumors in which massive edema is present (a common finding in metastatic lesions). Although organic mental changes are very common in tumor patients, some patients have clinical symptoms that are predominately emotional. It is common for textbooks and newspaper articles to point out the number of patients dying in mental institutions who at autopsy are found to harbor an undiagnosed brain tumor. However, the actual percentage of such cases is small and is growing smaller as the awareness that organic disease can mimic psychiatric states increases. Yet the salient fact remains that the slowly growing cerebral neoplasm is quite capable of producing mental states that resemble functional psychiatric diseases in almost every way. As we have previously said, many of these cases will have evidence of organic features if they are carefully evaluated (some authors claim figures as high as 80 to 95%)[1,7] but, unfortunately, in the patient hospitalized with a psychiatric diagnosis, many subtle organic features are unappreciated.

Approximately 50 percent of all patients with brain tumors will have some psychiatric symptoms,[12] but only about 15 percent actually are hospitalized with a primary psychiatric diagnosis.[10] Those patients with predominately psychiatric features are usually those with tumors involving the limbic portions of the frontal and temporal lobes.[5,8,10] In fact, it has been reported that as many as 88 percent of patients whose psychiatric syndromes were associated with a tumor had lesions in those areas.[10] The actual psychiatric features are varied.[5,8,9,11] Depression, for example, is found in half of the reported cases; schizophreniform psychosis in 10 to 40 percent (greater in temporal than frontal loci); anxiety in 5 to 15 percent; with paranoia, mania[4], and personality change being less frequently reported. Some patients may have had overt or incipient psychiatric illness prior to the onset of their tumor, and still others may, in some way, develop psychiatric symptoms as a reaction to other symptoms caused by the tumor, but it appears to us that many of these major behavioral changes are a direct effect of the mass lesion localized within limbic structures.

Frontal lobe tumors probably are those which most frequently produce psychiatric symptoms. Depression, apathy, euphoria, social impropriety, and marked changes in basic personality are all well-known symptoms of frontal lobe damage. Hallucinations (olfactory, gustatory, auditory, and visual) and delusions may also be present albeit less frequently. Problems of bladder and bowel incontinence are quite common in cases of frontal tumor (35%) and are certainly major clues to the organicity in an individual case.[13]

Temporal lobe tumors are clinically somewhat different, because epileptic phenomena play an important part in the overall presentation. Temporal lobe ictal and interictal behavioral phenomena are seen in almost all patients with temporal lobe tumors and, therefore, can serve as important diagnostic features.[8] Hallucinations, which are probably frequently epileptic phenomena, are somewhat more common in patients with temporal lobe tumors; however, the only specific and localizing type are those in which a half field formed visual hallucination is experienced.[6] In such instances, the hallucination is pathognomonic of a lesion within the contralateral posterior temporal region.

There is no specific psychiatric syndrome seen exclusively with temporal lobe tumors. Depression is seen as frequently in this group as it is seen in patients with frontal tumors. A rather high incidence (45%) of schizophreniform psychosis has been reported;[8] however, clinically this does not include any specific features that differentiate it from the schizophrenic syndrome seen with tumors in other locations. Subtle personality change is also common (50%) and has been noted to be the earliest symptom in over 20 percent of temporal lobe tumor cases presenting with behavioral change.[6] Because of the memory circuits and language centers in the temporal lobe, it is frequently possible to elicit evidence of memory difficulty and aphasia in these patients. Basically it is the associated focal behavioral features of aphasia, amnesia, hemihallucinations, and temporal lobe epileptic manifestations and not the specific character of the psychiatric symptoms alone that help the clinician to localize a tumor to the temporal lobe.

EVALUATION

The clinical evaluation of a patient with a brain tumor is similar to that of any patient presenting with complaints of a progressive behavioral change. The history and physical examination must include specific elements that will help identify those patients with tumor. One abiding principle is that a tumor must be suspected in any person of middle age or older who develops any behavioral change with slow progression whether it be cognitive or emotional. This is particularly true when the change arises in a patient who has never had any such symptoms in the past. The elements of the history that must be carefully assessed are:

Element in History	Abnormality in Presence of Tumor
1. Speed of onset	Unless associated with hemorrhage into the tumor, the onset is gradual
2. Character of course	Usually steady progression, but can show an intermittent course
3. Seizures	Quite frequent, particularly with temporal lobe tumors
4. Headache	Common (85%), usually mild, sometimes localized, often worse at night and in morning
5. Visual complaints	Visual blurring or diplopia occur as intracranial pressure increases
6. Hallucinations	All varieties can be seen with tumors, but they are relatively uncommon
7. Specific neurobehavior and psychiatric symptoms	Changes in memory, language, affect, personality, and a host of other similar areas of symptomatology must be explored
8. History of carcinoma or symptoms of active cancer	Metastatic cancer to the brain is very frequent with such common cancers as lung, breast, and melanoma
9. Neurologic symptoms	Specific motor, sensory or cranial nerve abnormalities often are present, though the behavioral change usually precedes this

The examination should, as in all behavioral cases, include a complete neurologic and mental status examination. Funduscopic examination is of critical importance since papilledema is a very common finding with cerebral neoplasm.

DIFFERENTIAL DIAGNOSIS

The differential diagnosis depends upon the mode of presentation of the tumor; if focal, then brain abscess or vascular lesions are considered. Usually the slowness of onset clearly distinguishes an expanding mass from a vascular event, but within the spectrum of mass lesions the features are similar. The tumors presenting with confusional behavior or dementia must be identified and differentiated from the myriad other causes of those conditions (see Chaps. 4 and 5).

If the patient presents with the symptoms of a psychiatric syndrome, it behooves the physician and the psychiatrist to exhaustively seek any organic or neurologic signs before beginning extensive and expensive psychiatric treatment. The dire consequences of an incorrect diagnosis in these ofttimes confusing cases are obvious.

LABORATORY INVESTIGATION

The CT scan of the brain has made recognition of brain tumors considerably easier. This is certainly the exam of choice if a tumor is suspected. If the patient presents with confusional behavior or dementia, the appropriate laboratory studies for that diagnosis should be carried out (see Chaps. 4 and 5). One of the major questions is always, how much screening laboratory work is necessary in cases of routine psychiatric disease? Is it financially justifiable to order an EEG and a CT scan on all psychiatric cases? The answer to this question is not easy. Obviously a 35-year-old male who has had a diagnosis of simple schizophrenia since age 19 is not very likely to have a brain tumor; neither is the 50-year-old female with a 20 year history of bipolar manic-depressive illness. However, middle-aged or older patients with no previous history of psychiatric illness probably deserve a neurologic examination and at least an EEG but preferably a CT scan before the institution of lengthy psychotherapy. The cost, both financial and emotional, of long-term psychiatric therapy or hospitalization is far greater than that involved in a brief, yet thorough, evaluation for organic disease during the diagnostic phase of the psychiatric consultation.

MANAGEMENT AND PATHOLOGY

The surgical management and neuropathology of brain tumors are topics that are not germane to the central theme of this book and the reader is referred to the standard texts of neurosurgery and neuropathology.

REFERENCES

1. Fisher, R.G.: The psychiatric symptoms of patients having neurosurgical lesions. J. Med. Soc. N.J. 11:963, 1976.
2. Hobbs, G.E.: Brain tumors simulating psychiatric disease. Can. Med. Assoc. J. 88:186, 1963.
3. Jackson, J.H.: Lectures on the diagnosis of tumors of the brain in Taylor, J. (ed.): Selected Writings of John Hughlings Jackson, Vol. 2. Basic Books, Inc., New York, 1958, pp. 270–286.
4. Jamieson, R.C., and Wells, C.E.: Case studies in neuropsychiatry: manic psychosis in a patient with multiple metastatic brain tumors. J. Clin. Psychiatry 40:280, 1979.
5. Kanakaratnam, G., and Direkze, M.: Aspects of primary tumors of the frontal lobe. Br. J. Clin. Pract. 30:220, 1976.
6. Keschner, M., Bender, M.B., and Strauss, I.: Mental symptoms in cases of tumor of the temporal lobe. Arch. Neurol. Psychiatry 35:572, 1936.
7. Levin, S.: Brain tumors in mental hospital patients. Am. J. Psychiatry 105:897, 1949.
8. Malmud, N.: Psychiatric disorders with intracranial tumors of the limbic system. Arch. Neurol. 17:113, 1967.
9. Pool, J.L., and Correll, J.W.: Psychiatric symptoms masking brain tumor. J. Med. Soc. N.J. 55:4, 1958.
10. Redlich, F.C., Dunsmore, R.H., and Brody, E.B.: Delays and errors in the diagnosis of brain tumor. N. Engl. J. Med. 339:945, 1948.
11. Remington, F.B., and Rubert, S.L.: Why patients with brain tumors come to the psychiatric hospital: a thirty year survey. Am. J. Psychol. 119: 256, 1962.
12. Soniat, T.L.L.: Psychiatric symptoms associated with intracranial neoplasm. Am. J. Psychiatry 108:19, 1951.
13. Strauss, I., and Keschner, M.: Mental symptoms in cases of tumor of the frontal lobe. Arch. Neurol. Psychiatry 33:986, 1935.
14. Williams, S.E., Bell, D.S., and Gye, R.S.: Neurosurgical disease encountered in a psychiatric service. J. Neurol. Neurosurg. Psychiatry 37:112, 1974.

SECTION IV

BORDERLAND ORGANIC BRAIN SYNDROMES

14

OTHER NEUROBEHAVIORAL SYNDROMES AND NEUROLOGIC ASPECTS OF PSYCHIATRIC DISEASE

After discussion of delirium, dementia, focal brain lesions and the encephalopathies of trauma, toxins, and infection; the border between neurology and psychiatry is recognized as being indistinct. Conditions such as schizophrenia, sleep disorders, and Gilles de la Tourette's syndrome currently are placed within a borderland category of psychiatric diseases which may well have organic etiologies. Most of the classic neurobehavioral concepts are based on an anatomic or structural model and someday it may be possible to reduce all behavior to basic biologic explanations. In this chapter we will briefly enumerate and review some of the diseases in this borderland category to provide a full concept of the field of neurobehavior as currently defined.

SLEEP DISORDERS

During the past decade there has been a growing interest in a wide range of sleep disorders which includes insomnia, narcolepsy, somnambulism, and sleep apnea. Sleep laboratories have been established in major medical centers and the pathophysiology of these disorders is slowly being elucidated. With the understanding of the basic mechanisms of these disorders, patient management has become more satisfactory. The conditions with the most interesting neurobehavioral symptoms are the narcoleptic syndrome and the syndrome of periodic hypersomnia and bulimia (Kleine-Levin syndrome).

Narcolepsy

Narcolepsy is a relatively common and very curious syndrome. Patients with this disease present with a variety of very interesting symptoms in different combinations. The principal symptom is the sleep attack or narcoleptic spell itself. This attack is characterized by a sudden inopportune dropping off to sleep. This can occur at most inappropriate times; we have one patient who is a professional roofer and has been known to fall asleep while sitting on the edge of a roof. Although these episodes are sensitive to environmental ennui and such stress as a high carbohydrate meal, they can occur at any time. They tend to have incidences ranging from several to many times per day, last approximately 15 minutes, and electroencephalographically are associated with the almost immediate onset of rapid eye movement (REM) sleep.

The second cardinal feature of narcolepsy and the one that separates this syndrome from mere hypersomnia is the cataplectic attack. In cataplexy, the patient experiences a sudden loss of voluntary muscle control and falls precipitously to the ground. Such episodes are routinely brought on by a sudden expression of emotion such as laughter or excitement. They are short lived and do not involve a loss of consciousness. Seventy percent of all true narcoleptics have a combination of sleep attacks and cataplexy.[50] For this reason, it is very important to inquire carefully about episodes of sudden emotion-induced hypotonia when examining the patient with a complaint of hypersomnia.

The third symptom is sleep paralysis: an inability to move and sometimes breath when first falling asleep or, less frequently, upon awakening. This symptom is experienced by 50 percent of all narcoleptic patients but is present as the sole manifestation of the syndrome in only 5 percent of the cases.[50] The fourth clinical feature is hypnagogic hallucinations. These may be auditory or visual, are often vivid and frightening, and by definition, occur at the onset or termination of sleep.

A final, and very fascinating behavioral feature of this syndrome is what has been called automatic behavior.[22,38,53] Clinically, this behavior is very similar to the episodes experienced with transient global amnesia. The patient becomes absentminded and is totally unable to appreciate the passage of time but is able to carry out routine, yet not demanding, tasks and on occasion will have involuntary outbursts of meaningless words. These episodes may last from a few minutes to several hours, and the patients are usually at least partially, if not completely, amnesic for the duration of the episode.

The onset of narcolepsy has been reported to range from age 4 to age 72 years, but these age extremes are rare.[38] Its usual onset is before the age of 30 (most frequently in adolescence or shortly thereafter), and it may continue throughout the patient's life. There are some families in which the condition is dominantly inherited but most cases are genetically sporadic.

Treatment of hypersomnia has been quite successful, with methylphenidate (Ritalin) being the drug of choice for most patients.[51] Dosage varies with patient response, but daily doses of more than 100 mg. may be needed. The drug is best given 45 minutes before meals to insure adequate absorption and should not be given after 5 P.M. to preclude interference with the patient's sleep. Methylphenidate, unfortunately, will not usually help the cataplectic component of the problem, so the cautious addition of imipramine (25 mg. t.i.d.) is usually necessary in those cases in which both symptoms are present.

The pathophysiology of narcolepsy is not yet fully understood, but sleep research and neuropharmocologic studies suggest a basic imbalance in the biogenic amines in the brain stem.[11] Since serotonin augments REM sleep and noradrenalin inhibits it, the assumption that a defect in these neurotransmitters is the basis of the syndrome seems quite feasible.

Kleine-Levin Syndrome

Another clinically interesting episodic sleep disorder is the Kleine-Levin syndrome, a rare condition in which patients experience symptoms of periodic hibernation. The condition is predominately seen in males and is first manifested in adolescence. The clinical course follows a fairly regular sequence. From their usual level of functioning, such patients enter an initial phase of personality change. They become hyperactive, irritable, giddy, hostile, and sometimes confusional; this phase may last from a few hours to two weeks. The patients then become more hostile, withdrawn, and frequently nauseated. Other autonomic signs such as cold extremities can occur and hallucinations have been reported.[38] This phase is also of variable length, usually lasting days to two weeks.[19] The third phase is a period of hibernation, during which the patient sleeps and eats excessively (bulimia or megaphagia). This final phase also lasts for a few days to two weeks but can last for months; the patients often gain considerable weight (e.g., 20 to 30 pounds) in a very short time and sexual interest may increase and irritability may be present.[6] After the attack ceases, the patient returns to his normal mode and level of functioning. The episodes recur on an average of once every 5 months[9] but occur monthly in some patients.

The laboratory evaluation of these cases has not revealed any consistent medical, endocrine, or neurologic dysfunction. During the hibernation phase, the EEG is often slow and disorganized, with some patients demonstrating sleep onset REM sleep, but these findings are far from uniform.[52] From the clinical features of abnormal sleep patterns, disturbed eating habits, and other autonomic symptoms, it is logical to assume that some form of hypothalamic or brain stem dysfunction is present, but it has been impossible thus far to clinically or pathologically identify it.

Treatment has been attempted with various psychotropics, but little success has been achieved. The hypersomnic phase has been helped by the use of methylphenidate (Ritalin) in some cases,[6] but in other patients this medication has exacerbated some of the negative behavioral effects.[49] Fortunately, the disorder is usually self-limited and the symptoms typically remit permanently by age 30.

Sleep Apnea

Sleep apnea or, more appropriately, the sleep apnea syndromes are characterized by an involuntary cessation of airflow at the nostrils and mouth lasting for at least ten seconds.[22,23] These are a group of relatively rare, yet very real, disorders, which may often produce behavioral abnormalities. Although sleep apnea has traditionally been reported in association with rare otolaryngologic and neurologic disorders (e.g., Shy-Drager syndrome, muscular dystrophy, or Ondine's curse), it has received increasing attention during the past decade as a problem which may present without other complications to the general practitioner or psychiatrist. The uncomplicated disorder has been differentiated into those syndromes due to an obstruction of the upper airway and those syndromes of central apnea with transient discontinuation of all respiratory motor activity.[13] Medically, these disorders are important, as identification and appropriate therapeutic approaches in many cases may prevent acute hypoxia, chronic cardiorespiratory failure, or sudden death.[12] The sleep apnea syndromes do produce a wide range of behavioral changes including daytime hypersomnia, altered states of awareness, periods of automatic behavior, hallucinations, increased irritability, and a deterioration in the general quality of daily performance.[22] The social impact of these behavioral factors upon the patient's day to day life is obvious. The evaluation of such patients has become increasingly accurate with polygraphic recording of EEG, airflow and respiratory movement, and monitoring of arterial Po_2 and Pco_2. As most adult cases of sleep apnea have proven to be of obstructive etiology, surgical intervention is the most frequently employed treatment. It is possible to speculate that demand ventilation and diaphragm pacing may, at some future point, be utilized with those patients with central nonobstructive apnea.[20]

PERIODIC PSYCHOSIS

Other episodic pathologic behavioral disorders have been reported in the literature. One such syndrome is a periodic psychosis that has been seen in association with the menstrual cycle.[16] The patients begin to experience the episodes at the age of puberty. Many have had some minor emotional problems prior to the onset of the disorder but nothing to compare with the symptoms experienced during these attacks. The episodes have a typical pattern: in the 5 to 10 day period before menstruation, the patients acutely display symptoms that are not merely those of exaggerated premenstrual tension but are characterized by delusions, illusions, and actual hallucinations. Autonomic disturbances are also present, including nausea, flushing, and anorexia.[16] With the onset of the menstrual period, the symptoms quickly recede and behavior returns to the patient's baseline functioning. This cycle has been reported to repeat as many as 3 to 14 times and then to cease permanently. Electroencephalographic abnormalities are often seen during the attacks and there are some alterations in the rhythmic excretion of hormones; however, no major endocrinologic disease has ever been found. It appears that this condition represents one type of organic disease in which there is a temporary imbalance of endocrine and transmitter function which is present in the early menstrual years. Why this occurs and the exact mechanism of the symptom production are not yet known.

EPISODIC DYSCONTROL

Episodic violence is yet another paroxysmal behavioral disorder which includes both neurologic and psychiatric features. In Chapter 11, we touched briefly upon the organically induced violence seen with temporal lobe epilepsy, but that is only one aspect of this problem. The spectrum of violent behavior is wide ranging, from psychopathic violence of wholly environmental etiology to the strictly organic violence occurring with the Klüver-Bucy syndrome, hypothalamic tumors, or temporal lobe epilepsy. Between these extremes is a syndrome which has been called the "episodic dyscontrol syndrome." Patients thus afflicted are given to sudden, destructive outbursts that are in stark contrast to their normal personalities and emotional functioning.

The attacks themselves are usually provoked by a very minimal environmental stress and on many occasions are totally unprovoked. The first symptoms take the form of an aura, with rising anxiety, drowsiness, headache, visual illusions, hyperacusis, extremity numbness, and in many patients, staring.[1,33] Some clinicians have noted that many individuals with this disorder sense an increasing feeling of tension prior to the overt behavioral outburst and may attempt to abort the episode by avoiding interpersonal contact and isolating themselves either in a room or by walks or driving.[2] The attack itself lasts from 15 minutes to 2 hours and is very violent. Aggression is directed against objects, family members, and in one series of patients actually lead to homicide by 5 of the 22 patients reported upon.[33] After termination of the attack, many patients claim amnesia for the attacks and remorse for the havoc wreaked. In the immediate postviolent period, they frequently feel very fatigued and often sleep heavily.

Physical assaultiveness is not the only component of this syndrome, many patients also have: (1) a great sensitivity to alcohol with associated pathologic intoxication, (2) multiple inexplicable traffic accidents and moving violations, and (3) a history of sexual impulsiveness which is occasionally violent.[34] Neurologic examination often reveals minor neurologic signs and the EEG can be abnormal. In one large series of patients with episodic violent behavior, however, the incidence of EEG abnormalities did not differ from that of the normal population.[54]

Although the etiology of this condition is probably varied, there are many predisposing factors in the past histories of these patients. Sixty percent were known to have been hyperactive children,[1,33] a large number have had significant birth injury or early central nervous system disease, mental subnormality is common, previous psychiatric problems are found in 50 percent,[33] and lastly there is often a history of disrupted present and past households with violence being present in many. As is true with the general problem of violence, this group of individuals seems to represent a mosaic of social and organic factors. Many cases probably are the result of early damage to the temporal limbic structures; some are associated with actual temporal lobe epilepsy; some are associated with irritative areas in the temporal lobes that are electrophysiologically demonstrable yet do not cause overt seizures; and in others the episodic abnormal electrical phenomena are only discovered by the use of depth electrodes and extensive study.

Some cases may represent extremes on the normal spectrum of constitutional temperament. These include those individuals who are not consistently seriously violent, yet are overwhelmed by impulses of anger at the least provocation. We personally have seen one excellent clinical example of this type of patient: her response to medication was sufficiently rewarding to report the details of the case here.

The patient is a 25-year-old woman who was referred because of temporal dysrhythmia on an EEG which was obtained to evaluate the possible etiology of a headache that she had suffered following pelvic surgery. The patient did not report any evidence of overt temporal lobe seizures but did state that she had always been a rebellious girl who had run away from home, gotten into frequent arguments and fights at home, and generally had demonstrated very poor impulse control. Her husband, a very calm physics graduate student had always resignedly adapted to this behavior though certainly not relishing it. Following evaluation, the patient was begun on diphenylhydantoin (Dilantin), 300 mg. daily, and has undergone a virtual personality transformation. She no longer allows insignificant problems to upset her, she does not fight with her husband, and she has actually begun to relate well with her family for the first time in 10 years. She feels physically and emotionally well, saying that it seems as if she were a new person.

We do not mean to intimate by this case that all such temperamental differences and all violent patients have a simple remediable electrical disturbance in the limbic areas of the temporal lobes; however, some may, and it is important to consider this possibility when evaluating the violent patient.

For appropriate patients, treatment is best initiated with diphenylhydantoin (Dilantin), but carbamazepine (Tegretol) has also been used efficaciously.[47] In Maletsky's series, 70 percent of the patients were cured by diphenylhydantoin and an additional 16 percent were reported to be markedly improved.[33] Thioridazine (Mellaril) can also be used, but the benzodiazepines (Valium and Librium) can often worsen the symptoms and should be avoided. In many cases, however, it is important to utilize a combined approach of pharmacologic agents and psychiatric therapy. Some clinics have devised "crisis lines" for their patients to use when they feel the aura of anxiety developing[1] and others utilize family therapy, particularly for their adolescent patients with episodic dyscontrol.[24]

There are no good prognostic statistics yet, since many patients resist and drift out of treatment, but the current contention is that this condition burns itself out by age 50, since few if any cases have been reported in individuals over that age.[33] The life history of hyperactivity as a child, episodic violence during adulthood, and gradual diminution during late middle age suggests a basic constitutional, biological alteration that may well be influenced by hormonal changes or brain damage. Some cases are obviously related to both ictal and interictal seizure phenonema, while others probably represent subclinical behavioral seizures.

We realize the difficulties encountered in carrying out research on the violent individual, especially that including behavior controlling neurosurgical operations, but violence is a serious threat to many individuals' day to day freedom and thereby should not be ignored by the scientific community. Many violent persons could and should be helped; accordingly, all clinicians must take this situation seriously and refer these patients for full evaluation and possible help.

GENERALIZED TIC

There is a group of conditions, Gilles de la Tourette's syndrome being the most celebrated, in which involuntary motor tics are the primary clinical feature. Some tic disorders are due to well established organic factors (e.g., high dose phenothiazine use and following encephalitis), while others seem primarily of psychogenic origin such as the facial tics and grimaces seen in young children.[48] The Gilles de la Tourette's or Tourette's syndrome is one in which the etiology is less clear and the behavioral manifestations more dramatic.[45] The syndrome is well illustrated by the following case.

A local physician consulted one of us (RLS) in the hospital corridor one day to discuss some extremely upsetting symptoms that the family had noticed in their eldest daughter, then 23 years of age. The young woman was a school teacher and lived at home with her parents and younger siblings. She did not have difficulty while at school, but in the evenings she would arrive home, park her car in front of the house, and could be heard coming up the walk spontaneously uttering vulgar oaths. The family would retreat to the furthest recesses of the house in hopes that it was merely a passerby. At the dinner table, particularly when stressed by her father, the patient would grunt, curse, and make low "barking" noises. The father reported that this behavior had been present to some degree since high school but was steadily worsening. Subsequent neurologic examination was completely normal and the patient was started on haloperidol (Haldol), 2 mg. twice daily. She has clinically done quite well but has been reluctant to take her medication and appears to resent her father's interference in what she perceives to be her own personal matter.

Tourette's syndrome is most likely an organic disorder that is sensitive to environmental stress, rather than one caused exclusively by psychogenic factors. The condition typically has onset in childhood, usually by 6 or 7 years of age. It is a progressive disease, with remissions and exacerbation of symptoms being a common feature. There does not seem to be any common psychopathology, but there is a well-documented familial, genetic tendency.[15,17]

Clinically, the initial symptom is usually an involuntary, facial twitch or tic. As the condition progresses, the tics become more general including the arm and then the leg. Respiratory grunting and involuntary utterances which are frequently profane (coprolalia) are eventually seen in most cases. In some advanced cases, jumping, kicking, gritting of teeth, and bizarre barking are experienced.[14] The symptoms exacerbate during stress and abate during periods of relative emotional calm. Unfortunately some patients progress to the point of a serious mental disorder (occasionally schizophrenia) but do not become demented.[48]

On neurologic examination, there are no gross abnormalities, however, minor motor clumsiness has been demonstrated in 50 percent of the cases carefully studied.[44,46] Of these patients, 35 percent are left handed,[46] 50 to 70 percent have abnormal EEGs and 75 percent showed organic signs on neuropsychologic testing.[44,46] This data strongly supports the hypothesis that this is primarily an organic syndrome with unusual behavioral symptoms that resemble so many of the abnormal involuntary movements seen with basal gangliar disease. Although pathologic studies have demonstrated only suspicious abnormalities in the cell populations in the corpus striatum, pharmacologic evidence has been more encouraging. Dopamine blocking drugs such as haloperidol (Haldol) have been very effective in treating the clinical symptoms of Tourette's syndrome, while the use of levodopa has caused exacerbations. Such observations suggest that there is a basic instability in the dopamine system which is probably a type of hyperactivity or hypersensitivity. It is hoped that the use of these drugs over longer periods of time can control the progression of this disease. At present, however, no long-term statistics are available.

DEVELOPMENTAL DISORDERS

A very large and common group of neurobehavioral disorders that we will discuss more fully in a subsequent volume is the developmental disorders seen in children.[4] This is a very interesting and important collection of conditions because they are both very common and also poorly understood by most physicians. Included within the category of developmental disorders are learning disorders, minimal brain dysfunction, developmental language disorders, and mental retardation. These are very complicated disorders to deal with clinically since they usually appear as a slowness in the developmental process (e.g., slowness in acquisition of language or reading skills). After the appearance of the initial developmental delay, secondary psychologic problems often occur which cloud the general clinical picture. The diagnostic and therapeutic approach to these children is necessarily multidisciplinary, involving the services of psychologists, special education teachers, speech pathologists, social workers, physicians, and neurologic and psychiatric consultants. These pediatric conditions are only mentioned here because we feel there is a strong organic aspect to many of these cases and they must be approached with this in mind. This area has received an increasing amount of professional attention in the literature.[27,43]

CLASSIC PSYCHIATRIC ILLNESSES THAT MAY HAVE AN ORGANIC BASIS

The major psychoses, schizophrenia, and manic-depressive illness have long been considered to be primarily functional (i.e., environmentally produced) diseases. However, in recent years, genetic, neurologic, and neurochemical research has begun to provide very convincing evidence that these psychoses not only have organic aspects but possibly organic etiologies.

Some of the most impressive evidence for the hypothesis of organicity comes from the genetic studies in schizophrenia. (In the discussion to follow, we will be concerned with the slowly developing process schizophrenias rather than reactive schizophrenia.) Studies of twins show a very high concordance rate for schizophrenia (60%) in monozygotic twins and a significantly lesser (12%) rate in dizygotic twins.[21] Nontwin siblings also showed a 12 percent schizophrenia rate in families with one schizophrenic twin. In these schizophrenic twins, the disease was considered severe in over 75 percent of the cases.[21] The usefulness of this data has been challenged because the twins were reared in the same home environment and therefore had an increased functionally related risk of becoming schizophrenic. In response to this criticism, several studies compared the offspring of schizophrenic mothers who had subsequently been adopted by normal families with normal children adopted by schizophrenic mothers.[29,32] Approximately 15 percent of the children of schizophrenic parents developed schizophrenia regardless of the environment in which they were raised, while normal children (adopted by schizophrenic mothers) developed schizophrenia at the same rate as the general population (0.25–0.50%). These studies suggest that environment plays a limited role in the production of schizophrenia, whereas heredity appears to be a significant factor.

Genetic predisposition is obviously not the only factor, as concordance rates do not approximate 100 percent. Pollin and Stabenau[39] noted that the twin that became schizophrenic was quite often the one with the lower birth weight or with other factors providing suspicion of prenatal or perinatal brain damage. Their contention was that both the elements of genetic predisposition and very early brain injury may be necessary to actually produce the full clinical syndrome of schizophrenia.

In pursuit of the concept that brain dysfunction may be an important element in schizophrenia, several investigators have performed careful neurologic examinations on groups of schizophrenic patients in search of subtle neurologic abnormalities. In as many as 65 percent of the schizophrenics thus tested, subtle signs of tremor and impaired equilibrium, gait, coordination, and stereognosis were elicited.[39,42] In a matched group of depressed patients, very few such signs were present. On otoneurologic testing, schizophrenics have also demonstrated abnormal vestibular function, particularly in response to caloric stimulation.

Providing supporting evidence for these observations of brain dysfunction are several studies that have shown that the cerebral ventricles of 60 percent of chronic schizophrenics studied are significantly dilated.[25,31] This finding does not appear related to a concomitant dementing illness, medication use, or trauma.[30] The atrophy in schizophrenics is also progressive with the progression of the disease; therefore, it does not appear to be secondary to premorbid brain damage alone.[25] The reader, however, should be cautioned that such findings are not uniformly verified by autopsies of schizophrenics.

EEG studies of schizophrenic patients have not always been consistent but many have shown a high incidence of basic abnormalities.[39,41] Heath and his coworkers, using depth electrodes within the limbic structures of schizophrenic patients, have shown very impressive repetitive spiking discharges from the septal area and anterior hippocampus during periods of active psychosis.[26] These discharges were never demonstrable with standard scalp electrodes, only on depth studies. When treated and with remission of the acute psychotic phase, the abnormal limbic discharge subsided. Whereas not suggesting that all schizophrenia is an epileptic-related condition, this data demonstrates the degree of organic disturbance that is kindled in the limbic structures of the schizophrenic during those times when he is most actively psychotic.

A final avenue of investigation that has further bolstered the organic hypothesis in relation to the psychoses is the pharmacologic and neurochemical studies of neurotransmitter function in schizophrenia.[55] Drugs that restrict dopamine release, such as the phenothiazines and butyrophenones, are very effective in controlling the symptoms of schizophrenic psychosis. Conversely, the amphetamines, which release dopamine, if used in sufficient quantity, can actually produce a clinical psychosis that resembles a paranoid schizophrenia in many ways. Following the direction suggested by these observations, basic neurochemical research has shown that schizophrenics do not have a primary defect in dopamine production as was originally thought but rather have hypersensitive or excessive numbers of dopamine receptor sites.[10,28] This postsynaptic receptor hypersensitivity is seen most prominently in the nucleus accumbens (septal area), the putamen, and also the caudate nucleus.[37] Whether the dopamine receptor alone represents the essential defect in schizophrenia is not yet known, but such biochemical evidence has been very encouraging thusfar.

In reviewing the information currently available, it appears likely that schizophrenia results from a constitutional and often genetic defect in the neurotransmitter systems, particularly that for dopamine, in the subcortical limbic structures. Structurally, there are reports that schizophreniform syndromes have been produced by such diseases as temporal lobe epilepsy and focal temporal lobe encephalitis. Chemically, the limbic and basal gangliar structures seem to be those structures in schizophrenics with transmitter abnormalities; accordingly, research has begun to concentrate evidence in favor of this hypothesized limbic-chemical defect in schizophrenia.

The catatonic form of schizophrenia should be discussed separately because the outstanding clinical feature, rigidity or waxy flexibility, is also seen as a symptom in a variety of treatable medical illnesses. Therefore, this symptom is not necessarily pathognomonic of schizophrenia. The associated autonomic features which are frequently seen in severe cases are also interesting.

Catatonic schizophrenia has an onset in young adulthood and, unlike simple process schizophrenia, can evolve abruptly. Accompanying the schizophrenic withdrawal and thought disorder is a significant disorder of motility: some patients become hyperkinetic, excited, and often violent; while others become mute, immobile, and rigid. Sudden shifts from immobility to excitability are common. In severe cases, the limbs become rigid and remain in unusual postures for extended periods. Many patients refuse food, lie motionless for weeks, and eventually develop a fever of very uncertain origin.[36,40] The disease is often progressive and can produce a dementia-like state. During the severe withdrawn state, intravenous amylobarbitone can often be used to therapeutically mobilize the patient, but frequently electroconvulsive therapy is necessary in an attempt to save the patient's life.[36]

Catatonic schizophrenia is an interesting example of the interaction of abnormalities in motor, autonomic, and mental behavior. With the full-blown syndrome, the patients demonstrate basal gangliar, hypothalamic, and arousal dysfunction. It is very tempting to postulate a basic defect in subcortical transmitter systems such as that of dopamine as the explanation of this unusual syndrome.

Catatonic schizophrenia must be differentiated from other conditions that may mimic it.[18] The manic form of manic-depressive illness often has catatonic features yet has a much better prognosis. Hysterical coma or psychiatric unresponsiveness is another psychiatric condition that can produce catatonic-like behavior. Drug overdose with phencyclidine (PCP or "angel dust"), mescaline, amphetamines, and phenothiazines must all be part of the differential diagnosis. Frontal lobe lesions, general paresis, diabetic ketoacidosis, porphyria, hyperparathyroidism, petit mal status, acute systemic lupus erythematosus, viral encephalitis, and Wernicke's encephalopathy can all present with catatonic features. Therefore, it is very important to (1) look carefully for true signs of a schizophrenic thought disorder, (2) take a complete history and perform a complete physical examination and laboratory screening, and (3) utilize the intravenous amylobarbitone test (the schizophrenic should become more responsive, whereas the organic patient will become increasingly lethargic).

MANIC-DEPRESSIVE ILLNESS

Manic-depressive illness is an endogenous, cyclical disease in which the patient exhibits swings of mood which are of psychotic proportion. Some patients have only depressive or only manic episodes (unipolar), while others manifest both extremes during the course of a lifetime (bipolar). This illness typically has an onset in adulthood and has a greater than 60 percent recovery rate with treatment.[35] The disease has a strong familial tendency and the affected members of each family tend to demonstrate the same general type of illness, either monopolar or bipolar.

Many types of depression including neurotic depression, reactive depression, acute psychotic depression, and involutional depression seem to be largely functional diseases brought on by the patient's interaction with the stress of his environment. However, there is both genetic and pharmocologic evidence that suggests that manic-depressive illness has basic organic components. The concept that depression was related to a neurochemical process arose quite serendipitously. The first clue came when depressed tuberculosis patients improved mentally when they were given the monoamine oxidase inhibitor, iproniazid. This drug is known to prevent the breakdown of neurotransmitters (serotonin, dopamine, and norepinephrine), thus the conclusion was reached that the depression was caused by a deficiency in these biogenic amines or neurotransmitters. A bit of corroborative information came from the observation that hypertensive patients treated with reserpine (a drug that exhausts catecholamines) frequently became depressed. The concept that a deficit in neurotransmitters was the cause of depression was appealing since the hypothesis also explained many of the vegetative signs (e.g., sleep, sexual activity, and eating disturbances). It is known that these functions are controlled by the same biogenic amines in the hypothalamus and brain stem.

Various theories have been postulated as to which transmitter substance is responsible for these conditions, but no firm proof has yet been given for any. It is generally agreed that decreased levels of transmitter substance are responsible for the depressive phase and that increased levels cause the manic phase, but whether these alterations in transmitter levels are the cause or the effect of the disease is still not known. Some investigators feel that serotonin abnormalities alone can cause these conditions,[8] while others strongly hold that catecholamines (dopamine or norepinephrine) are the primary transmitters involved.[5] Most of the evidence thus far has been based either upon the measurement of metabolites of the various transmitters in the serum or cerebrospinal fluid or upon the patient's response to the administration of various transmitter precursors or other pharmacologic agents.

As in the case of schizophrenia, the answer will undoubtedly be complex. There may be various subtypes of manic-depressive illness which are based on different metabolic defects, or conversely there may be a very complicated interaction among many hormonal, neurochemical, genetic, and environmental factors which is at the root of the disease process. It is a fascinating new area of study and one that demonstrates how firmly many of the psychiatric diseases are established within the borderland between social and physical science.

PSYCHIATRIC DISEASES
THAT MIMIC NEUROLOGIC DISEASE

In certain instances, functional psychiatric disease can present in the guise of a neurologic problem. We have previously discussed (Chap. 5) depressive pseudodementia in which the depressed patient demonstrates the apathy, memory dysfunction, and general cognitive impairment so typical of Alzheimer's/senile dementia. The importance of appropriately diagnosing this type of patient cannot be overstressed. Hysterical neurosis with conversion symptoms or dissociative symptoms is another condition which may simulate neurologic disease. Patients with conversion reactions classically demonstrate special sensory or voluntary motor problems such as blindness, hemiparesis, paraparesis, or anesthesia but can have behavioral features as well. An uncommon hysterical conversion behavior seen in hospitalized patients is simulated coma also known as psychiatric unresponsiveness. This condition is usually fairly easy to distinguish from a true coma by a complete physical, neurologic, and laboratory screening. The psychiatric coma patient has a completely normal exam and overtly looks "too healthy" for his depressed level of consciousness. It is not prudent to make this diagnosis too quickly, however, since the misdiagnosis of an organic coma as hysteric is a considerably more serious error than the reverse.

A dissociative episode (amnesia) is another hysterical syndrome that can at times appear to be of organic etiology to the naive examiner. As pointed out in Chapter 7, patients in dissociative episodes or fugues are able to actively learn during their amnesic periods, whereas organic amnesics cannot. The psychiatric amnesia seen most commonly is that of memory problems associated with anxiety. People under stress can become so preoccupied with their life situation and their anxiety about it that they frequently lose track of day-to-day details. This type of forgetfulness is usually alleviated by (1) demonstrating the patient's memory competence to them by asking questions about personal details and current events (be careful about requesting that patients learn new material since the anxiety will interfer with that type of test), (2) pointing out the emotional stress that the patient is subjected to and reassuring them about the relationship between the anxiety and their perceived memory symptoms, and (3) using tranquilization and/or directive psychotherapy to ameliorate the underlying anxiety.

Another interesting condition that is frequently associated with emotional factors yet simulates a dementia is the Diogenes syndrome.[3,7] Patients with this syndrome are usually elderly and live very peculiarly; they are physically unkempt, their homes are filthy, they are compulsive hoarders, (syllogomania), and they neglect their health and nutrition. On initial observation one would assume that they were either demented or chronically schizophrenic, but in fact most are not. Intelligence quotients are typically high normal (an average of 115 in one study),[7] they are not financially destitute, and many were members of responsible professions during their working years. The etiology of the syndrome is not known, but it seems in most cases to be a type of emotional reaction to the stresses of old age, marginal health, and loneliness. In younger patients, it may reflect more serious psychopathology.[3]

NEUROLOGIC DISEASE THAT RESEMBLES PSYCHIATRIC DISORDERS

These conditions have been previously mentioned; however, we feel that is important to reemphasize the fact that classic psychiatric disease must always be evaluated very carefully for a possible organic etiology. Frontal and temporal lobe tumors, systemic lupus erythematosus, temporal lobe epilepsy, dementia, hydrocephalus, other focal lesions from stroke or abscess, infection, and occasionally a confusional state can all initially demonstrate the clinical features of standard psychiatric disease. In fact, one of the principal purposes of this book has been to acquaint the reader not only with the classic organic syndromes but also those organic syndromes that simulate psychiatric disease.

COMBINATION SYNDROMES

A single diagnosis that can explain all the patient's symptoms is usually the best, but the reader is cautioned that two conditions do occasionally occur in the same patient. Demented patients suffer strokes, neurotics develop tumors, and the senile frequently develop confusional states. The clinician must become very astute in his diagnostic acumen if he is to appreciate these subtle and complicated neurobehavioral syndromes.

The physicians treating patients with organic brain syndromes must also be aware of the possibility of emotional reactions superimposed on the basic disease process. These reactions can be treated and often remarkable restitution of social and integrative function can occur. This is particularly true when the anxiety or depression in an early demented or brain damaged patient is adequately controlled. The physician working with problems within this borderland between neurology and psychiatry must borrow heavily from both disciplines if he is to truly understand these fascinating diseases and offer effective help to patients who are thus afflicted.

REFERENCES

1. Bach-Y-Rita, G., Lion, J.R., Clement, C.E., and Ervin, F.R.: Episodic dyscontrol: A study of 130 violent patients. Am. J. Psychiatry 127:1473, 1971.
2. Benson, D.F.: Personal communication. October, 1978.
3. Berlyne, N.: Diogenes syndrome. Lancet 1:515, 1975.
4. Black, F.W., and Strub, R.L.: The developmental disorders of childhood. F.A. Davis Company, Philadelphia, 1981, in preparation.
5. Brodie, H.K.H., Murphy, D.L., Goodwin, F.K., and Bunney, W.E.J.: Catecholamines and mania: the effect of alpha-methyl-p-tyrosine on manic behavior and catecholamine metabolism. Clin. Pharmacol. Ther. 12: 218, 1971.
6. Chiles, J.A., and Wilkus, R.J.: Behavioral manifestations of the Kleine-Levin syndrome. Dis. Nerv. Syst. 37:646, 1976.
7. Clark, A.N.G., Mankikar, G.D., and Gray, L.: Diogenes syndrome: A clinical study of gross neglect in old age. Lancet 1:366, 1975.
8. Coppen, A., Prange, A.L., Jr., Whybrow, P.C., and Noguera, R.: Abnormalities of indoleamines in affective disorders. Arch. Gen. Psychiatry 26: 474, 1972.
9. Critchley, M., and Hoffman, H.L.: The syndrome of periodic somnolence and morbid hunger (Kleine-Levin syndrome) Br. Med. J. 1:137, 1942.
10. Crow, T.J., Deskin, J.F.W., Johnston, E.C., and Longden, A.: Dopamine and schizophrenia. Lancet 2:563, 1976.
11. Editorial: Narcolepsy and cataplexy. Lancet 1:845, 1975.
12. Editorial: Sleeping and breathing. New Engl. J. Med. 299:1009, 1978.
13. Editorial: Sleep apnoea syndromes. Lancet 1:25, 1979.
14. Eisenberg, L., Ascher, E., and Kanner, L.: A clinical study of Gilles de la Tourette's disease (maladie des tics) in children. Am. J. Psychiatry 115:715, 1953.
15. Eldridge, R., Sweet, R.O., Lake, R., Ziegler, M., and Shaprio, A.K.: Gilles de la Tourette's syndrome: clinical, genetic, psychologic, and biochemical aspects in 21 selected families. Neurology 27:115, 1977.
16. Endo, M., Daiguji, M., Asano, Y., Yamashita, L., and Takahashi, S.: Periodic psychosis recurring in association with menstrual cycle. J. Clin. Psychiatry 39:456, 1978.

17. Fernando, S.J.M.: Six cases of Gilles de la Tourette's syndrome. Brit. J. Psychiatry 128:436, 1976.
18. Gelenberg, A.J.: The catatonic syndrome. Lancet 1:1339, 1976.
19. Gilbert, G.J.: Periodic hypersomnia and bulimia: The Kleine-Levin syndrome. Neurology 14:844, 1964.
20. Glenn, W.W.L., Phelps, M., and Gersten, L.M.: Diaphragm pacing in the management of central alveolar hyperventilation, in Guilleminault, C., and Dement, W.C. (eds.): Sleep Apnea Syndromes. Alan R. Liss, Inc., New York, 1978, pp. 333–345.
21. Gottesman, I.I., and Shields, J.: Schizophrenia in twins: 16 years consecutive admissions to a psychiatric clinic. Br. J. Psychiatry 112:809, 1966.
22. Guilleminault, C., Billiard, M., Montplaisir, J., and Dement, W.C.: Altered states of consciousness in disorders of daytime sleepiness. J. Neurol. Sci. 26:377, 1975.
23. Guilleminault, C., and Dement, W.C. (eds.): Sleep Apnea Syndromes. Alan R. Liss, Inc., New York, 1978.
24. Harbin, H.T.: Episodic dyscontrol and family dynamics. Am. J. Psychiatry 134:1113, 1977.
25. Haug, J.O.: Pneumoencephalographic investigation of psychiatric patients. Acta Psychiatr. Neurol. Scand. [Suppl.] 38:1, 1962.
26. Heath, R.G.: Studies in Schizophrenia: A multidisciplinary approach to mind-body relationships. Harvard University Press, Cambridge, Massachusetts, 1954.
27. Henderson, P.: Disability in Childhood and Youth. Oxford University Press, London, 1974.
28. Henn, F.A.: Dopamine and schizophrenia: a theory revisited and revised. Lancet 2:293, 1978.
29. Heston, L.L.: Psychiatric disorders in foster home reared children of schizophrenic mothers. Br. J. Psychiatry 112:819, 1966.
30. Hill, D.: Cerebral atrophy and cognitive impairment in chronic schizophrenia. Lancet 2:1132, 1976.
31. Johnstone, E.C., Crow, T.J., Frith, C.D., Husband, J., and Kreel, L.: Cerebral ventricular size and cognitive impairment in chronic schizophrenia. Lancet 2:924, 1976.
32. Kety, S.: Genetic aspects of schizophrenia. Psychiatr. Ann. 6:11, 1976.
33. Maletzky, B.M.: The episodic dyscontrol syndrome. Dis. Nerv. System 34:178, 1973.
34. Mark, V.H., and Ervin, F.R.: Violence and the Brain. Harper and Row, New York, 1970, pp. 125–135.
35. Morrison, J.R., Winokur, G., Crowe, R., and Clancy, J.: The Iowa 500. Arch. Gen. Psychiatry 29:678, 1973.
36. O'Toole, J.K., and Dyke, G.: Report of psychogenic fever in catatonia responding to electroconvulsive therapy. Dis. Nerv. Syst. 38:852, 1977.
37. Owen, F., Cross, A.J., Crow, T.J., Longden, A., Poulter, M., and Riley, G.L.: Increased dopamine-receptor sensitivity in schizophrenia. Lancet 2:223, 1978.
38. Parkes, J.D.: The sleepy patient. Lancet 1:990, 1977.
39. Pollin, W., and Stabenau J.: Biological, psychological, and historical differences in a series of monozygotic twins discordant for schizophrenia, in Rosenthal, D., and Kety, S. (eds.): Transmission of Schizophrenia. Pergamon, London, 1968.

40. Powers, P., Douglass, T.S., and Waziri, R.: Hyperpyrexia in catatonic states. Dis. Nerv. Syst. 37:359, 1976.
41. Rieder, R., Rosenthal, D., Wender, P., and Blumenthal, H.: The offspring of schizophrenics. Arch. Gen. Psychiatry 32:200, 1975.
42. Rochford, J.M., Detre, T., Tucker, G.J., and Harrow, M.: Neuropsychological impairments in functional psychiatric disease. Arch. Gen. Psychiatry 22:114, 1970.
43. Schain, R.J.: Neurology of Childhood Learning Disorders. Williams & Wilkins, Co., Baltimore, 1977.
44. Shapiro, A.K., Shapiro, E.S., Wayne, H., and Clarkin, J.: Organic factors in Gilles de la Tourette's syndrome. Br. J. Psychiatry 122:659, 1973.
45. Shapiro, A.K., Shapiro, E.S., Bruun, R.D., and Sweet, R.D.: Gilles de la Tourette Syndrome. Raven Press, New York, 1978.
46. Sweet, R.D., Solomon, G.E., Wayne, H., Shapiro, E.S., and Shapiro, A.K.: Neurological features of Gilles de la Tourette's syndrome. J. Neurol. Neurosurg. Psychiatry 36:1, 1973.
47. Tunks, E.R., and Dermer, S.W.: Carbamazepine in the dyscontrol syndrome associated with limbic system dysfunction. J. Nerv. Ment. Dis. 164:56, 1977.
48. Weingarten, K.: Tics, in Vinken, P.J., and Bruyn, G.W., (eds.): Diseases of the Basal Ganglia, Vol. 6 in Handbook of Clinical Neurology. Elsevier-North Holland Publishing Co., New York, 1968, pp. 782–808.
49. Yassa, R., and Nair, N.P.V.: The Kleine-Levin-a variant? J. Clin. Psychiatry 39:254, 1978.
50. Yoss, R.E., and Daly, D.D.: Narcolepsy. Arch. Int. Med. 106:168, 1960.
51. Yoss, R.E., and Daly, D.D.: On the treatment of narcolepsy. Med. Clin. N.A. 52:781, 1968.
52. Reynolds, C.F., Black, R.S., Coble, P., Holzer, B., and Kupfer, D.J.: Similarities in EEG sleep findings for Kleine-Levin syndrome and unipolar depression. Am. J. Psychiatry 137:116, 1980.
53. Zorick, F.J., Salis, P.J., Roth, T., and Kramer, M.: Narcolepsy and automatic behavior: A case report. J. Clin. Psychiatry 40:194, 1979.
54. Riley, T.L.: The electroencephalogram in patients with rage attacks or episodic violent behavior. Milit. Med. 144:515, 1979.
55. Fredrickson, P., and Richelson, E.: Mayo seminars in psychiatry: Dopamine and schizophrenia—a review. J. Clin. Psychiatry 40:399, 1979.

INDEX

409

Attention
  acute confusional state and, 95, 116
  Alzheimer's/senile dementia and,
    127, 134
  assessment of ability to sustain,
    47–49
Auditory agnosia, 234
Auditory function
  cortex and, 28
  temporal lobe and, 237–238
Aura
  definition of, 339
  psychic, automatic behavior in epi-
    lepsy and, 344
Automatic behavior
  narcolepsy and, 392
  psychic aura and, in epilepsy, 344

BARBITURATES, acute confusional
    state and, 101
Battery, Halstead-Reitan, 67–68
Bechterew, nuclei of Gudden and,
    18
Behavior
  acute confusional state and fluctua-
    tions in, 96
  anatomy of, 9–38
  automatic
    narcolepsy and, 392
    psychic aura in epilepsy and, 344
  changes in
    closed head trauma and, 270
    epilepsy and, 340
      ictal, 342–345
      postictal, 345–347
      preictal, 341–342
    frontal lobe and, 242–244
    severe closed head trauma and,
      282
  confusional. See Confusional behav-
    ior; Confusional state.
  emotional, 9
    limbic system and, 23–25
  evaluation of, mental status exami-
    nation and, 49–52
  fighting and fleeing, 22–23
  intellectual, 9
  sexual, temporal lobe epilepsy and
    alterations in, 359–360
Behavioral findings, neuropsychologi-
    cal report and, 75–76
Bender Gestalt Test, 71–72
Benton Visual Retention Test, 72

Binswanger, subcortical arterioscle-
    rotic encephalopathy of, 186
Blindness
  acute cortical, 236–237
  color, 236
Blood tests, differential diagnosis of
    Alzheimer's/senile dementia
    and, 146
Brain abscess, 318–319
Brain damage
  drug misuse and, 308
  handedness and early, 216
  hemispheric compensation for, 252
Brain lesion
  focal. See Focal brain lesion.
  neuropsychologic evaluation and
    known, 65
Brain scan
  acute confusional state and, 110–
    111
  differential diagnosis of Alz-
    heimer's/senile dementia and,
    148
Brain stem reticular formation, 11
  input to, 12–14
Brain tumor, 381–388
  dementia and, 174–175
  differential diagnosis in, 387
  differential diagnosis of Alzheim-
    er's/senile dementia and, 143
  evaluation of, 385–386
  laboratory investigation in, 387
  management and pathology in, 387
Broca's aphasia, 218–220
Bulimia, Kleine-Levin syndrome and,
    393

CALCULATIONS test, 61
Carcinoma, dementia and, 203
Cardiac surgery, confusional state
    and, 108
Carotid artery disease, acute confu-
    sional state and, 107
Carotid stenosis, anoxia without in-
    farction and, dementia second-
    ary to, 187–188
Carphologia, Alzheimer's/senile de-
    mentia and, 127
Cataplectic attack, narcolepsy and,
    392
Catastrophic anxiety reaction, hemis-
    pheric differences and, 253
Catatonic schizophrenia, 402–403

411

Incontinence
  Alzheimer's/senile dementia and, 127
  hydrocephalus and, 171
Infarctions
  cerebral
    acute confusional state and, 106
    dementia and, 185–187
    cortical and subcortical, dementia and, 186
Infection(s)
  acute confusional state and, 103
  central nervous system, 315–333
Inhalation, organic solvent, 300–302
Inhibiting system, ascending, 15
Injury. See Trauma.
Instincts
  basic, limbic system and, 21–23
  feeding, hypothalamus and, 21
Intellect
  alcoholism and impairment of, 307
  Alzheimer's/senile dementia and deficits in, 124
  cortical localization of higher processes of, 32
  severe closed head trauma and functioning of, 282
Intellectual behavior, 9
Intelligence
  aging and, 139–140
  epilepsy and, 348–350
Intelligence Quotient, 69
Intelligence Scale, Wechsler Adult, 68–70
  organic disease and, 70
  verbal-performance discrepancies and, 74–75
Intensive care unit psychosis, 108
Interictal, definition of, 339
Intoxication. See also Poisoning.
  alcoholic idiosyncratic, 303
  clinical picture of acute, 301
  heavy metal, 302–303
  pathologic, 303
Intracranial pressure, acute confusional state and, 104
IQ, 69
Ischemic attacks, transient, 372

KLEINE-Levin syndrome, 393–394
Klüver-Bucy syndrome, 249

Korsakoff's syndrome, 246
  alcohol abuse and, 305–306
Kuru, 329

LANGUAGE
  Alzheimer's/senile dementia and, 125, 134–135
  cerebral dominance for, handedness and, 216
  cortical localization of, 30–31
  evaluation of speech and, 81–83
  hemispheric specialization and, 29–30, 214–215, 252
  mental status examination and assessment of, 52–56
  problems with speech and, speech pathologist and, 80–81
L-dopa
  confusional state in Parkinson's disease and, 95, 101
  dementia in Parkinson's disease and, 197–198
Learning, testing of new, 57–59
Left-handed individual, aphasia in, 227–228
Left hemisphere. See also entries beginning Hemispheric.
  handedness and dominance of, 29–30
Lethargy, definition of, 45–46
Leukoencephalopathy, progressive multifocal, 327–328
Limbic syndromes, 245–249
Limbic system, 15–27
  anatomy of, 16–20
  function of, 21–27
Litigation, neuropsychologic evaluation and, 65
Lupus erythematosus
  acute confusional state and, 106
  dementia and, 176–177

MAMILLARY bodies, memory and, 26
Mamillothalamic tract of Vicq d'Azyr, 19
Manic-depressive illness, 403–404
Marijuana, effect of, 308
Marinesco, senile plaque of, 159
Masked facies, Alzheimer's/senile dementia and, 128
Mathematics, Alzheimer's/senile dementia and, 136–137

417

Mating, limbic structures and, 23
Measles, subacute sclerosing panencephalitis and, 325–327
Medial forebrain bundle, 20
Medical and social history, 41–44
    outline for, 43–44
Medical practice, organic brain syndromes in, 7–8
Medication(s). *See also names of specific medications;* Drugs.
    acute confusional state and, 101–102, 113
    psychosis and anticonvulsant, 354–355
Megaphagia, Kleine-Levin syndrome and, 393
Memory. *See also* Amnesia; *names of other specific memory disorders.*
    aging and, 140–141
    Alzheimer's/senile dementia and, 124, 135
    limbic system and, 26–27
    minor head trauma and, 275
    rehabilitation in focal brain lesions and, 258–259
    testing of, 56–59
    testing of remote, 59
    testing of short-term. *See* Digit repetition test.
    visual, testing of, 58–59
Memory Quotient, 71
Memory Scale, Wechsler, 71
Meningitis, 319–320
    chronic, dementia and, 182–183
Menstrual cycle, periodic psychosis and, 394–395
Mental status examination, 44–62. *See also names of specific functions and conditions for which mental status examination conducted.*
    screening, patients who should receive, 41
Mercury poisoning, 302–303
Metabolic disorders
    acute confusional state and, 102–103
    dementia and, 177–182
Metabolism, copper
    acute confusional state and, 103
    dementia and, 180–181
Metal intoxication, heavy, 302–303

Minnesota Multiphasic Personality Inventory, 74
Mirror sign, Alzheimer's/senile dementia and, 127
Mood, assessment of emotional status and, mental status examination and, 50–52
Motor areas, primary cortical, 28
Multi-infarct dementia, 185–187
    differential diagnosis of Alzheimer's/senile dementia and, 143
Multiple sclerosis, dementia and, 202–203
Musical function, temporal lobe syndromes and, 237–238
Mutism, akinetic, 374–375
Myxedema
    acute confusional state and, 103
    dementia and, 177–178

NAMING, object, language testing and assessment of, 54–55
Narcolepsy, 391–393
Neglect
    rehabilitation in focal brain lesions and, 258
    unilateral, 241–242
Neologisms, in Wernicke's aphasia and schizophrenia and, 222
Neurologic disease
    acute confusional state and, 104–105
    psychiatric diseases that mimic, 404–405
    that resembles psychiatric disorders, 405
Neurology, consultation and, 62–63. *See also names of specific conditions for which neurologic consultation obtained.*
Neuropsychologic evaluation, 63–76
    components of, 67–74. *See also names of specific tests.*
    criteria for referral for, 64–65
Neurosis(es)
    disorders resembling epilepsy and, 351–352
    pretraumatic, post-traumatic syndrome and, 277
Neurosyphilis, parenchymatous, dementia and, 183–184
Niacin deficiency, dementia and, 181

Postictal behavioral change, 345–347
Postictal period, definition of, 339
Postoperative period, acute confusional state and, 107–109
Post-traumatic syndrome, 276–278
Problem solving ability, Alzheimer's/senile dementia and, 124
Prodromal states, epilepsy and, 341–345
Prodrome, definition of, 339
Progressive supranuclear palsy, dementia and, 199
Prosopagnosia, 235–236
Prostatectomy, postoperative confusional state and, 108
Proverb interpretation
    Alzheimer's/senile dementia and, 137
    test of, 61, 73
Pseudobulbar effect, Alzheimer's/senile dementia and, 128
Pseudobulbar syndrome, severe closed head trauma and, 283
Pseudodementia, depressive, differential diagnosis of Alzheimer's/senile dementia and, 141–143
Pseudoparesis, alcoholic, 188
Psychiatric disease(s)
    neurologic disease that resembles, 405
    organic basis and, 399–403
    that mimic neurologic disease, 404–405
Psychiatric evaluation, patients referred for, 76
Psychiatric unresponsiveness, 404
Psychiatry
    consultation and, 76–79
    in Alzheimer's/senile dementia, 151–152
Psychologist, Alzheimer's/senile dementia and consultation with, 150–151
Psychomotor attacks, definition of, 339
Psychomotor expressions of seizure discharge, 343–345
Psychosis
    epilepsy and disorders resembling, 352–355
    intensive care unit, 108
    periodic, 394–395

schizophreniform
    brain tumor and, 384
    temporal lobe epilepsy and, 357
Psychotic-like episodes, epileptic seizures and, 343
Psychotropic drugs, acute confusional state and, 102
Punch drunk syndrome, 279–280

READING
    corpus callosum and, 249
    focal brain lesions and, 230–231
    writing and, language testing and, 56
Recall, immediate
    testing of. See Digit repetition test.
    verbal story for, 58
Receiving areas, cortical, primary sensory, 28
Receptive aphasia, 220
Recovery, neuropsychologic evaluation and, 65
Reduplication of place, 241
Reflexes, Alzheimer's/senile dementia and, 127
Repetition test, mental status examination and, 55–56
Reproduction drawing, testing of, 60
Restlessness, Alzheimer's/senile dementia and, 134
Retardation, epilepsy and mental, 348
Reticular formation, brain stem, 11
    input to, 12–14
Reticular systems, ascending, 10–15

SCHIZOPHRENIA
    differential diagnosis of Wernicke's aphasia and, 221–223
    organicity and, 400–403
Schizophreniform psychosis
    brain tumor and, 384
    temporal lobe epilepsy and, 357
Scopolamine, acute confusional state and, 101
Seizure discharge, psychomotor expressions of, 343–345
Seizures
    acute confusional state and, 104
    Alzheimer's/senile dementia and, 128
    epileptic
        classification of, 337, 338

420

Vasculitis
cerebral, acute confusional state and, 106
dementia and, 176–177
Vegetative state, severe closed head trauma and, 284
Ventricles, cerebral, studies for visualization of, differential diagnosis of Alzheimer's/senile dementia and, 148–150
Verbal apraxia, 233
Verbal material, parietal lobe and, 239
Verbal Scale IQ, 69
Vicq d'Azyr, mamillothalamic tract of, 19
Vigilance. *See also* Concentration.
"A" test for, 49
definition of, 47
Violence
episodic dyscontrol and, 395–397
postictal behavior and, 346–347
temporal lobe epilepsy and, 358–359
Viral dementia, transmissible, 328–330
Viral encephalitis, 323–330
Viral encephalopathies, subacute spongiform, 328–330
Virus(es), progressive multifocal leukoencephalopathy and, 327–328
Visual agnosia, 234–235
Visual memory test, 58–59
Visual perception
cortex and, 28, 31
parietal lobe and, 239

Visual processing, temporal lobe and, 238
Visual Retention Test, Benton, 72
Visual spatial orientation, hemispheric specialization and, 215
Visual symptoms, bizarre, 236
Vitamin deficiencies
acute confusional state and, 103
dementia and, 181–182
Vocation
outline for history of, 44
severe closed head trauma and, 285–286
Vocational services, rehabilitation in focal brain disease and, 259

WECHSLER Adult Intelligence Scale, 68–70
organic disease and, 70
verbal-performance discrepancies and, 74–75
Wechsler Memory Scale, 71
Wernicke-Korsakoff syndrome, 304–306
Wernicke's aphasia, 220–223
Wernicke's encephalopathy, alcohol abuse and, 305
Wide Range Achievement Test, 74
Wilson's disease
acute confusional state and, 103
dementia and, 180–181
Word deafness, 226–227
Writing
focal brain lesions and ability of, 231–232
reading and, language testing and, 56